Decision Making in Small Animal Oncology

Decision Making in Small Animal Oncology

David J. Argyle
B.V.M.S., Ph.D., D.E.C.V.I.M.-C.A. (Oncology) M.R.C.V.S.

Malcolm J. Brearley
M.A., Vet.M.B., M.Sc. (Clinical Oncology), DipE.C.V.I.M.-C.A. (Oncology), F.R.C.V.S.

Michelle M. Turek
D.V.M., D.A.C.V.R. (Radiation Oncology), D.A.C.V.I.M. (Oncology)

WILEY-BLACKWELL

A John Wiley & Sons, Inc., Publication

Edition first published 2008
©2008 Wiley-Blackwell

Blackwell Publishing was acquired by John Wiley & Sons in February 2007. Blackwell's publishing program has been merged with Wiley's global Scientific, Technical, and Medical business to form Wiley-Blackwell.

Editorial Office
2121 State Avenue, Ames, Iowa 50014-8300, USA

For details of our global editorial offices, for customer services, and for information about how to apply for permission to reuse the copyright material in this book, please see our website at www.wiley.com/wiley-blackwell.

Library of Congress Cataloguing-in-Publication Data

Argyle, David J.
    Decision making in small animal oncology / David J. Argyle, Malcolm J. Brearley, Michelle M. Turek.—1st ed.
        p.; cm.
    Includes bibliographical references and index.
    ISBN 978-0-8138-2275-4 (alk. paper)
    1. Dogs—Diseases—Diagnosis—Decision making.   2. Cats—Diseases—Diagnosis—Decision making.   3. Tumors in animals.   4. Veterinary oncology.   I. Brearley, Malcolm J.   II. Turek, Michelle M.   III. Title.
        [DNLM: 1. Neoplasms—veterinary.   2. Algorithms.   3. Cat Diseases—diagnosis.   4. Cat Diseases—therapy.
    5. Decision Support Techniques.   6. Dog Diseases—diagnosis.   7. Dog Diseases—therapy.   SF 910.T8 A695d 2008]

    SF992.C35A74 2008
    636.089'6994—dc22

                                                                                                2008007429

A catalogue record for this book is available from the U.S. Library of Congress.

Set in 9 on 11.5 pt Sabon by SNP Best-set Typesetter Ltd., Hong Kong

1   2008

To Sally, Blythe and Sam. For all your love and support, this is what I was doing upstairs for all those weeks.

David J. Argyle

To Gregg, for his loving support of my endeavors. And to Mom, Dad and John for their lasting wisdom and encouragement.

Michelle M. Turek

I should like to dedicate this book to my early mentors, Dave Bostock and the late Larry Owen, who inspired me into clinical oncology. Also to my colleagues over the years with whom I have continued to learn, and finally to the oncologists of the future – if I have helped inspire them in any way then I consider that a great honor.

Malcolm J. Brearley

Contents

Contributors

David J. Argyle BVMS PhD DECVIM-CA
(Oncology) MRCVS
RCVS and European Specialist in Veterinary
Oncology
William Dick Professor of Veterinary
Clinical Studies
Royal (Dick) School of Veterinary Studies
The University of Edinburgh
Hospital for Small Animals
Easter Bush Veterinary Centre
Roslin, Midlothian
EH25 9RG

Laura Blackwood BVMS PhD MVM CertVR
DipECVIM-CA (Oncology) MRCVS
RCVS & European Specialist in Veterinary Oncology
Senior Lecturer in Medicine (Oncology)
Small Animal Teaching Hospital
The Leahurst Campus
Chester High Road
Neston
Wirral
CH64 7TE

Malcolm J. Brearley, MA VetMB MSc(Clin Onc)
DipECVIM-CA(Oncology) FRCVS
European & RCVS Recognised Specialist in
Veterinary Oncology
Principal Clinical Oncologist
The Queen's Veterinary School Hospital
University of Cambridge
Madingley Road
Cambridge CB3 0ES
UK

Alison Hayes BVMS CertVR MSC(Clin Onc) Dip
ECVIM-CA(Oncology) MRCVS
RCVS Recognised Specialist in Veterinary Oncology
European Specialist in Veterinary Oncology
Senior Clinical Oncologist
Animal Health Trust
Lanwades Park
Kentford, Suffolk
UK, CB8 7UU

Valerie MacDonald, BSc, DVM
Diplomate ACVIM (Oncology)
Associate Professor
Western College of Veterinary Medicine
University of Saskatchewan
52 Campus Drive, Saskatoon, SK S7N 5B4

Elspeth Milne BVM&S PhD DipECVCP DipRCPath
FRCVS
Head of Division of Veterinary Clinical Sciences
Royal (Dick) School of Veterinary Studies
Easter Bush Veterinary Centre
Roslin
Midlothian
EH25 9RG

Suzanne Murphy BVM&S MSc (Clin Onc) Dip
ECVIM-CA (Oncology) MRCVS
European and Royal College Recognised Specialist in
Small Animal Oncology
Head, Oncology Unit
Animal Health Trust
Lanwades Park
Kentford, Suffolk
UK, CB8 7UU

Melissa C. Paoloni, DVM, DACVIM (Oncology)
National Institutes of Health, National Cancer
Institute
Center for Cancer Research, Comparative Oncology
Program
NIH/NCI
37 Convent Dr., RM 2144
Bethesda, MD 20892

Mala G. Renwick BSc. Bvet.Med MSc. (Clinical
Oncology) MRCVS
Lecturer in Clinical Oncology
Royal (Dick) School of Veterinary Studies
The University of Edinburgh
Hospital for Small Animals
Easter Bush Veterinary Centre
Roslin, Midlothian
EH25 9RG

Linda Roberts Dip AVN (Medical) RVN
Royal Canin Cancer & Wellness Nurse
Royal (Dick) School of Veterinary Studies
Hospital for Small Animals
Easter Bush Veterinary Centre
Roslin, Midlothian
EH25 9RG

Corey Saba, DVM, DACVIM (Oncology)
Assistant Professor of Oncology
University of Georgia
College of Veterinary Medicine
501 DW Brooks Drive
Athens, GA 30606

Michelle M. Turek, DVM, DACVIM (Oncology),
DACVR (Radiation Oncology),
Staff oncologist
Angell Animal Medical Center's Cancer Care Center,
Boston, MA

Foreword

Cancer is a major cause of morbidity and mortality in domestic animals. Recent reports suggest that there is an increase in the prevalence of diagnosed cases of cancer in dogs and cats, partly because of the increased life span through improved nutrition, vaccination, and control of infectious disease. As a consequence there is increased demand on the practitioner to diagnose and manage cancer patients in general practice.

This book is not a comprehensive oncology text. It was specifically written to
- Provide veterinary students with the cancer knowledge they need in general practice.
- Provide general practitioners with a readable practice manual for rapid reference.
- Answer the common questions that specialist oncologists are asked by practitioners every day.

We have tried to arrange the material in the form of easy-to-follow algorithms that allow the clinician to make appropriate decisions when faced with a cancer patient. We have also stressed the need for practitioners to work with their pathologists and local specialist oncologists to provide the best care for their patients.

The reader must acknowledge that this is a rapidly changing field and best practice and knowledge may change over time. Consequently, the authors recommend that readers should check the most up-to-date information on procedures and drugs (including formulation, dose, and method of administration) prior to embarking on therapy.

David J. Argyle
Malcolm J. Brearley
Michelle M. Turek

Decision Making in Small Animal Oncology

1
INTRODUCTION: CANCER BIOLOGY AND TERMINOLOGY

David J. Argyle

A Definition of Tumor

- A tumor is any tissue mass or swelling and may or may not be neoplastic.
- Neoplasia is the abnormal growth of a tissue into a mass. It is usually phenotypically recognized by the fact that its cells show abnormal growth patterns and are no longer under the control of normal homeostatic growth-controlling mechanisms.
- Neoplasms can be considered as either benign or malignant tumors. Although the range of mechanisms involved in the development of tumors and the spectrum of tissues from which tumors are derived is diverse, they can be classified into three broad types:
    1. **Benign Tumors:** Broadly speaking, these tumors arise in any of the tissues of the body and grow locally. They can grow to a large size but are not invasive. Their clinical significance is their ability to cause local pressure, cause obstruction, or form a space-occupying lesion such as a benign brain tumor. Benign tumors do not metastasize.
    2. **In situ Tumors:** These are often small tumors that arise in the epithelium. Histologically, the lesion appears to contain cancer cells, but the tumor remains in the epithelial layer and does not invade the basement membrane or the supporting mesenchyme. A typical example of this is preinvasive squamous cell carcinoma affecting the nasal planum of cats.
    3. **Cancer:** This refers to a malignant tumor, which has the capacity for both local invasion and distant spread by the process of metastasis.

A Definition of Cancer

- Cancer is a disease of all vertebrate species and is well documented throughout history, with fossil records indicating dinosaurs of the Jurassic period suffered from the disease.
- The Greek physician Galen is accredited with describing human tumors of having the shape of a crab, with leglike tendrils invading deep into surrounding tissues—hence, the term cancer.

> **Key Point**
> We define cancer as any malignant growth or tumor caused by abnormal and uncontrolled cell division, able to invade tissues locally and able to spread to other parts of the body through the lymphatic system or the bloodstream. This is obviously a simplistic attempt at describing a complex disease that can utilize a myriad of biological pathways to sustain growth and proliferation.

Nomenclature

The nomenclature of tumors is based upon two concepts:
- First, tumors can be considered as either benign or malignant. For simplicity, the pathobiological differences between benign and malignant are outlined in Table 1.1.
- The second concept is concerned with the tissue or cell of origin (Tables 1.2, 1.3).

Cancer Biology

- Fundamental to our basic understanding of mammalian physiology is the concept of homeostasis.
- If we consider the body as a multicellular unit, cells within this unit form part of a specialized society that cooperates to promote survival of the organism. In terms of homeostasis, cell division, proliferation, and differentiation are strictly controlled and a balance exists between normal cell birth and the natural cell death (Argyle and Khanna, 2006).
- Cancer can be considered as a breakdown in cellular homeostasis leading to uncontrolled cell division and proliferation, which ultimately leads to a disease state.

The Pathways to Cancer

- For many years, cancer researchers have considered a stochastic model of cancer development (McCance and Roberts, 1997).

Table 1.1. The biological differences between benign and malignant tumors

Feature	Benign	Malignant
Degree of differentiation	Cells of benign tumors demonstrate a stage of development at which they have their mature morphological and functional characteristics: and are thus considered to be **well differentiated.**	Malignant tumors demonstrate a range of differentiation from very good to very poor. A severe lack of differentiation is referred to as **anaplasia.**
Growth rate	Benign tumors often grow slowly and have periods of dormancy when no growth is recognized.	Malignant tumors have a wide range of growth rates.
Mode of growth	The mode of growth is considered to be by **expansion**, and tumors are usually encapsulated.	The mode of growth is initially by expansion, but eventually by **invasion**. There is no capsule containing the tumor and the borders are ill defined. Once malignant cells have infiltrated outside their normal confines, they travel along the natural cleavage plains and interstices of tissue.
Metastatic potential	The ability for tumor cells to spread and grow in distant organs (metastasis) is **NOT** a feature of benign tumors.	Malignant tumors have varying capability to metastasize. This can be via the hematogenous, lymphatic, or trans-serosal routes.
Host consequences	The effect on the host is usually through the presence of a **space-occupying lesion**. Consequently, this can be a minimal effect (benign lipoma in the subcutaneous tissue); or can be life threatening (benign brain tumor).	Often **life threatening** based on the tumor's destructive effects on tissues and vital organs, and its ability to metastasize.

Table 1.2.   The nomenclature of benign tumors

Tissue or Cell of Origin	Naming
Mesenchymal	Named by the addition of the suffix **oma** to the cell type of origin: • Fibrous tissue = fibroma • Fat tissue = lipoma • Cartilage = chondroma
Glandular epithelium	Referred to as **adenoma:** • A benign tumor of the sweat gland epithelium would be a *sweat gland adenoma.*
Protective epithelium (squamous or transitional)	Referred to as **papilloma:** • Squamous papilloma of the skin (wart) • Transitional papilloma of the urinary bladder
Nervous tissue	Named by the addition of the suffix **oma** to the cell type of origin: • A benign tumor of the astrocytes would be an *astrocytoma.*

Table 1.3.   The nomenclature of malignant tumors

Tissue or Cell of Origin	Naming
Mesenchymal	Named by the addition of the suffix **sarcoma** to the cell type of origin: • Fibrous tissue = fibrosarcoma • Fat tissue = liposarcoma • Cartilage = chondrosarcoma
Glandular epithelium	Referred to as **adenocarcinoma:** • A malignant tumor of the sweat gland epithelium would be a *sweat gland* or *apocrine adenocarcinoma.*
Protective epithelium (squamous or transitional)	A malignant tumor of squamous epithelium would be a *squamous cell carcinoma.* A malignant tumor of transitional epithelium would be a *transitional cell carcinoma.*
Round cell tumors	Lymphoma and other lymphoid neoplasia Plasmacytoma and multiple myeloma Histiocytoma and other histiocytic diseases Mast cell tumor Transmissible venereal tumor With the exception of the transmissible venereal tumor, round cell tumors affect cell lines of hemolymphatic origin

- In this, cancer formation is the phenotypic end result of a whole series of changes that may have taken a long period of time to develop.
- Following an initiation step produced by a cancer-forming agent on a cell, there follows a period of tumor promotion (Figure 1.1). The initiating step is a rapid step and affects the genetic material of the cell. If the cell does not repair this damage, promoting factors may progress the cell toward a malignant phenotype. In contrast to initiation, progression may be a very slow process, and may not even manifest in the lifetime of the animal.
- Over the past 4 decades, cancer research has generated a rich and complex body of information revealing that cancer is a disease involving dynamic changes in the genome. Each stage of multistep carcinogenesis reflects genetic changes in the cell with a selection advantage that drives the progression toward a highly malignant cell. The age-dependent incidence of cancer suggests a requirement for between four and seven rate-limiting, stochastic events to produce the malignant phenotype.

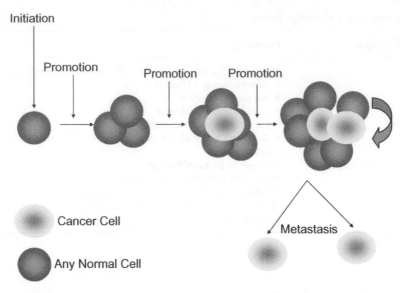

Figure 1.1. The stochastic model of carcinogenesis: Cancer formation is the phenotypic end result of a whole series of changes that may have taken a long period of time to develop. They can occur in any cell type in the body. After an initiation step produced by a cancer-forming agent on a cell is a period of tumor promotion. Each stage of multistep carcinogenesis reflects genetic changes in the cell with a selection advantage that drives the progression toward a highly malignant cell. The age-dependent incidence of cancer suggests a requirement for between four and seven rate-limiting, stochastic events to produce the malignant phenotype. Reprinted from "From Viruses to cancer stem cells: Dissecting the pathways to malignancy" by Argyle D.J. and Blacking T.M. (The Veterinary Journal, 2007) with kind permission from Elsevier.

Oncogenes

- Seminal to our understanding of cancer biology has been the discovery of the so-called "cancer genes," or oncogenes, and tumor suppressor genes.
- The term *proto-oncogene* is used to describe a gene that, in its native state, does not have transforming potential to form tumors but that can be altered to promote malignancy. Once altered, the gene is referred to as an *oncogene*.
- Most proto-oncogenes are key genes involved in the control of **cell growth** and **proliferation** and their roles are complex.
- For simplicity, the mode of action of proto-oncogenes in the normal cell can be divided as follows (Table 1.4, Figure 1.2):
  - Growth factors
  - Growth factor receptors
  - Protein kinases
  - Signal Transducers
  - Nuclear proteins
  - Transcription factors
- The conversion of a proto-oncogene to an oncogene is a result of **somatic events (mutations) in the genetic material of the affected cell.** The activated (mutated) allele of the oncogene **dominates** the wild-type (nonmutated) allele and results in a **dominant gain of function.**
- **The mechanisms of oncogene activation include the following (Figure 1.3):**
  - **Chromosomal translocation:** Where proto-oncogenes are translocated within the genome (i.e., from one chromosome to another), their function can be altered. In human chronic myeloid leukemia (CML) a chromosomal breakpoint produces a translocation of the c-abl oncogene on chromosome nine to a gene on chromosome twenty-two (bcr). The bcr/abl hybrid gene produces a novel transcript whose protein product has tyrosine kinase activity and can contribute to uncontrolled cellular proliferation. This tyrosine

Table 1.4. Oncogenes can be growth factors, growth factor receptors, protein kinases, signal transducers, nuclear proteins, and transcription factors

Oncogene Class	Examples
Growth factors	Platelet-derived growth factor (PDGF)
	Epidermal Growth Factor (EGF)
	Insulin Like Growth Factor-1 (ILGF-1)
	Vascular Endothelial Growth Factor (VEGF)
	Transforming Growth Factor-β (TGF-β)
	Interleukin-2 (IL-2)
Growth factor receptors	PDGF-Receptor (PDGF-R)
	EGFR-Receptor (erbB-1)
	ILGF-1 Receptor (ILGF-R)
	VEGF-Receptor (VEGFR)
	IL-2 receptor (IL-2R)
	Hepatocyte Growth Factor Receptor (met)
	Heregulin Receptor (neu/erbB-2)
	Stem Cell Factor Receptor (kit)
Protein kinases	Tyrosine Kinase, e.g.: bcr-abl, src
	Serine-Threonine Kinase, e.g.: raf/mil, mos
G-protein signal transducers	GTPase, e.g.: H-*ras*, K-*ras*, N-*ras*
Nuclear proteins	Transcription factors, e.g.: ets, jun, fos, myb, myc, rel

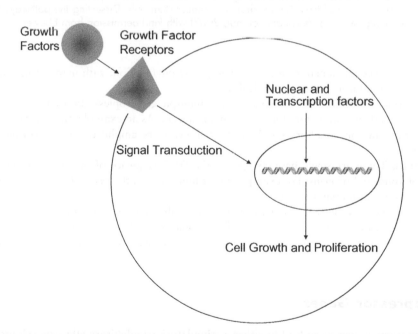

Figure 1.2. Oncogenes are normal cellular genes involved in cell growth and proliferation: Most proto-oncogenes are key genes involved in the control of cell growth and proliferation and include growth factors, growth factor receptors, protein kinases, signal transducers, nuclear proteins, and transcription factors. The conversion of a proto-oncogene to an oncogene is a result of somatic events in the genetic material of the target tissue. The activated allele of the oncogene dominates the wild-type allele and results in a dominant gain of function. The mechanisms of oncogene activation include chromosomal translocation, gene amplification, point mutations, and viral insertions. Reprinted from "From Viruses to cancer stem cells: Dissecting the pathways to malignancy" by Argyle D.J. and Blacking T.M. (The Veterinary Journal, 2007) with kind permission from Elsevier.

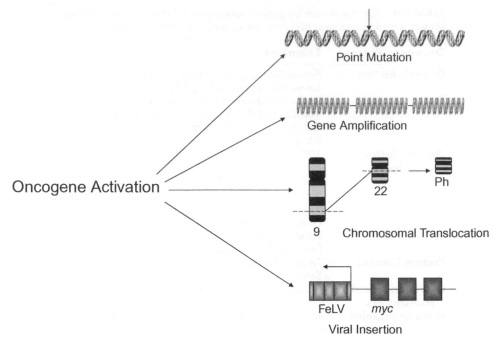

Figure 1.3. Oncogenes may become activated through point mutations, gene amplifications, chromosomal rearrangements, and viral insertions. Reprinted from "From Viruses to cancer stem cells: Dissecting the pathways to malignancy" by Argyle D.J. and Blacking T.M. (The Veterinary Journal, 2007) with kind permission from Elsevier.

kinase activity has become a major target for therapeutic intervention, with many drugs such as Imatinib (a tyrosine kinase inhibitor) in human clinical trials.

- **Gene amplification:** Amplification of oncogenes (i.e., multiple gene copies) can occur in a number of tumor types and has been demonstrated in domestic animal cancers. As an example, the MDM2 proto-oncogene has been identified in dogs and horses and has been shown to be amplified in a proportion of canine soft-tissue sarcomas.
- **Point mutations:** These are single base changes in the DNA sequence of proto-oncogenes leading to the production of abnormal proteins. For example, point mutations in the *ras* proto-oncogene are a consistent finding in a number of human tumors.
- **Viral insertions:** Studies of the tumor-causing viruses allowed for the discovery of oncogenes. The insertion of tumor-causing viral elements into the genome of a cell leads to alteration of proto-oncogene function, transforming the proto-oncogene into an oncogene. This results in the development of a tumor.

Tumor Suppressor Genes

- Changes or mutations in genes can lead to either a stimulatory or inhibitory effect on cell growth and proliferation.
- The stimulatory effects are provided by the proto-oncogenes described above. Mutations of these genes produce positive growth and proliferative signals leading to uncontrolled cellular growth.
- In contrast, tumor formation can result from a loss of inhibitory functions associated with mutation of another class of cellular genes called the *tumor suppressor genes*. In their wild-type, or non-mutated state, the role of tumor suppressor genes is to inhibit cellular proliferation and growth.
- The retinoblastoma gene (Rb) was the first gene that led to the understanding of the mechanisms of tumor suppressor genes.

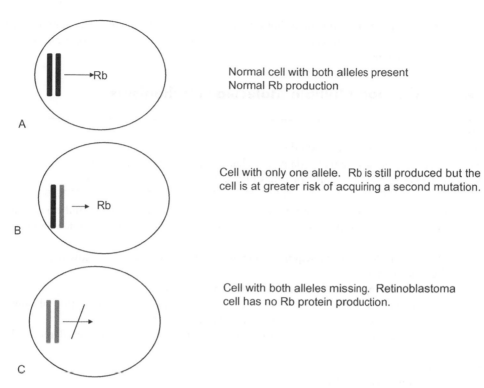

Figure 1.4. In contrast to oncogene mutations, suppressor effects are recessive. Normal cell (A). Mutation in 1 copy (B) usually has no effect but the cell is at risk. Cells with both alleles affected produce no tumor suppressor effects (C). Reprinted from "From Viruses to cancer stem cells: Dissecting the pathways to malignancy" by Argyle D.J. and Blacking T.M. (The Veterinary Journal, 2007) with kind permission from Elsevier.

- Rb plays a central role in regulating cell cycle progression. Alteration of Rb function has been found to be a common feature of many human cancers as well as the classical retinoblastoma tumor, a childhood cancer that arises from the retina. Rb function can be abrogated by point mutations, deletions, or by complex formation with viral oncoproteins. These genetic changes lead to uncontrolled cell cycle progression and cellular proliferation.
- In a cell with one normal, nonmutated allele of a tumor suppressor gene such as Rb, that allele usually produces enough tumor suppressor product to maintain normal function of the gene and control of cellular proliferation. Mutations in tumor suppressor genes behave very differently from oncogene mutations. Whereas activating oncogene mutations in a single allele are dominant to wild-type (i.e., only one mutated allele is required for expression of the proliferating signals), tumor suppressor gene mutations are **recessive** and both alleles must be mutated for the loss of inhibitory function to be expressed.
- Mutation in one tumor suppressor gene copy usually has no effect on wild-type function of the gene, as long as a reasonable amount of wild-type protein remains as a result of the nonmutated allele (Figure 1.4).
- **P53** is a tumor suppressor gene whose product is also intimately involved in cell cycle control.
- P53 has been described as the guardian of the genome, by virtue of its ability to promote cell cycle arrest or apoptosis depending on the degree of DNA damage. Consequently, the p53 tumor suppressor gene plays an important role in cell cycle progression, regulation of gene expression, and the cellular response mechanisms to DNA damage.
- Failure by p53 to activate such cellular functions may ultimately result in abnormal uncontrolled cell growth leading to tumorigenic transformation.

- P53 is the most frequently inactivated gene in human neoplasia with functional loss commonly occurring through gene mutational events, including nonsense, missense, and splice site mutations; allelic loss; rearrangements; and deletions.

Cancer Arises Through Multiple Molecular Mechanisms

Key Points

From the preceding section we can conclude that
- Cancer is a genetic disease, involving fundamental changes in the cell at the genetic level.
- Changes in oncogenes or tumor suppressor genes may contribute to carcinogenesis.

- Cancer research has demonstrated that, despite the many potential causes of cancer and carcinogenic pathways, transformation of a normal cell into a malignant cell actually requires very few molecular, biochemical, and cellular changes.
- These changes can be considered as **the acquired capabilities of a cancer cell** that allow it to be regarded as displaying a malignant phenotype.
- These acquired capabilities appear to be common to all types of cancer.
- Consequently, we can consider that the vast array of cancer phenotypes is a manifestation of only seven alterations in cellular physiology that collectively dictate malignant growth.
- These characteristics are acquired during the process of carcinogenesis and can be considered as the following (Figure 1.5):
  - A self sufficiency in growth
  - An insensitivity to antigrowth signals
  - An ability to evade programmed cell death (apoptosis)
  - Limitless replicative potential (mainly through reactivation of telomerase)
  - An ability to sustain angiogenesis
  - An ability to invade and metastasize
  - An ability to evade host immunity

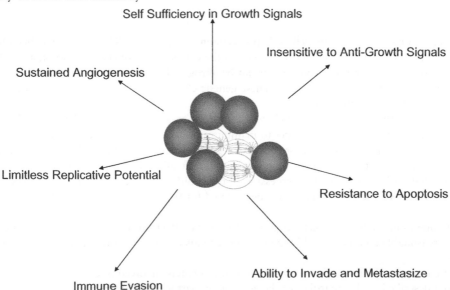

Figure 1.5. The pathways to cancer. Despite the complexity of cancer as a disease, it can be defined on the basis of the acquisition of seven fundamental characteristics: self sufficiency in growth, an insensitivity to antigrowth signals, an ability to evade programmed cell death (apoptosis), limitless replicative potential (mainly through reactivation of telomerase), an ability to sustain angiogenesis, an ability to invade and metastasize, and an ability to evade host immunity. Reprinted from "From Viruses to cancer stem cells: Dissecting the pathways to malignancy" by Argyle D.J. and Blacking T.M. (The Veterinary Journal, 2007) with kind permission from Elsevier.

Key Points
- The pathways for cells becoming malignant are highly variable.
- Mutations in certain oncogenes can occur early in the progression of some tumors, and late in others.
- As a consequence, the acquisition of the essential cancer characteristics may appear at different times in the progression of different cancers.
- Irrespective of the path taken, the hallmark capabilities of cancer will remain common for multiple cancer types and will help clarify mechanisms, prognosis, and the development of new treatments.

The Importance of the Microenvironment

- Tumor formation is a consequence of genetic changes in the target cell.
- However, the formation of a tumor is also directly reliant on an appropriate environment for tumor growth.
- Several studies have demonstrated that the supporting stroma (e.g., fibroblasts), blood vessels and local environmental conditions (e.g., tissue hypoxia), have a direct effect on the ability of a tumor to grow and survive.
- Consequently, the tumor microenvironment also represents a target for therapy.

A Challenge to the Accepted Model of Carcinogenesis: The Cancer Stem Cell Theory

For completeness we mention here a challenge to the accepted model of carcinogenesis:
- The accepted model of carcinogenesis has been a stochastic model whereby any cell in the body has the potential for malignant transformation. A challenge to the stochastic model is the cancer stem cell theory, which suggests that cancer is, in fact, a true stem cell disease.
- The cancer stem cell theory states that malignant transformation occurs in the adult stem cell and gives rise to a cancer stem cell. This would reconcile how a cell would survive long enough to acquire the appropriate number of genetic changes, as stem cells are long-lived.
- This has given rise to the concept that tumors are composed of both cancer stem cells, which have a large proliferative capacity, and a daughter population of cells, with a limited proliferative potential.
- If a population of cancer stem cells is responsible for the propagation of a tumor, this has immense implications for therapy. The evidence suggests that daughter cells, which make up the bulk population of tumors, may be sensitive to the effects of conventional treatments such as radiation and/or chemotherapy. However, stem cell populations tend to harbor strong resistance mechanisms, entering periods of quiescence during which they are resistant to strategies aimed at eradicating cycling cells.
- If conventional therapies are not appropriate for killing cancer stem cells, it would follow that alternative pathways in these cells need to be identified (Figure 1.6).
- The identification of cancer stem cells in both humans and dogs has been a defining moment in cancer research. If the theory is correct, future efforts must be made to characterize these cells with a view to identifying therapeutic targets.

The Causes of Cancer

- In many circumstances, exposure to one tumor-inducing agent or carcinogen provides only one hit toward the development of the malignant phenotype.
- The nature of tumor-inducing agents has been crucial to our understanding of cancer formation because they all have the common property of being able to affect host DNA via genetic or epigenetic means.
- In particular, seminal experiments in animal retroviruses led to the discovery of oncogenes, which was a turning point in our understanding of cancer biology.

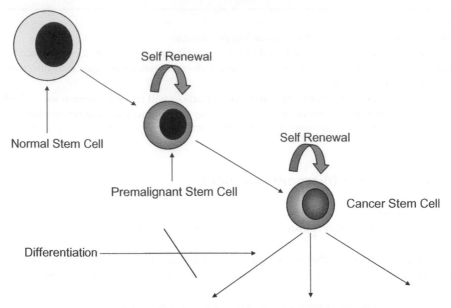

Figure 1.6. The cancer stem cell theory. This theory challenges the stochastic model presented in Fig. 1.1 and suggests that malignant transformation is restricted to adult stem cells. Progression to a full malignant cell then leads to the formation of an asymmetrically dividing cancer cell capable of self-renewal and the production of daughter cells. In a similar way to the production of committed cells from normal stem cells, daughter cancer cells have a limited proliferative capacity. Reprinted from "From Viruses to cancer stem cells: Dissecting the pathways to malignancy" by Argyle D. J. and Blacking T.M. (The Veterinary Journal, 2007) with kind permission from Elsevier.

- These cancer-causing agents can be broadly divided into
  - The oncogenic viruses
  - Chemical carcinogens
  - Physical agents such as radiation

The Oncogenic Viruses

- Oncogenenic viruses provided the first evidence that genetic factors play a role in the development of cancer.
- These viruses are a diverse group of pathogens that include all the major families of the DNA viruses and a class of RNA viruses known as *retroviruses*.
- Although diverse, one almost universal feature is the importance of a DNA stage in the replication of the viral genome.

Retroviruses and Cancer

- Retroviruses are important oncogenic viruses of cats, cattle, and chickens, the studies of which have been seminal to our understanding of viral and nonviral oncogenesis.
- The structure and basic replication cycle of a typical retrovirus is shown in Figure 1.7.
- Retroviruses become integrated into the genome of the cell and can promote carcinogenesis through the activation of cellular oncogenes adjacent to them.
- For example, *myc* is an oncogene intimately associated with cell cycle progression and proliferation. When there is viral insertion close to the *myc* locus, the gene becomes controlled by the powerful viral promoters

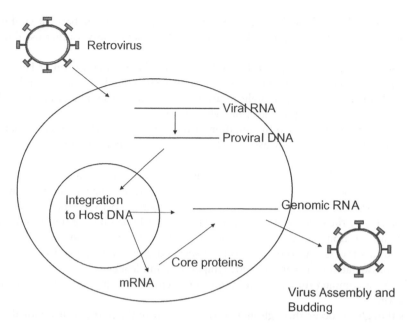

Figure 1.7. The structure and replication life cycle of a typical retrovirus. The retrovirus is a double-stranded RNA virus, which, on entry to the cell, reverse transcribes into proviral DNA. This DNA can integrate into the host genome. Reprinted from "From Viruses to cancer stem cells: Dissecting the pathways to malignancy" by Argyle D. J. and Blacking T.M. (The Veterinary Journal, 2007) with kind permission from Elsevier.

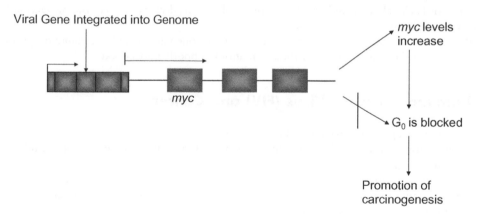

Figure 1.8. Oncogenesis through insertional mutagenesis. In this scenario, the *myc* gene comes under control of the integrated retroviral promoters. There is a failure of cells to enter G$_0$ of the cell cycle, leading to uncontrolled proliferation. Reprinted from "From Viruses to cancer stem cells: Dissecting the pathways to malignancy" by Argyle D.J. and Blacking T.M. (The Veterinary Journal, 2007) with kind permission from Elsevier.

leading to unregulated *myc* expression. Uncontrolled *myc* protein production prevents cells from entering G$_0$, the resting phase of the cell cycle, and thereby promotes unregulated cellular proliferation, a common occurrence in FeLV-associated lymphoma in cats (Figure 1.8).

Feline Leukemia Virus (FeLV)

- Hemopoietic tumors are the most commonly diagnosed neoplasms of the cat accounting for around 30–40% of all tumors and this is directly related to FeLV infection.

- FeLV isolates are classified into three distinct subgroups (A, B, and C) on the basis of viral interference with superinfection. These subgroups most likely define viral envelope subtypes that use different cellular receptor molecules for viral entry.
- FeLV A is ecotropic (can infect only feline cells) and represents the dominant form of FeLV.
- FeLV B is polytropic (can also infect human cells) and is overrepresented in cases of virally induced lymphoma in cats. FeLV B isolates are thought to arise de novo, from recombination events between FeLV A and feline endogenous sequences present in the feline genome.
- FeLV C is also thought to arise de novo by mutation of the *env* gene in FeLV A and are not transmitted in nature. They are uniquely associated with the development of pure red cell aplasia (PRCA) in cats.
- Persistently viremic cats are the main source of infection. The virus is secreted continuously in the saliva and is spread by intimate social contact. The virus can also be spread congenitally from an infected queen to her kittens. In the first few weeks after viral exposure, interactions between the virus and the host's immune system determine the outcome of infection. The potential outcomes of infection include persistent viral infection, latent infection, and the establishment of complete immunity and viral clearance. It is the persistently viremic cats that go on to develop FeLV-associated diseases (Chapter 10).
- Malignant diseases associated with FeLV include lymphomas and leukemias.
- Lymphoma is the most common tumor of cats and can present most commonly in thymic, multicentric, and alimentary forms.
- Tumorigenesis is thought to occur through immunosuppression of the host and insertional effects of proviral DNA on cellular oncogenes such as *myc*.
- However, it is important to note that FeLV is not isolated from all cats with lymphoma. Only 80% of cats with thymic lymphoma are viremic; only 60% and 30% are viremic in the multicentric and alimentary forms, respectively. There is some evidence to suggest that these viruses may be involved as an initiating event before being cleared by the animal's immune system.
- The incidence of FeLV-related lymphoproliferative neoplasia has decreased since routing vaccination protocols were implemented in the 1980s.
- FeLV is also associated with nonmalignant diseases such as bone marrow failure, immunosuppression, and reproductive failure. The pathogenesis of these conditions is poorly understood.

Feline Immunodeficiency Virus (FIV) and Cancer

- In contrast to the oncogenic retroviruses, FIV is a lentivirus.
- These are retroviruses that classically cause diseases with a slow incubation period and include FIV, HIV, maedi visna, and equine infectious anemia.
- FIV has also been associated with neoplastic disease in cats, especially lymphomas. These can largely be explained by the immunosuppression caused by the virus, however, a direct effect associated with viral insertional mutagenesis has been postulated.

The DNA Viruses

- Many DNA viruses have been associated with the development of cancer in animals and humans. In particular, the papilloma viruses (which are small DNA viruses) have long been known to cause wart lesions, which can become malignant depending on a number of several other predisposing factors.
- Most often, wart lesions are overcome by the immune system and disappear from the animal over a 6-month period. The life cycle of the virus is tightly coupled with the differentiation process of the epithelial cell and, in certain circumstances, the benign wart can persist and ultimately become transformed to become a malignant tumor, squamous cell carcinoma.
- The most extensively studied of the papilloma viruses are the bovine papilloma viruses (BPV). Papilloma viruses have been used as model systems to study the role of co-carcinogens in the development of cancer.

- In contrast to the papilloma viruses, herpes viruses are large DNA viruses and are known to cause Mareks disease in chickens. The herpes viruses are the subject of extensive studies in man through their involvement in Epstein-Barr virus (EBV) – associated lymphomas and Kaposi's sarcoma.

Chemical Carcinogenesis

- In 1775 Sir Percival Potts perceived the relationship between the high incidence of scrotal cancer in chimney sweeps and their chronic exposure to soot. He also noted that skin cancer in the general population was a disease of middle to late age, whereas the chimney sweep boys, who often were exposed to soot at the age of 4 years, developed cancer in their teens.
- These observations demonstrated the link between chemicals such as hydrocarbons and the development of cancer. Since this time, the role of chemical carcinogens has been extensively studied in human and, to a lesser extent, in veterinary medicine.
- The role of tobacco smoke and asbestos are well documented from epidemiological studies in human cancer patients, but their role in veterinary cancer medicine is still unclear.
- Examples of chemically induced carcinogenesis playing a role in veterinary cancers include the following:
  - Bracken fern has been shown to provide a cofactor for malignant transformation with papilloma viruses in cattle.
  - Some epidemiological studies have linked the use of herbicides with the development of canine lymphoma. However, the data presented for the latter has been questioned and the role of herbicides and pesticides in domestic animal cancers still remains unclear.
  - Food substances can also be carcinogenic and notable is aflatoxin, an alkaloid produced by Aspergillus species, which grows on badly stored peanuts. A classical veterinary case involved an epizootic of liver cancer in trout reaching up to 60% incidence in Denmark and Kenya. The trout had been fed on a batch of moldy peanuts in hatcheries in Denmark.
  - Of major importance is the use of chemicals that induce **chronic inflammation**. The use of cyclophosphamide for treatment of cancer patients can lead to chronic inflammation of the bladder due to renal excretion of a metabolite of cyclophosphamide called *acrolein*. Although not common, there are case reports of transitional cell carcinoma of the bladder in dogs after treatment with cyclophosphamide.

Chronic Inflammation, Bacteria, and Cancer

- There is still little known about the role of inflammation, chronic irritation, or trauma in the development of cancer, and many reports have largely been anecdotal. However, there are a number of important observations that have been made that warrant further investigation:
  - There is epidemiological evidence to suggest that primary bone neoplasia may occur at the site of a previous fracture or repair. In most documented cases, there has been a complication of surgery such as low-grade osteomyelitis that may contribute to the development of cancer. In addition, the presence of microfractures through increased mechanical stress in the growing long bones of the giant breeds may contribute to the higher incidence of bone cancer in these dogs.
  - There have been case reports that have described the development of squamous cell carcinomas at the sites of both burns and scar tissue in horses. The development of tumors at the site of previous burns in humans is well recognized.
  - It has been suggested that the development of cutaneous epitheliotropic lymphoma (mycosis fungoides) in dogs may be through persistent antigenic stimulation in the skin. Although c-type retroviral particles have been isolated from canine lymphoma cells in culture, their role in tumorigenesis is still speculative. It is possible that persistent stimulation of lymphoid cells in the skin may allow the selection of malignant cells and the establishment of the tumor. A similar situation occurs in human gastric lymphoma associated with helicobactor pylori infection.
  - There is still uncertainty surrounding the carcinogenic trigger in injection-site sarcomas in cats. Numerous theories have been suggested, including the role of the adjuvant and the vaccine itself (chemical carcinogenesis). However, malignant transformation may not be a reflection of what is injected or applied, but

rather may result from the local irritation/inflammation that is adding another "hit" to a cell that is on its way to malignancy.

- Although not well studied in animals, *Helicobactor pylori* has emerged as a highly important pathogen of man, especially in its association with gastric ulcer disease and gastric carcinoma. The role of this bacteria in this disease is now undisputed and it is regarded as a causal agent of cancer in man. Further, it is also associated with the development of gastric lymphoma in man, through chronic inflammation. It is incredible that simple treatment of these tumors with antibiotics can lead to regression.

Parasitic Infections

- A paucity of information exists regarding the role of parasites in carcinogenesis.
- The most quoted example is that of the helminth infection *Spirocerca Lupi*. This parasite is endemic in Africa and Southeast U.S. and causes esophageal tumors (fibrosarcoma or osteosarcoma) in dogs and foxes). Worm eggs develop into larvae in an intermediate host. In the dog, ingested larvae migrate to the esophagus via the aorta and form highly vascular fibroblastic nodules. These nodules can undergo malignant transformation to form either fibrosarcomas or osteosarcomas.

Physical Agents

- Radiation is a well-known carcinogen in animals and man. This is due to DNA damage that is caused directly by the radiation or indirectly through radiation-mediated intracellular production of oxygen free radicals. DNA damage can lead to genetic mutations that play a role in tumorigenesis. For this reason, the use of diagnostic and therapeutic radiation should be thoughtful and planned. Unnecessary exposure to radiation should be unconditionally avoided.
- In terms of ultraviolet radiation, the association between sunlight and the development of malignancies has been recognized for over a hundred years and has been one of the most extensively studied physical causes of cancer.
- In man, the association between the frequency and severity of sunburns during childhood and the eventual development of malignant melanoma has been proven in epidemiological studies.
- In domestic animals, the best-documented examples of this kind are in the development of squamous cell carcinomas in white cats, whiteface cattle, and possibly in gray horses.
- In white cats, the pinnae and the nasal planum are susceptible to chronic inflammatory dermatitis that may be initiated by excessive exposure to direct sunlight containing UV radiation (especially UVB). A photon of UVB can cause malignant transformation of skin cells by its subcellular effects on DNA.
- It has also been suggested that a contributing mechanism may be immunosuppression as a consequence of UV exposure. In this, UV-B photons can convert transurocyanic acid in the skin to cisurocyanic acid that can have profound effects on antigen-presenting cell function and T cell activity.

Hormones and Cancer

- In man, cancer of the breast, endometrium, ovary, and prostate occur in hormone-responsive tissues, and these tumors may require hormones for their continued growth.
- Hormones can influence cancer development by enhancing cellular replication in cells that may have already acquired a number of genetic hits toward malignancy.
- Estrogen in bitches is known to influence the development of benign vaginal fibromas that regress after a season or ovariohysterectomy.
- It is well documented that early ovariohysterectomy in bitches is protective for mammary carcinoma. The hormonal influences on breast cancer are far better defined for women than dogs. The complete role of estrogens and progesterones, and the significance of receptor expression on canine mammary tumors are still under investigation.

Genetic Predisposition to Cancer

- In man, there are a number of inherited syndromes that give rise to familial cancer syndromes. The best characterized are Li-Fraumeni syndrome (inheritance of an abnormal copy of a p53 allele) and retinoblastoma (inheritance of an abnormal copy of a Rb allele). In both of these cases, the defect occurs in a tumor suppressor gene and therefore both alleles must be affected for abnormal function of the gene to be expressed. Affected individuals are more likely to develop cancers at a younger age.
- Other inherited cancers include Wilm's tumor (WT1), familial adenomatous polyposis (FAP), and breast cancer (BCRA 1 and BCRA 2).
- It is well recognized that certain breeds of dogs have a predisposition to certain cancers.
- The publication of the canine genome, and the development of appropriate linkage maps, is now allowing the opportunity to identify specific genetic changes in breeds that allow their susceptibility to certain cancers.

References and Suggested Further Reading

Adams G.E., Cox R. 1997. Radiation carcinogenesis. *In* The Molecular and Cellular Biology of Cancer, Third Edition, edited by Franks and Teich. Oxford University Press, pp. 130–148.

Argyle D.J., Blacking T.M. 2007. From viruses to cancer stem cells: Dissecting the pathways to malignancy. The Veterinary Journal (*In press*).

Argyle D.J., Khanna C. 2006. Tumour biology and metastasis, *In* Small Animal Clinical Oncology (Withrow and Vail). Elsevier, Amsterdam, pp. 31–53.

Blacking T.M., Wilson H., Argyle D.J. 2007. Is cancer a stem cell disease? Theory evidence and implications. Veterinary and Comparative Oncology 5(2):76–89.

Hanahan D., Weinberg R.A. 2000. The hallmarks of cancer. Cell Jan 7(100:1):57–70.

Jarrett O., Onions D. 1992. Leukaemogenic viruses. *In* Leukaemia, Second Edition, edited by J.A. Whittaker. Blackwell Scientific Publications, Oxford, pp. 34–63.

Lane D.P. 1992. P53: Guardian of the genome. Nature 358:15–16.

McCance K.L., Roberts L.K. 1997. Cellular biology. *In* Pathophysiology, The Biological Basis of Disease in Adults and Children, Third Edition, edited by K.L. McCance and S.E. Huether. Mosbey College Publishing, St. Louis, Missouri, pp. 1–43.

Neil J.C., Hughs D., McFarlane R. et al. 1984. Transduction and rearrangement of the *myc* gene by feline leukaemia virus in naturally occurring T cell leukameias. Nature 308:814–820.

O'Byrne K.J., Dalgleish A.G. 2001. Chronic immune activation and inflammation as the cause of malignancy. British Journal of Cancer, Aug 17(85:4):473–483.

Onions D.E., Jarrett O. 1987. Naturally occurring tumours in animals as a model for human disease. Cancer Surveys 6:1–181.

Onions D.E., Lees G., Forrest D. et al. 1987. Recombinant feline viruses containing the *myc* gene rapidly produce clonal tumours expressing T-cell antigen receptor gene transcripts. International Journal of Cancer 40:40–45.

Tennent R., Wigley C., Balmain A. 1997. Chemical Carcinogenesis. *In* The Molecular and Cellular Biology of Cancer, Third Edition, edited by Franks and Teich. Oxford University Press, pp. 106–129.

Vousden K.H. 1994. Cell Transformation by human papillomaviruses. *In* Viruses and Cancer, edited by Minsen). Cambridge University Press, Cambridge U.K., pp. 27–46.

Wyke J. 1997. Viruses and cancer. *In* The Molecular and Cellular Biology of Cancer, Third Edition, edited by Franks and Teich. Oxford University Press, pp. 151–168.

2
PARANEOPLASTIC SYNDROMES

Mala G. Renwick and David J. Argyle

This chapter describes the main clinical and pathological features of paraneoplastic syndromes (PNS) in dogs and cats, including algorithms for treatment. The main aims of this chapter are
1. An appreciation of the diversity, complexity, and clinical relevance of PNS
2. Recognition and treatment options for the most common PNS

Key Points
- PNS represent diverse clinical syndromes resulting from systemic effects of neoplasia (Tables 2.1, 2.2).
- The effects occur at sites distant from the tumor and can affect many end-target organs.
- Syndromes include hormonal, metabolic, hematologic, neuromuscular, dermatologic, musculoskeletal, renal, gastrointestinal, and cardiovascular disorders.
- PNS may occur as a result of
  - Immune-mediated mechanisms
  - Peptide, protein, ectopic, or eutopic hormone secretion
  - Protein hormone precursor or cytokine secretion
  - Production of enzymes or other biochemical mechanisms that interfere with normal metabolic pathways

---

The presence of PNS may affect the following:
- **Diagnosis:**
  - Detection may indicate occult malignancy.
  - Recognition may suggest the type of tumor.
- **Management:**
  - It may represent a true oncologic emergency.
  - Successful treatment requires a parallel approach to both PNS and the tumor.
  - It may be difficult to differentiate from adverse effects of therapy.
- **Prognosis:**
  - Co-morbid disease is often a negative prognostic factor.
  - Reduced performance status may preclude specific therapy with impact on survival.
- **Quality of life:**
  - It may increase morbidity and deleterious long-term effects.
  - It may cause an impact on recovery and hospitalization times.

Tumor response may parallel that of the PNS in two ways:
- As a marker of clinical remission
- With recrudescence often heralding relapse

19

Table 2.1. Canine and feline paraneoplastic syndromes and commonly associated tumors

	Paraneoplastic Syndrome	Common Associations
Metabolic	Fever	Lymphomas; leukemias; histiocytic disease; sarcomas; hepatic, renal, gut tumors and others
	Anorexia, cachexia	Many tumors
Endocrine	Hyperthyroidism	Feline adenoma/hyperplasia, 20% canine thyroid carcinomas
	Hyperadrenocorticism, Cushing's syndrome (glucocorticoid excess)	Pituitary adenoma (dogs), adrenal carcinoma
	Hypercalcemia	Lymphomas, anal sac apocrine gland adenocarcinoma, parathyroid adenoma/carcinoma, multiple myeloma, mammary carcinoma, thyroid carcinoma, thymoma, other tumors
	Acromegaly	Pituitary adenoma (cats)
	Hypoglycemia	(Pancreatic β cell) insulinoma, hepatic and smooth muscle tumors, some hemopoietic tumors
	Feminization syndrome	Testicular tumors
	Hypertension	Adrenal medullary tumor – pheochromocytoma
	Hypergastrinemia, Zollinger-Ellison syndrome	(Pancreatic islet cell) gastrinoma
	Hyperaldosteronism, Conn's syndrome	Adrenocortical tumor – rare
	Inappropriate secretion of ADH	Rare
	Diabetes insipidus	Rarely paraneoplastic
Hematologic	Anemia	Many tumors and mechanisms
	Erythrocytosis	Renal and lung tumors, hepatic tumors
	Thrombocytopenia	Hemopoietic tumors, histiocytic disease
	Thrombocytosis	Lung, mammary, gut, reproductive tumors
	Leucocytosis	
	• Neutrophilia	Lymphomas; lung, mammary, gut renal tumors
	• Eosinophilia	Lymphomas, mast cell tumors, thymoma, lymphomatoid granulomatosis
	• Basophilia	Mast cell tumor
	Bleeding diathesis/coagulopathy DIC	Hemopoietic, epithelial and mesenchymal tumors, mast cell and histiocytic tumors, end stage many tumors
	Aplastic anemia	Hyperestrogenism – testicular and ovarian tumors
Hyperviscosity	Hyperviscosity	Multiple myeloma, lymphomas, leukemias
Dermatologic	Alopecia	Feline pancreatic adenocarcinoma, biliary carcinoma
	Exfoliative dermatitis	Feline thymoma
	Nodular dermatofibrosis	German shepherd dog renal cystadenocarcinoma
	Superficial necrolytic dermatitis	Glucagonoma – rare
	Flushing/erythema	Hemangiosarcoma, mast cell tumor, pheochromocytoma
	Feminization syndrome	Testicular tumors
	Hypertrichosis	Insulinoma
	Pemphigus complex	Lymphoma, sarcomas
Renal	Renal protein loss	Lymphomas; leukemias; melanoma; lung, thyroid, gut, mammary, pancreatic tumors
	Glomerulonephritis, nephrotic syndrome	Myeloma, lymphomas, leukemias, polycythemia vera, renal carcinoma
Neuromuscular	Myasthenia gravis	Thymoma, osteosarcoma
	Peripheral neuropathy	Insulinoma
Musculoskeletal	Hypertrophic osteopathy, Marie's disease	Primary lung and other intrathoracic tumors
	Polyarthropathy	Lymphomas; leukemias; histiocytic disease; gut, prostate, and mesenchymal tumors
	Polymyositis	Lymphomas; lung, stomach, breast, uterine tumors

Table 2.2.   Investigation of the patient with suspected PNS

Investigation	Specifics	Comments
Signalment and history	Species, breed, age, sex	Disease associations
	Duration and progression of signs	Acute, chronic, insidious
Clinical examination	Demeanor, body condition score, physical exam	Constellation of signs, rule in/out neoplasia
CBC, smear examination	RBC parameters and morphology	ACD, IMHA, MAHA, IDA, erythrocytosis
	WBC parameters and morphology	
	Platelet count	Neutrophilia, eosinophilia – inflammation/infection/neoplasia
		Thrombocytopenia, thrombocytosis, DIC
Serum chemistries	Renal parameters, calcium, ionized calcium, electrolytes, proteins, enzymes, bile acids, tT4 PTH, PTH-rp, paired insulin and glucose	Hypercalcemia, gammopathy, hypoglycemia, renal protein loss, endocrinopathy, organ function
Coagulation profile	PT, APTT / KCCT, fibrinogen, FDPs, AT-III, D-dimers	Bleeding, thromboembolism, DIC, hyperviscosity
Urinalysis	SG, sediment exam, quantify proteinuria with UPCr	Renal protein loss, nephropathy
Protein electrophoresis	Serum, urine, CSF	Monoclonal or polyclonal gammopathy, nephropathy, neuropathy
Serum autoantibodies	AChR antibodies	Myasthenia gravis
Marrow examination	Hypercalcemia, gammopathy, cytopenias, increased cell numbers, aberrant cells, PUO	Myelodysplasia, hemopoietic neoplasia, metastatic disease
CSF evaluation	Neuropathy, pyrexia hypercalcemia, gammopathy	
Imaging	Survey, local and locoregional radiography, ultrasonography – abdomen, mediastinum, neck, masses, endoscopy procedures, CT, MRI	Rule in/out/localize neoplasia, tissue sampling
Cytology, histology	Tissue biopsy – FNA, needle core, blade	Rule in/out neoplasia, cytology, histopathology
Exploratory surgery	Laparotomy, thoracotomy, neck exploration, masses	Histopathology

CBC, complete blood count; RBC, red blood cells; WBC, white blood cells; ACD, anemia of chronic disease; IMHA, immune-mediated hemolytic anemia; MAHA, microangiopathic hemolytic anemia; IDA, iron deficiency anemia; DIC, disseminated intravascular coagulopathy; PTH, parathyroid hormone; PTH-rp, parathyroid hormone related peptide; PT, prothrombin time; APTT, activated partial thromboplastin time; KCCT, kaolin cephalin coagulation time; FDPs, fibrin degradation products; AT-III, antithrombin III; SG, urine specific gravity; UPCr, urine protein creatinine ratio; AChR, acetylcholine receptor antibodies; PUO, pyrexia of unknown origin; CT, computed tomography scan; MRI, magnetic resonance imaging; FNA, fine needle aspirate.

Specific Syndromes

Hypercalcemia

- Hypercalcemia is a consequence of deregulation of homeostatic mechanisms between parathyroid hormone (PTH), calcitonin, and active vitamin D (calcitriol) $1,25\text{-}(OH)_2D_3$ (Figure 2.1).
- PNS hypercalcemia is the most common metabolic emergency in canine and feline cancer patients.
- The most frequent causes of hypercalcemia are
  - Malignancy and hypoadrenocorticism in dogs
  - Malignancy, renal failure, or idiopathic in cats

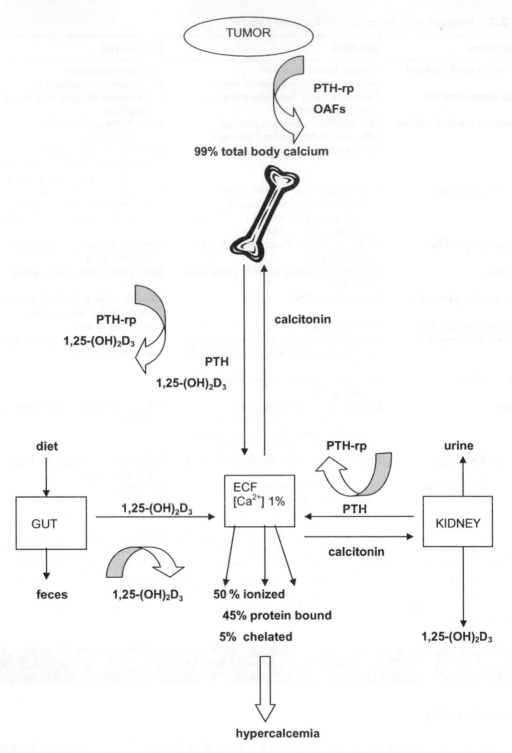

Figure 2.1. Calcium regulation and pathophysiology of hypercalcemia of malignancy.

- Nearly half of total serum calcium is albumin-bound, so measured total calcium is affected by serum albumin.
- To avoid artificially low calcium levels, total calcium is interpreted with respect to serum albumin by using the corrected calcium value in dogs:

$$\text{corrected total } Ca^{2+} = \{[(\text{total } Ca^{2+} \text{mmol}/L \times 4) - (\text{albumin g}/L \times 0.1)] + 3.5\} \times 0.25$$

- Biologically active ionized calcium is increased by acidosis and decreased by alkalosis and should be assessed using anaerobic samples.

Humoral hypercalcemia of malignancy (HHM) 80%

- In nonskeletal solid tumors as a result of tumor-derived parathyroid hormone–related protein (PTH-rp), and cytokines such as transforming growth factors (TGF) ά and β, interleukins IL-1 and 6, epidermal growth factor (EGF), tumor necrosis factor (TNF), and estrogen functioning as osteoclast activating factors (OAFs)—e.g., T-cell lymphoma, anal gland adenocarcinoma, thyroid carcinoma, thymoma, malignant melanoma, squamous cell carcinoma.
- Increased plasma PTH-rp concentration in a hypercalcemic patient in the absence of renal failure gives a strong index of suspicion for neoplasia.

Osteolytic hypercalcemia 10–20%

Results from direct bone destruction in primary (myeloma, leukemia, bone tumor) or metastatic (mammary and thyroid carcinoma) tumor.

1,25-(OH)$_2$D$_3$

Secretion of calcitriol by some hemopoietic tumors.

Main clinical features of hypercalcemia

The most common clinical signs are
- In the dog, polyuria and polydipsia
- In the cat, lethargy and anorexia
  The severity of clinical signs depends on
- The absolute magnitude
- The rate of rise
- The underlying cause
- Metastatic disease
- The duration of the hypercalcemia
  Clinical signs may be vague and nonspecific, or represent severe life-threatening illness (Figures 2.2–2.4). Hypercalcemic nephropathy and renal failure are common sequelae.
- In general, verified total calcium greater than 3 mmol/L or ionized calcium greater than 1.4–1.5 mmol/L associated with clinical signs represents a medical emergency warranting aggressive treatment, monitoring and investigation (Table 2.3, Figures 2.2–2.4).
- If ionized calcium measurements are not available, a calcium phosphate product greater than 4.5–6.0 mmol/L implies a high risk of soft-tissue calcification.

Hypoglycemia

Factors implicated in PNS hypoglycemia include (Figure 2.6)
- Autonomous insulin production from pancreatic islet β cell tumors:
  - Tumor glucose metabolism (Figure 2.6)
  - Increased hepatic glucose metabolism
  - Inappropriate hepatic gluconeogenesis and glycogenelysis
  - Increased activity of insulin-like growth factor IGF-II in non-islet cell tumor induced hypoglycemia, NICTH

Table 2.3. Management of hypercalcemia

Treatment	Mode of Action	Moderate to Severe ± Clinical Signs	Comment
IVFT 0.9% NaCl	Restore ECF volume, ↑GFR, ↑calciuresis	100–150 ml/kg/day	Effect in hours; volume overload risk (cardiac, renal dysfunction, hypoalbuminemia); supplement potassium
Frusemide[a]	↓tubular Ca^{2+} reabsorption at the Loop of Henle	2–4 mg/kg bid/tid IV/SQ/PO	Effect in hours; ensure volume expansion before use; supplement potassium
Corticosteroid • Dexamethasone • Prednisolone	Inhibits OAF and vitamin D;↓gut absorption, bone resorption and ↑renal Ca^{2+} excretion	0.1–0.25 mg/kg bid IV/SQ 1 mg/kg sid/bid PO	Effect in hours; may hamper diagnosis by early use; may induce multidrug resistance
Calcitonin	Salmon-derived or synthetic; ↓ bone resorption	D: 4–8 IU/kg bid/tid SQ C: 4 IV/kg bid SQ	Effect in hours; short-acting; emesis and refractoriness are common; hypersensitivity
Bisphosphonates • Pamidronate • Zoledronate • Clodronate	Bind Ca^{2+} to hydroxyappetite crystals; ↓ bone resorption; some analgesic ± anti-tumor effect	D: 0.75–2.0 mg/kg IV in saline 2 hr c.r.i. D: 0.25 mg/kg IV in saline 15 min c.r.i. D: 20–40 mg/kg/daily PO	Onset in 24 hours; risk hypo $Ca^{2+}/PO_4/K^+/Mg^{2+}$, renal failure
Sodium bicarbonate	Promotes alkalosis; ↑ protein bound Ca^{2+} fraction	1 mEq/kg IV slow bolus/infusion; then 0.3× base deficit × weight in kg/day	Blood gas analysis indicated; only mild Ca^{2+} reduction; short-lived effect
H₂ receptor antagonist • Ranitidine • Famotidine		D: 2 mg/kg bid IV/PO C: 3.5 mg/kg bid IV/PO 0.5–1.0 mg/kg sid PO	
Dopamine	Inotrope; Restore urine output, treat oliguric renal failure	D: 2–10 ug/kg/min IV c.r.i C: 1–5 ug/kg/min IV c.r.i	

Note: D = dog; C = cat; C.R.I. = Continuous Rate Infusion

Main clinical features of hypoglycemia

Clinical signs of hypoglycemia may be associated with (Figures 2.7; Table 2.4):

• exercise by increased glucose use
• fasting by decreased glucose availability
• feeding by stimulation of insulin secretion

Clinical signs may be

• neuroglycopenic, or
• compensatory adrenergic due to catecholamine release

Although neuroglycopenica signs may be anticipated with blood glucose less than 2 mmol/lg, the severity of clinical signs depends on

• The absolute level
• The rate of fall
• The underlying cause
• Metastatic disease
• The duration of hypoglycemia

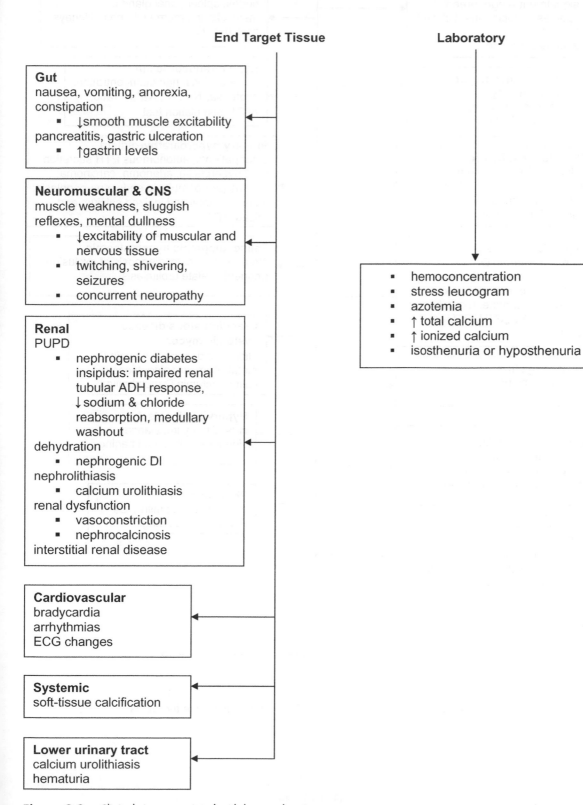

End Target Tissue

Gut
nausea, vomiting, anorexia, constipation
- ↓smooth muscle excitability
pancreatitis, gastric ulceration
- ↑gastrin levels

Neuromuscular & CNS
muscle weakness, sluggish reflexes, mental dullness
- ↓excitability of muscular and nervous tissue
- twitching, shivering, seizures
- concurrent neuropathy

Renal
PUPD
- nephrogenic diabetes insipidus: impaired renal tubular ADH response, ↓sodium & chloride reabsorption, medullary washout
dehydration
- nephrogenic DI
nephrolithiasis
- calcium urolithiasis
renal dysfunction
- vasoconstriction
- nephrocalcinosis
interstitial renal disease

Cardiovascular
bradycardia
arrhythmias
ECG changes

Systemic
soft-tissue calcification

Lower urinary tract
calcium urolithiasis
hematuria

Laboratory

- hemoconcentration
- stress leucogram
- azotemia
- ↑ total calcium
- ↑ ionized calcium
- isosthenuria or hyposthenuria

Figure 2.2. Clinical signs associated with hypercalcemia.

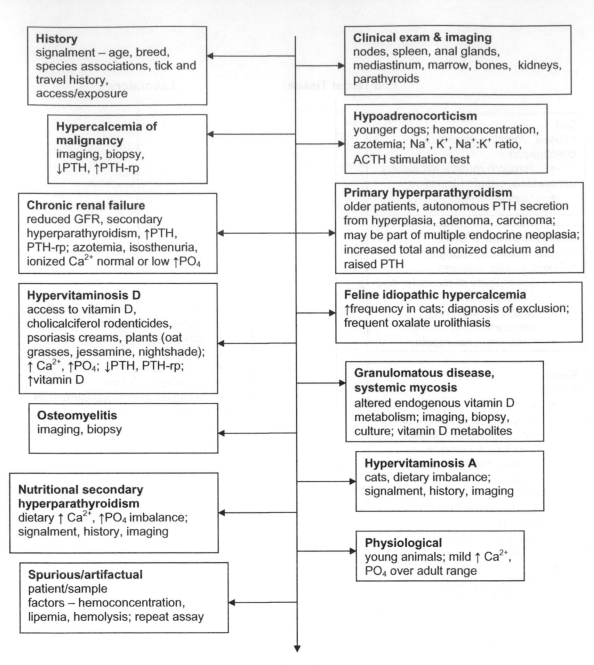

Figure 2.3. Initial screening tests for paraneoplastic hypercalcemia.

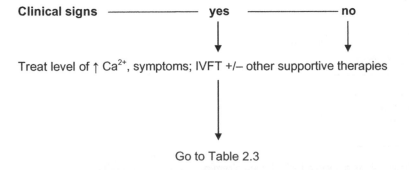

Figure 2.4. Management of hypercalcemia treatment decision tree.

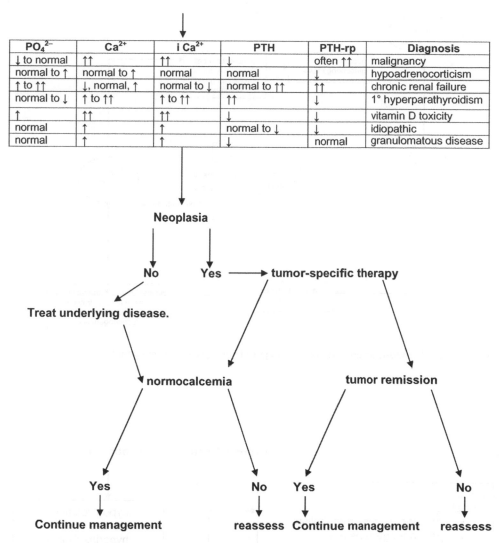

PO$_4^{2-}$	Ca^{2+}	i Ca^{2+}	PTH	PTH-rp	Diagnosis
↓ to normal	↑↑	↑↑	↓	often ↑↑	malignancy
normal to ↑	normal to ↑	normal	normal	↓	hypoadrenocorticism
↑ to ↑↑	↓, normal, ↑	normal to ↓	normal to ↑↑	↑↑	chronic renal failure
normal to ↓	↑ to ↑↑	↑ to ↑↑	↑↑	↓	1° hyperparathyroidism
↑	↑↑	↑↑	↓	↓	vitamin D toxicity
normal	↑	↑	normal to ↓	↓	idiopathic
normal	↑	↑	↓	normal	granulomatous disease

Figure 2.5. Discrimination between PNS and non-PNS hypercalcemia.

Diagnosis and treatment of hypoglycemia (Figures 2.8 and 2.9; Table 2.4)

- Irrespective of the etiology, supportive therapy and investigations are initiated in a parallel approach to management of hypoglycemia and the underlying tumor.
- Surgery is the treatment of choice, partial pancreatectomy for insulinoma with metasectomy as required, and radical resection for other tumors.
- Prognosis is good for uncommon benign tumors and where neurological damage is reversible.

Hypertrophic Osteopathy (HO)

- Hypertrophic osteopathy (HO) features progressive, palisading periosteal hyperostosis of the distal extremities.
- HO is more common in dogs than cats.

Main clinical features of HO (Table 2.5)

- HO is often insidious in onset and most commonly represents a PNS, although some non-malignant diseases are implicated.
- The tumor is often occult at presentation; signs are attributable to progressive limb lesions before signs of malignant disease.

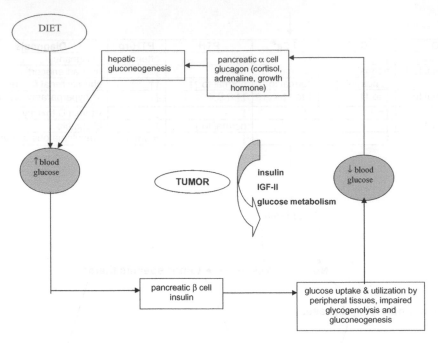

Figure 2.6. Glucose homeostasis and pathophysiology of hypoglycemia of malignancy.

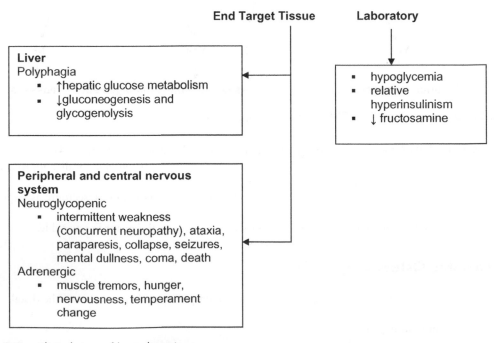

Figure 2.7. Clinical signs of hypoglycemia.

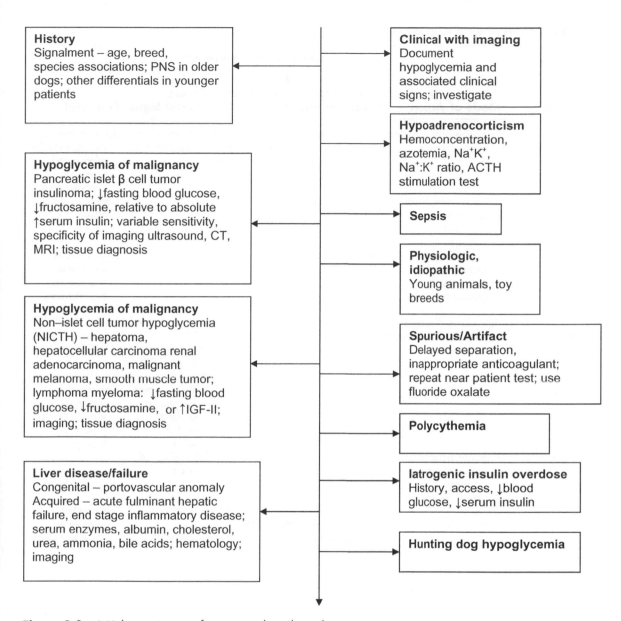

| | History
Signalment – age, breed, species associations; PNS in older dogs; other differentials in younger patients | | Clinical with imaging
Document hypoglycemia and associated clinical signs; investigate |

Figure 2.8. Initial screening tests for paraneoplastic hypoglycemia.

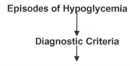

Episodes of Hypoglycemia

Diagnostic Criteria

		? cell tumor	NICTH	Non-malignant hypoglycemia
Whipple's triad	hypoglycemia	yes	yes	yes
	symptomatic with hypoglycemia	yes	yes	yes
	symptoms resolve with euglycemia	yes	yes	yes
relative or absolute hyperinsulinism (paired insulin and glucose)		yes	no	no
↑IGF-II		no	yes	no

Figure 2.9. Diagnosis of hypoglycemia.

Table 2.4. Management of hypoglycemia

| Treatment | Mode of Action | Level of Hypoglycemia | | | Comment |
		Mild and/or Asymptomatic	Moderate ± Mild Clinical Signs	Severe ± Severe Clinical Signs	
Diet	Minimize post prandial hyperglycemia	4–6 meals per day; high protein, fat, and complex carbohydrates; low simple sugars or starches; plus feed in response to clinical signs			Sugar feeding can stimulate insulin release and precipitate hypoglycemia
Prednisolone	Promotes peripheral insulin resistance, promotes glycogenotysis	0.5–1.0 mg/kg bid PO			Corticosteroid side effects
Diazoxide	Inhibits insulin secretion, promotes gluconeogenesis	5 mg/kg bid PO			Emesis, blood dyscrasias tachycardia, hypertension, refractoriness
Hydrochlorthiazide Somatostatin analog (Ocreotide)	Potentiates diazoxide Inhibits insulin synthesis and release	2–4 mg bid PO		5–20 mg bid/tid PO 10–20 ug per dog bid SQ	Needs specific tissue receptors; variable effiacy
Dextrose 5% Dextrose 50%			IV c.r.i.	IV c.r.i. 1 ml/kg IV over 10 minutes to effect, diluted 1:3 in saline	Can stimulate insulin production and precipitate hypoglycemia
Dexamethasone	Promatis peripheral insulin resistance, promotes glycogenolysis			0.5 mg/kg bid IV c.r.i.	
Streptozotocin	Selective β cell cytotoxic	Indicated only for management of insulinoma, primary or metastatic disease 500 mg/m² IV q 21 days with diuretic protocol			Nephrotoxic, emetogenic, renal tumors in man
Glucagon	Promotes glycogenolysis and gluconeogenesis				

- HO results in severe disability, pain, and reduced quality of life.
- Recognition should prompt early investigation for the underlying lesion.
- Successful management of the underlying lesion can produce rapid resolution.

Dermatological Paraneoplastic Syndromes (Table 2.6)

Hematologic Paraneoplastic Syndromes (Tables 2.7–2.13)

Investigation of anemia, thrombocytopenia

- complete blood count, smear examination, reticulocyte count – regeneration
- serum proteins, urea, creatinine, liver enzymes, bile acids – blood loss, g.i. involvement, liver function

Table 2.5. Hypertrophic osteopathy

Etiology	Pathophysiology	Associations	Differential Diagnosis	Clinical Signs	Diagnostic Tests	Management
Intrathoracic (pulmonary) tumors	Implicated factors include effects of proteins produced by the lesion: i. Vasoactive estrogen or GH ii. Changes in the peripheral vascular supply iii. Vagal and intercostal irritation and hyperactivity iv. Irritation of periosteum and synovial membranes by toxins v. Enhanced blood flow to the extremities vi. Fibrovascular	Primary pulmonary neoplasia, pulmonary metastatic disease in association with primary bone tumor are most common	Osteoarthritis Osteomyelitis Primary bone tumor Hypertrophic osteodystrophy Panosteitis Hypervitaminosis A (cat) Musopolyscccharidosis (cat)	Nonedematous, symmetrical, extremity soft tissue: • Swelling • Pain • Heat • Tightness of the skin • Lameness • Immobility	Clinical signs and radiographic assessment. Limb localization Radiography – symmetrical, proliferative periosteal, distal extremity reaction. Changes support intrathoracic neoplasia. Routine laboratory assessment. Further imaging.	i. Pain relief, antiinflammatory medication ii. Surgical extirpation of the underlying lesion; resolution in clinical and radiographic changes in weeks to months
Extrathoracic tumors		Hepatic and UGT tumors without pulmonary metastatic disease				
Chronic inflammatory intrathoracic disease	connective tissue proliferation through chondroid metaplasia to new bone formation					

Note: GH, growth hormone; UGT, urogenital tract.

31

Table 2.6 Canine and feline dermatological paraneoplastic syndromes

Paraneoplastic Syndrome	Tumor Associations	Etiology	Clinical Findings	Comment	Treatment
Flushing	MCT, HSA, carcinoid, pheochromocytoma	tumor secretion of vasocative hormones, PGs & histamine	intermittent skin flushing/redness and heat	may be hypertensive; systemic signs reflect metastatic disease or other PNS (DIC, mast cell degranulation)	surgery; chemotherapy; palliative management with H1, H2 blockers, anti-serotonin agents (ondansetron, cyproheptidine)
Feminization syndrome	30% of Sertoli cell tumors; other testicular tumors	sex hormone imbalance/hyperestrogenism	bilaterally symmetrical non-pruritic alopecia, linear preputial dermatosis, pendulous prepuce; gynecomastia	systemic signs reflect myelosuppression, behavior change, attractiveness to male dogs, squamous prostatic metaplasia (prostatomegaly); <10% metastatic rate	castration; coeliotomy if cryptorchid; castration is curative in the absence of metastases or pancytopenia
Nodular dermatofibrosis	Renal cystadenoma, cystadenocarcinoma	increased local tissue cytokine TGFβ1; collagenous fibrosis	concurrent multiple dermal and subcutaneous masses, limbs and head; systemic signs reflect renal involvement	autosomal dominant inherited cancer syndrome; tumor suppressor gene; GSD; skin signs precede systemic illness; also smooth muscle tumors in bitches; chronic course	if signalment and skin signs are appropriate, monitor for renal lesions; surgery for skin lesions; spay to avoid uterine tumors and breeding; nephrectomy if unilateral
Exfoliative dermatitis	Thymoma	erythema multiforme type reaction	progressive, non-pruritic, alopecia, erythema, scaling, systemic signs relate to mediastinal mass	feline, older	surgery or radiotherapy, variable prognosis

(*Table 2.6 Continued.*)

Feline paraneoplastic alopecia	Exocrine pancreatic adenocarcinoma, biliary carcinoma	atrophy and miniaturization of follicles	progressive, non-pruritic, shiny skin, +/− footpad involvement, systemic signs include weight loss	association with *Malassezia* infection	temporary resolution with treatment of primary tumor; poor prognosis
Superficial necrolytic dermatitis	Glucagonoma	perivascular to lichenoid dermatitis	alopecia; pressure point crusting, erosions; foot pad hyperkeratosis	differentiate from hepatocutaneous syndrome, pemphigus, SLE, zinc responsive dermatosis	surgery is treatment of choice; often have metastatic disease at the time of diagnosis; somatostatin to reduce hormone levels; fatty acid and zinc supplements temporary resolution with treatment of primary tumor; poor prognosis
Adipose nodular necrosis, panniculitis	Exocrine pancreatic adenocarcinoma	necrosis of subcutaneous tissues due to release of lipases and lytic enzymes	nodular, draining tracts, oily fat, fat necrosis	may occur with pancreatitis	
Hypertrichosis Pemphigus complex	Insulinoma Sarcoma, LSA	anabolic effect immune mediated – pemphigus foliaceus and vulgaris	fluffy long coat multifocal peripheral erythematous vesicobullous lesions; erosive stomatitis of oropharynx & URT		good prognosis for resolution with remission of underlying tumor

MCT mast cell tumor; HSA hemangiosarcoma; LSA lymphoma; GSD German Shepherd Dog; SLE systemic lupus erythematosus; URT upper respiratory tract; PGs prostaglandins.

Table 2.7 Anemia

PNS	Tumor Associations	Etiology	Clinical Findings	Comment	Treatment
Anemia of chronic disease (ACD)	potentially all tumors	anti-EPO factor, reduced RBC lifespan, macrophage (acute phase protein) apoferritin-mediated poor iron utilization/blunted marrow response, membrane alterations in neoplasia lead to increased RBC phagocytosis	mild/moderate normocytic normochromic non-regenerative anemia	Hb and Hct may only be moderately affected but can affect quality of life; proteins, red cell morphology not affected	Tumor specific therapy, rarely PRBC transfusion
Immune-mediated hemolytic anemia (IMHA)	hemopoietic neoplasia	anti-RBC antibodies produced by lymphomatous clones or directed against novel antigens produced by other tumors	severe acute anemia, hemolysis, jaundice, hemoglobinuria, intravascular (IgM, complement fixation), extravascular (IgG)	plasma jaundiced or hemolysed, slide agglutination test or DCT positive, leukoeryhroblastic blood picture, spherocytosis, autoagglutination, PCV falls in spite of regeneration; differentiate IMHA secondary to drugs, toxins, inflammatory/infective disease/sepsis differentiate from IMHA	Combination immunosuppressive therapy, IVFT and PRBC or whole blood transfusion; stabilize and institute tumor specific therapy
Microangiopathic hemolytic anemia (MAHA)	hemangiosarcoma, tumors of liver, spleen, kidney	fibrin deposition in capillary walls; intimal damage in small vessels; mechanical hemolysis	red cell fragmentation/schistocytosis; highly associated with DIC		IVFT and PRBC or whole blood transfusion, surgery for primary tumor, high incidence of metastatic disease at diagnosis

(Table 2.7 Continued.)

Heinz body hemolytic anemia	gastrointestinal lymphoma	RBC oxidant damage	red cell inclusions	more common in non-neoplastic disease – drugs, toxins, zinc, diabetes mellitus	Often debilitated with signs due to tumor; may require IVFT, PRBC or whole blood transfusion and nutritional support prior to surgery or chemotherapy; Gastroprotectants, H1, H2 blockers, whole blood or PRBC transfusion for investigation, surgery, chemotherapy
Iron deficiency anemia (IDA)	mast cell tumor, gastrointestinal tumors	chronic external blood loss; indirect with cytokine involvement eg. histamine; coagulopathy	regenerative, may become non-regenerative	microcytic hypochromic blood picture, hypoproteinemia	Whole blood or PRBC transfusion for investigation, surgery, chemotherapy; IVFT, antibiotic and medical supportive measures
Myelophthisis	lymphoma, leukemia, myeloma, metastatic disease	marrow infiltration, chronologically may occur much later than leukopenia, thrombocytopenia	variable cytopenias, may present as sepsis, or disorder of primary hemostasis	differentiate from marrow failure, myelodysplasia, myelofibrosis, ACD, megaloblastic anemia, effects of chemotherapy, radiation therapy	Whole blood, PRBC or platelet rich plama transfusions for investigation; IVFT, parenteral antibiotic and medical supportive measures; sertoli cell tumor – castration, <10% metastatic rate but poor prognosis for pancytopenia, 80% mortality; granulosa cell tumor – ovariectomy/ ovariohysterectomy, moderate metastatic rate, high mortality associated with pancytopenia
Marrow failure	Sertoli cell tumor, granulosa cell tumor	hyperestrogenism	aplastic anemia, may present as sepsis, or disorder of primary hemostasis	differentiate from myelophthisis, myelodysplasia, myelofibrosis, ACD, megaloblastic anemia, effects of chemotherapy, radiation therapy	
Hemophagocytic syndrome	lymphoma, histiocytic neoplasia	oversecretion of cytokines causing macrophage activation, poorly understood	regenerative, may become non-regenerative; bicytopenia or pancytopenia in marrow	differentiate from IMHA, myelodysplasia	Whole blood or PRBC transfusion for investigation, surgery, chemotherapy; poor prognosis

Table 2.8 Thrombocytopenia (TBC)

PNS	Tumor associations	Etiology	Clinical Findings	Comment	Treatment
Shortened platelet lifespan	hemangiosarcoma, hemopoietic neoplasia	abnormal tumor vessel endothelium, microaggregation due to tumor proteins	may present as sepsis, or disorder of primary hemostasis	Differentiate from thrombocytopathy	Whole blood, PRBC or platelet rich plama transfusion for investigation; vincristine can improve circulating platelet count prior to surgery, chemotherapy
Immune-mediated thrombocytopenia (IMT)	hemopoietic neoplasia, carcinomas	tumor-produced anti-platelet antibody, cross reactive tumor and platelet antigens, antigen-antibody complex binding	may present as sepsis, or disorder of primary hemostasis	Differentiate from indiopathic, drug associated (NSAIDs, sulphonamides, anticonvulsants, cytotoxics), infectous (FeLV, Ehrlichia, Leishmania), sepsis, IBD, SLE	Combination immunosuppressive therapy, IVFT and PRBC, whole blood or platelet rich plasma transfusion; vincristine can improve circulating platelet count and stabilize prior to surgery, chemotherapy
Consumption, sequestration	many tumors esp. liver, spleen & advanced disease	bleeding, thrombophlebitis, DIC	may present as sepsis, or disorder of primary hemostasis, hemoperitoneum often present, possibly thromboembolic disease.	Differentiate from hemorrhage, DIC, vascular injury, cardiac disease, hepatosplenomegaly, vasodilation	Whole blood, PRBC or platelet rich plasma transfusion for investigation, surgery, chemotherapy; splenic or right atrial mass common; many sites of metastasis
Myelophthisis	lymphoma, leukemia, myeloma, metastatic disease	marrow infiltration	variable cytopenias, may present as sepsis, or disorder of primary hemostasis	Differentiate from aplastic anemia, myelodysplasia, megakaryocytic leukemia	Whole blood, PRBC or platelet rich plasma transfusion for investigation; chemotherapy; IVFT, antibiotic and medical supportive measures; chemotherapy for primary tumor
Marrow failure	sertoli cell tumor, granulosa cell tumor	hyperestrogenism	aplastic anemia may present as sepsis, or disorder of primary hemostasis	Differentiate from myelophthisis, myelodysplasia, megakaryocytic leukemia	Whole blood, PRBC or platelet rich plasma transfusions for investigation; IVFT, parenteral antibiotic and medical supportive measures; sertoli cell tumor – castration, <10% metastatic rate but poor prognosis for pancytopenia, 80% mortality; granulosa cell tumor – ovariectomy/ovariohysterectomy, moderate metastatic rate, high mortality associated with pancytopenia

Risk of spontaneous clinical signs with platelet count <20X109^l, or higher depending on rate of fall and vascular integrity.
Disorder of primary hemostasis most often presents with petechiae, ecchymoses, epistaxis, intra-articluar hemorrhage.

Table 2.9 Erythrocytosis

PNS	Tumor associations	Etiology	Clinical findings	Differentials	Investigation	Treatment
Absolute (inappropriate) secondary erythrocytosis	Primary renal, lung, hepatic, intestinal tumors	ectopic neoplastic cell EPO production; increased renal EPO secretion as a result of compression by a tumor and local renal hypoxia; increased production of hypoxia-inducible transcription factors promoting production; altered catabolism of EPO	Increased red cell mass (Hct, PCV) hyperviscosity, dilatation & decreased perfusion of small blood vessels; tissue hypoxia, bleeding and thrombosis; lethargy, anorexia, PUPD, bleeding diatheses (hematemesis, hematochezia, hematuria, retinal bleeding), azotemia, brick red mucous membranes lung, kidney, liver, adrenal, thymic, nasal, smooth muscle, CNS tumors	**primary erythrocytosis** myeloproliferative disorder (MPD): polycythemia vera (PV), erythroleukemia **appropriate secondary erythrocytosis** • benign intrathoracic lesions • benign renal lesions eg. PKD • cardiopulmonary disorders • venoarterial shunts • high altitude **relative (spurious) secondary erythrocytosis** hemoconcentration **Physiological erythrocytosis** Breed associations	renal parameters, proteins, urine SG; [a]arterial blood gas; [b]serum EPO; [c]imaging; tissue diagnosis	i) Erythrocytosis resolves after treatment of the underlying tumor/lesion [d]phlebotomy ii) [d]phlebotomy iii) hydroxurea iv) inhibitors of EPO transcription factors?

[a] Arterial blood gas – normal oxygenation suggests that hypoxia is not the cause of the increased red cell mass.
[b] Plasma EPO will be normal to high despite erythrocytosis vs low EPO with PV.
[c] Imaging should include radiography, echocardiography, abdominal ultrasonography.
[d] Periodic phlebotomy (every 1 to 2 weeks; 100 to 200 ml) with infusion of an equivalent volume of 0.9% NaCl saline used to maintain the PCV > 60 to 65%, may be successful up to 2 years.

Table 2.10 Effect of etiology on serum [EPO]

	[EPO]	[O$_2$]	Renal function	EMH
PV	↓	normal	normal*	no
PNS erythrocytosis	↑	normal	normal*	yes
tissue hypoxia	↑	↓	normal	yes

EMH extramedullary hematopoiesis.
*may become azotemic with progression/as a consequence of erythrocytosis.

- direct Coombs test, slide agglutination test, total bilirubin, urinalysis – immune-mediated hemolysis
- fecal occult blood test and urinalysis – blood loss
- coagulation screen – DIC – thrombocytopenia, hypofibrinogenemia, increased FDPs, prolonged PT, KCCT/APTT, increased D-dimers
- Buccal mucosal bleeding time (BMBT) – platelet function
- marrow cytology, histopathology – diagnose or eliminate neoplasia, myelophthisis, myelodysplasia, myelofibrosis, marrow failure, metastatic disease
- imaging – tumor diagnosis and staging – survey thoracic, skeletal and abdominal radiographs, abdominal and cardiac ultrasound, with fine needle aspiration or biopsy of suspected abnormalities

Gastrointestinal Ulceration

- Mast cell tumors are common in dogs (cutaneous) and cats (visceral).
- Normal and neoplastic mast cell intracytoplasmic granules contain histamine, heparin, other vasoactive amines, and proteolytic enzymes.
- Mast cell degranulation may be spontaneous, traumatic or iatrogenic, risking gastric ulceration, hypotension, poor wound healing, and coagulopathy (Table 2.13 and 2.14).
- Gastrinoma is a rare pancreatic islet cell tumor that secretes excessive gastrin stimulating gastric acid secretion by parietal cells.
- The underlying tumor may be occult, with presentation due to hyperacidity, gastric ulceration, hemorrhagic complications, and gastrointestinal signs (inappetance, vomiting, pain, hematemesis, shock).

Cancer Cachexia

- Cancer cachexia refers to a progressive wasting syndrome manifested by
  - Severe weight loss, muscle wasting and loss of adipose tissue
  - Debilitation in spite of normal food intake that is separate from anorexia, but which can be complicated by the latter
- Neoplasia affects the patient's metabolism and normal homeostatic mechanisms:
  - Alterations in carbohydrate, fat, and protein metabolism
  - Metabolic c hanges brought about by substances secreted by the host and the tumor
  - Proinflammatory cytokines IL-6, IL-1, TNF α, and IFN α
  - The effect of these molecules on fatty acid, glucose, and carbohydrate metabolism resulting in net energy loss and negative protein balance

Table 2.11 Leukcocytosis

PNS	Etiology	Tumor associations	Differentials	Investigation	Treatment
Neutrophilic leukcocytosis	stimulation of marrow by necrotic or infected tumor; marrow metastases; production of colony stimulating factor by the tumor	hemopoietic neoplasia, renal neoplasia (+ hypertrophic osteopathy)	**physiological** – young animals, stress, exercise **corticosteroid induced** – exogenous, stress, Cushings syndrome **inflammatory** – systemic infection **miscellaneous** – hemorrhage, hemolysis (leuckerythroblastic picture), drugs (corticosteroids, anabolics, G-CSF), CML	Rule out infection, sepsis, endocrinopathy with blood smear exam, serum chemistries, urinalysis, imaging, marrow exam; tissue diagnosis	Parenteral antibiotic cover; surgery for solid tumor, chemotherapy for hemopoietic neoplasia
Eosinophilic leukcocytosis basophilia		lymphoma, lymphomatoid granulomatosis, thymoma, mast cell tumor, fibrosarcoma	**Hypersensitivity** EGC, eosinophilic enteritis, PIE **Inflammation** myositis, panosteitis **Purulent inflammation** pyometra **Parasites** Angiostrongylus spp, Crenasoma spp, Dirofilaria spp **MPD** eosinophilic leukemia **Hypereosinophilic syndrome** **Hypoadrenocorticism** **Drugs** Tetracycline, IL-12	Rule out infection, inflammatory disease with blood smear exam, serum chemistries, urinalysis, imaging, marrow exam; tissue diagnosis	Surgery for solid tumor, chemotherapy for hemopoietic neoplasia

G-CSF granulocyte colony stimulating factor; CML chronic myeloid leukemia; EGC (ecasinophilic granuloma complex); PIE (pulmonary infiltrates with eosinophilia).

Table 2.12 Pancytopenia

PNS	Etiology	Tumor association	Clinical features	Investigation	Treatment
Pancytopenia	bone marrow depression – hyperestrogenism	sertoli cell tumor (SCT), granulosa cell tumor (GCT) squamous prostatic metaplasia, feminization – SCT; persistent oestrus, cystic endometrial hyperplasia, pyometra – GCT	chronological decline in WBC, platelet & red cell numbers; sepsis, hemorrhage, anemia; squamous prostatic metaplasia, feminization – SCT; persistent estrus, cystic endometrial hyperplasia, pyometra – GCT	Hematology, blood smear exam, marrow cytology and histopathology, abdominal ultrasound, tissue diagnosis	whole blood, PRBC, FFP transfusion support, parenteral antibiotics; SCT – castration, <10% metastatic rate but poor prognosis for pancytopenia, 80% mortality; GCT – ovariectomy/ ovariohysterectomy, moderate metastatic rate, high mortality associated with pancytopenia

Table 2.13 Hyperviscosity

PNS	Tumor associations	Etiology	Clinical findings	Comment	Treatment
Gammopathy	multiple myeloma, functional B cell lymphoma, chronic lymphocytic leukemia	increased monoclonal serum IgA, IgG, IgM increased blood viscocity, plasma osmolality, hypervolemia i) increased resistance to blood flow ii) reduced blood flow iii) decreased tissue & organ perfusion	cardiovascular – myocardial hypertrophy, lethargy, cardiomyopathy ocular – retinal bleeding & detachment, blindness renal – renal hypoxia, PUPD, renal failure neurological – CNS hypoxia, hemorrhage, lethargy, seizures hematologic – altered platelet & clotting factor function (paraprotein binding) – bleeding diatheses, primary & secondary coagulopathy myelophthisis – leukopenia (sepsis), thrombocytopenia (bleeding), anemia	hyperglobulinemia, azotemia, serum protein electrophoresis, urine protein electrophoresis – Bence Jones proteins (Ig fragments), renal protein loss, hematology, platelets, coagulation screen, marrow cytology/histology, imaging, tissue diagnosis	plasmapharesis – phlebotomy 20 ml/kg with retransfusion of RBC; chemotherapy for primary tumor
Increased red cell mass	primary erythrocytosis/polycythemia vera, erythroleukemia	increased blood viscocity, hypervolemia i) increased resistance to blood flow ii) reduced blood flow iii) decreased tissue & organ perfusion		chemistries, hyperglobulinemia, azotemia, hematology, coagulation screen, EPO assay, marrow cytology/histology, imaging, tissue diagnosis	phlebotomy 20 ml/kg with retransfusion of plasma; chemotherapy for primary tumor

Table 2.14 The consequences of mast cell degranulation

Constituent	Pathophysiology	Clinical Effect	Management	
			Hemodynamic	**Gastrointestinal**
Heparin	inhibits clotting factors	coagulopathy, hemorrhagic complications	Prophylactic H$_1$ blockers chlorpheniramine D:2–8 mg bid PO; 2.5–10 mg tid IM C: 2–4 mg bid PO; 2.5–5 mg bid IM IVFT 3 ml/kg/hr – 60 ml/kg/hr Transfuse whole blood, packed red cells, fresh frozen plasma as indicated	Prophylactic H$_2$ blockers ranitidine D:2 mg/kg bid IV/PO C:3.5 mg/kg bid IV/PO famotidine 0.5–1.0 mg/kg sid PO sucralfate 0.25–2 g tid PO
Histamine	hyperhistaminemia, activation of Type 2 receptors, gastric acid secretion	edema, erythema, pruritus; flushing, hypotension, hyperacidity, gastric ulceration, upper g.i.t. signs		
Other vasocative amines	vasodilation	hypotension, poor wound healing, g.i.t. capillary leakage		
Proteolytic enzymes		poor wound healing	Surgery, radiotherapy, chemotherapy as indicated by the treatment algorithm	Surgery, radiotherapy, chemotherapy as indicated by the treatment algorithm

- Appetite stimulants and nutritional supplementation are unable to control cancer cachexia
- Dysgeusia (altered taste sensation), nausea, and vomiting may also affect food intake.

Main clinical features
Clinical signs include weight loss, poor muscle mass, weakness, and loss of interest.
   Widespread effects include
- Immunosuppression
- Altered gastrointestinal function
- Poor wound healing.
   Cancer cachexia negatively impacts quality of life, performance status, treatment availability, treatment response, and survival time.
   Incidence varies with tumor phenotype; in dogs cachexia is common with gastric carcinoma and primary carcinoma of the lung.

Diagnosis and treatment of cachexia
The classification and detection of cachexia in dogs and cats has
i.   Diagnostic importance:
   a. Cachexia may be the first indicator of occult malignancy.
   b. Recognition may help direct the search for neoplasia.
ii. Therapeutic importance:
   a. Successful treatment requires parallel management of the cachexia and the tumor.
   b. Cachexia may be misinterpreted as an adverse effect of therapy.
   c. Cachexia may be complicated by adverse effects of therapy.

Table 2.15 Management of cachexia

Treatment	Mode of Action	Comment
Diet	Encourage voluntary feeding, enhance palatability, any food is better than none, aim for high bioavailability protein, 40–50% calories as fat (↑ omega 3 polyunsaturated fatty acids, fish oil high in eicosapentanoic acid), low levels of simple carbohydrates, moderate fibre	Individualized nutrition should be considered early rather than late
Enteral nutrition	Tube feeding, gradual increase to frequent small feeds, or continual low volume feeding	Individualized artificial nutrition should be considered early rather than late, blenderized foods or prescription enteral feeds
Prednisolone 0.5–1.0 mg/kg sid/bid PO	Stimulate a feeling of hunger	Corticosteroid side effects – PUPD; may further deplete muscle mass; hypokalemia; diabetogenic`
Dexamethasone 0.1–.2 mg/kg eod/sid SQ		
Megesterol acetate 2.5 mg sid PO 4 days then q 3 days	Downregulates synthesis and release of cytokines, inhibits action of TNF on fatty tissue, stimulates appetite	Diabetogenic, thrombotic complications; weight gain is primarily adipose and water, no effect on lean body mass
Cyproheptidine 0.1–0.5 mg/kg bid/tid PO	Antiserotonin, cytokine inhibitor, stimulates appetite	No net effect on progressive weight loss, even with improved appetite
Nandrolone decanoate	Anabolic steroid	May improve muscle bulk as well as appetite, increased risk of sodium and water retention with corticosteroid
Metoclopramide	Proximal gastrointestinal prokinetic, anti-emetic	Mentation and behavior changes at higher doses
Maropitant	Central and peripheral acting anti-emetic	Effective for chemotherapy induced emesis
Diazepam 0.05–0.5 mg/kg IV	Benzodiazepine, anxiolytic	Only suitable for acute use

iii. Prognostic importance:
    a. Reduced performance status may preclude patients from specific therapy with impact on survival.
    b. Cachexia is a negative prognostic indicator.
iv. Quality of life issues:
    a. Cachexia affects morbidity.
    b. Recovery and hospitalization times may be increased with increasing numbers and complexity of interventions.

Management of cachexia (Table 2.15)

Based on the following:
- Weight increase/maintaining body weight
- Appetite stimulation
- Managing issues that may inhibit appetite, e.g., pain and nausea associated with underlying disease or therapy
- Avoidance of lactate loading, which results in negative energy balance via tumor anaerobic metabolism

Pyrexia Associated with Neoplasia

While it is a fairly common paraneoplastic disorder, there is not a great deal known about the etiology of paraneoplastic fever.

Implicated factors include
- Host and tumor-derived endogenous pyrogens such as IL-1, IL-6, TNF, and IFNs
- Disordered metabolism, e.g., hepatic function and steroidogenesis
Neoplastic fever negatively impacts
- Quality of life
- Performance status
- Treatment availability

Differential diagnosis of pyrexia of unknown origin
- Infection
- Immune-mediated disease
- Neoplasia
There are no reliable specific sensitive markers to discriminate neoplastic from nonneoplastic fever, so each episode warrants thorough diagnostic intervention.

3
CLINICAL APPROACH TO THE CANCER PATIENT

David J. Argyle, Malcolm J. Brearley, and Michelle M. Turek

Key Points
- Cancer is one of the most common diseases encountered in small animal practice.
- As people's awareness of the disease has grown there is now greater demand for the general clinician to understand the disease and the current options available for treatment.
- When considering a small animal patient with a potential neoplasm, the diagnostic evaluation of the patient must take into consideration the following criteria:
  1. A histological diagnosis of the tumor must be made to determine the nature of the disease
  2. Determination of the histologic grade of the tumor is important for making treatment recommendations and establishing prognosis for many tumor types.
  3. The extent of the disease both locally and at distant sites should be determined.
  4. Any tumor-related complications must be recognized and treated.
  5. Any concurrent disease that may alter the prognosis or the patient's ability to tolerate treatment must be investigated.

Key Points
When presented with a small animal patient with a potential neoplasm there are essentially two questions that need to be answered
- **What type of tumor is it?**
- **What is the extent of disease?**
The first question requires either a **histological** or **cytological** diagnosis. The extent of disease is determined through **staging** procedures. Staging refers to the diagnostic procedures required to appreciate the full extent of disease.

Key Point
The **grade** of a tumor refers to a histological description of the tumor and is based upon several criteria (e.g., mitotic rate, tissue architecture, and pleomorphism). This should not be confused with tumor **stage**, which refers to the clinical extent of disease.

Determining the Type of Tumor

This requires the collection and microscopic examination of cells (**cytology**) or tissues (**histology**) from a tumor using a biopsy procedure (see next section).

Tumor Staging

Tumors are staged according to internationally accepted sets of rules, mostly developed by the World Health Organization (WHO), which give an alphanumeric value to a patient denoting the extent of disease. Different staging systems are used for a wide range of tumors. Most involve a consideration of primary tumor size, presence or absence of local lymph node metastasis, and presence or absence of distant metastases. Tumor stage should not be confused with tumor *grade*, which is a histopathological determination of how malignant the tumor appears microscopically. For many tumors, prognosis depends on stage and grade. However, stage is not always a precise indicator of prognosis.

Staging for Solitary Tumors

To stage solitary tumors we use the *TNM (tumor, node, metastasis) staging system.* In this system, the body is considered as three anatomical compartments that all have the potential to be invaded by neoplastic cells:
   T: Primary Tumor
   N: Regional lymph node
   M: Distant Metastasis
   Figure 3.1 diagrams the clinical assessment of a patient.

Evaluating the primary tumor (T)
The invasive nature of tumors necessitates the requirement for a detailed clinical assessment of the primary tumor. The exact methods and progression of evaluation will depend on the location of the tumor and how accessible it is. However, as a guide:
1. **Physical Examination**
   * Size of the tumor
   * Mobility with respect to underlying tissues and degree of fixation
   * Presence/absence and degree of erythema
   * Presence/absence and degree of ulceration
   * Relationship with associated anatomical structures
2. **Diagnostic Imaging**
   Diagnostic imaging is required for
   * Deep tumors that cannot be physically evaluated
   * Tumors involving vital structures/complex anatomical compartments
   * Tumors involving bone
   * Tumors adjacent to bone (e.g., invasive oral tumors)
   The indications for the different imaging modalities are given in Tables 3.1 and 3.2.
3. **Other Techniques**
   * Endoscopy or bronchoscopy in cases of suspected tumors of the gastrointestinal tract, respiratory tract, or urogenital system
4. **Biopsy** (as described in the next section)

The primary tumor (T) is allocated a numerical or alphabetical suffix denoting size and extent of the tumor as us

---

Evaluating the lymph node (N)
1. **Physical Examination**
   * Size of the lymph node
   * Mobility with respect to underlying tissues and degree of fixation
   * Texture and consistency
   * Relationship with associated anatomical structures

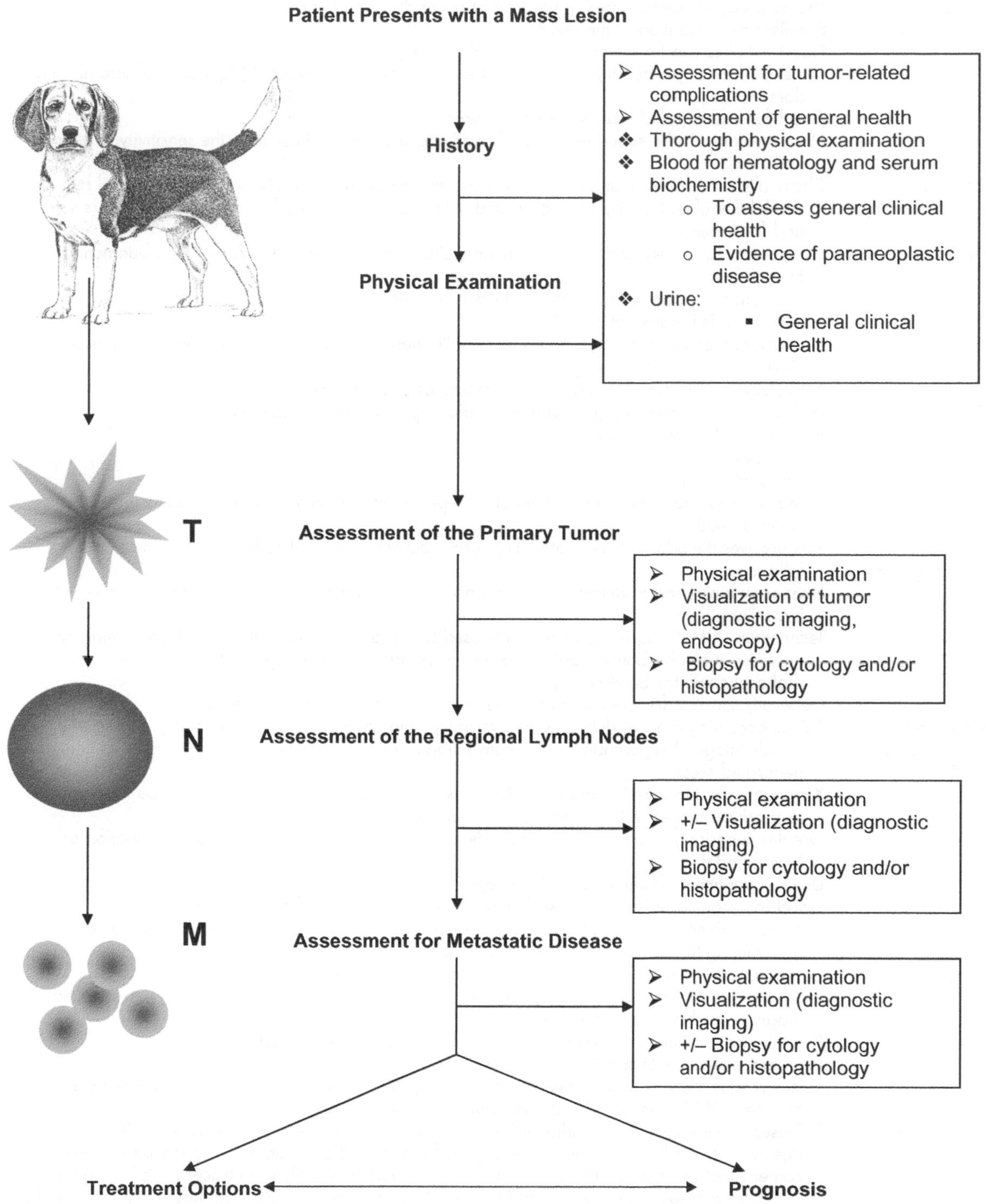

Patient Presents with a Mass Lesion

History

- ➢ Assessment for tumor-related complications
- ➢ Assessment of general health
- ❖ Thorough physical examination
- ❖ Blood for hematology and serum biochemistry
  - o To assess general clinical health
  - o Evidence of paraneoplastic disease
- ❖ Urine:
  - ▪ General clinical health

Physical Examination

T **Assessment of the Primary Tumor**

- ➢ Physical examination
- ➢ Visualization of tumor (diagnostic imaging, endoscopy)
- ➢ Biopsy for cytology and/or histopathology

N **Assessment of the Regional Lymph Nodes**

- ➢ Physical examination
- ➢ +/– Visualization (diagnostic imaging)
- ➢ Biopsy for cytology and/or histopathology

M **Assessment for Metastatic Disease**

- ➢ Physical examination
- ➢ Visualization (diagnostic imaging)
- ➢ +/– Biopsy for cytology and/or histopathology

Treatment Options ◄─────────────► **Prognosis**

Figure 3.1. Clinical assessment of patient.

Table 3.1. Imaging technologies and their indications in oncology

Technology	Indications
Plain radiography	The mainstay of cancer imaging because of accessibility and low cost. Excellent for evaluation of the skeleton. Good initial screen for metastatic disease of the lungs. For evaluation of pulmonary metastasis, three views are recommended (right and left lateral, and dorsoventral). Good for evaluation of size of abdominal organs. Main weakness is the superimposition of overlying structures, which limits the sensitivity of lesion detection.
Contrast radiography	Classically used for evaluation of the GI tract and the urinary tract. Now largely replaced by availability of endoscopy and ultrasound. Although can be used for myelography, MRI is safer and far superior.
Ultrasound	Ultrasound has largely replaced abdominal radiography for the evaluation of the abdomen. Essential for • Evaluation of abdominal organs for evidence of primary or metastatic disease. • Aid in guided biopsy of deep tumors. • Evaluation of internal lymph nodes (especially mesenteric and sublumbar nodes in cases of low GI and perianal tumors, respectively). • Evaluation of tumor invasion into vital structures (e.g., thyroid tumors).
Endoscopy	Endoscopy has largely replaced contrast radiography for the evaluation of • Upper and lower GI tract • Airways • Urogenital system In many cases, the technique is amendable to performing guided (endoscopic) biopsies of the systems listed above.
Nuclear scintigraphy	This involves the administration of radiopharmaceuticals that localize to areas of tumor or inflammation. Most commonly used to detect bone metastasis in dogs and functional thyroid tissue in cats with hyperthyroidism. Technetium-99M (^{99m}Tc) is most commonly used because of its short half-life and good imaging qualities. It can be bound easily to localizing pharmaceuticals (e.g., ^{99m}Tc-methylene diphosphonate for bone scans). Generally sensitive for disease lesions, but it is nonspecific for disease etiology.
Computerized tomography (CT)	This is becoming more widely used in veterinary medicine with greater availability. It gets over the disadvantage of superimposition in conventional radiography by portraying images as computer-generated slices. X-rays are used to acquire images in the transverse plane in real time. These can be reconstructed to produce images in the sagittal and dorsal planes. Greater superiority over radiography for detection of pulmonary metastasis and evaluation of lymph nodes. Used in treatment planning for radiotherapy. Good for imaging lesions of the skull (e.g., oral tumor and nasal tumor staging). Used in combination with contrast agents (contrast-enhanced CT), which can be invaluable in determining the extent of local tumor invasion.
Magnetic resonance imaging (MRI)	Can produce images in the transverse, sagittal, and dorsal planes in real time. Images generated through the properties of hydrogen atoms in the body when they are placed in a magnetic and radiofrequency field. Primary use in veterinary medicine is the evaluation of the central nervous system. Excellent evaluation of soft-tissue structures, less useful for cortical bone.
Positron-emission tomography (PET)	This is a sophisticated form of nuclear scintigraphy. Whereas CT and MRI are concerned with anatomy, PET is concerned with metabolic function. PET uses a positron-emitting radionuclide incorporated into a metabolically active molecule that is injected into the body. Gamma rays emitted from the radionuclide are detected by a gamma camera that reconstructs the images in 3-D. The most commonly used tracer in PET imaging is ^{18}F-fluorodeoxyglucose (FDG), a radioactive glucose molecule. FDG is preferentially taken up by tumor cells because tumor cells have increased glucose utilization through glycolysis. PET has greater sensitivity for detecting cancer cells than any other modality. It is particularly useful in detecting micrometastases. New machines combine CT and PET (PET-CT scanners), to provide optimal imaging (anatomy and function) of cancer patients. It has limited use in veterinary medicine to date due to limited availability.

2. **Diagnostic Imaging**
   Diagnostic imaging is required for
   - Internal, nonperipheral, lymph nodes that cannot be physically evaluated
3. **Biopsy** (as described in the next section)

The lymph node (L) is allocated a numerical value depending on the presence or absence of neoplastic disease.

Evaluating metastatic disease (M)

1. **Physical Examination/History**
   - This may give essential clues to the possibility of metastasis, including weight loss, coughing, or lameness.
2. **Diagnostic Imaging**
   - Imaging technologies will depend on the tumor type and its natural biological behavior. However, particular attention should be paid to lungs, liver, and bones.
3. **Biopsy**
   - May be required in some cases to confirm metastatic disease (versus nodular hyperplasia, for example).

The patient is allocated a numerical M value (metastasis) depending on the presence or absence of disease at distant sites.

Example 1: The TNM Classification System for Oral Tumors in Dogs and Cats

T	**Primary Tumor**
T_{is}	Preinvasive tumor (tumor in situ)
T_0	No evidence of tumor
T_1	Tumor <2 cm maximum diameter
	• T1a without bone invasion
	• T1b with bone invasion
T_2	Tumor 2–4 cm maximum diameter
	• T2a without bone invasion
	• T2b with bone invasion
T_3	Tumor >4 cm maximum diameter
	• T3a without bone invasion
	• T3b with bone invasion
N	**Regional Lymph Node**
N_0	No evidence of lymph node metastasis
N_1	Movable ipsilateral nodes
	• N_{1a}: Nodes not considered to contain cancer
	• N_{1b}: Nodes considered to contain cancer
N_2	Movable contralateral nodes or bilateral nodes
	• N_{2a}: Nodes not considered to contain cancer
	• N_{2b}: Nodes considered to contain cancer
N_3	• Fixed lymph nodes
M	**Distant Metastasis**
M_0	No evidence of distant metastasis
M_1	Distant metastasis detected

Table 3.2. WHO stage assignment for skin tumors

Tumor Size	Node Involvement	Metastases?	Stage
T1	N0, N1a, N2a	M0	I
T2	N0, N1a, N2a	M0	II
T3	N0, N1a, N2a	M0	III
Any T	N1b, N2b, N3	M0	IV
Any T	Any N	M1	

Staging for Systemic or Multicentric Disease

Diseases such as lymphoproliferative disorders often present as a disseminated form and thus the TNM classification is not appropriate. For diseases such as lymphoma, the disease may be staged according to the various organ systems involved and assigned a numerical figure (for example, refer to Chapters 9 and 10).

Assessment of General Clinical Health

As part of the staging procedure for tumors, it is essential that the clinician also
- Obtains a through history, including
  - i.   Onset of clinical signs
  - ii. Duration of disease
  - iii. Weight loss or weight gain
  - iv. Thirst and urination
  - v.   Vomiting or diarrhea
  - vi. Coughing or panting
- Performs a thorough physical examination
- Obtains blood for hematology and serum biochemistry
  - i.   To assess general clinical health
  - ii. To obtain evidence of paraneoplastic disease (Chapter 2)
- Obtains urine
  - i.   To determine general clinical health

> *Once staging has been completed we have essentially answered our two fundamental questions on the nature and the extent of the disease. This will allow us to make the appropriate treatment decisions and estimate prognosis.*

4
BIOPSY, TISSUE HANDLING, AND INTERPRETATION

David J. Argyle and Elspeth Milne

Key Points
- Biopsy is indispensable in the evaluation of every oncological case.
- Biopsy refers to the sampling of tissue for cytologic or histologic evaluation.
- The selection of the most appropriate treatment for an individual tumor is best made once a histopathological or cytological diagnosis has been established.
- Biopsies do not negatively influence survival.
- When taking biopsies for histological or cytological diagnosis, also consider submitting samples for bacterial culture and sensitivity is indicated.
- Biopsy technique should be thoughtful and planned so as not to contaminate the surrounding normal tissues with cancer cells, because this could complicate or compromise the success of a definitive procedure (surgical excision or radiotherapy).

Is Pretreatment Biopsy Necessary?

- Treatment without biopsy information will be speculative at best and can rarely be justified. However, exceptions to this rule do exist:

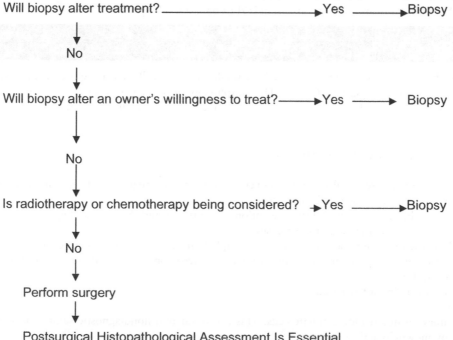

51

- Histopathologic evaluation is essential for
  - Identification of the histological type of the tumor, and tumor grade if applicable
  - Evaluation of surgical margins for assessment of completeness of excision
  - Treatment planning
  - Determination of prognosis
- Examples where the proposed treatment regime is unlikely to be modified by a presurgical biopsy include the management of mammary malignancy by mastectomy since mastectomy is the most appropriate approach.
- Contraindications to biopsy are rare. However, careful consideration should be given in cases where severe hemorrhage is a possibility. For example, a presurgical, percutaneous biopsy of a cavitated splenic mass may be contraindicated. Similarly, percutaneous biopsy of a thyroid mass should be approached with caution because hemorrhage is common.

Prebiopsy Considerations

Biopsy has the potential to provide the following information:
- **The detection** of neoplastic disease in either primary or secondary sites
- **The tumor type**
- **The histologic grade** of the tumor (requires a tissue biopsy)
- **The completeness** of surgical excision (margins) of an excisional biopsy
  Consequently, when deciding on an appropriate technique, the clinician must consider
- **The amount** of tissue that should be recovered in the biopsy
- **The position** within the tumor that tissue is to be recovered from (e.g., centrally in the case of a metastatic deposit in a lymph node or a bone tumor, or from the periphery of a tumor when the junction between normal and abnormal tissue is to be evaluated)
- **The type** of tissue to be biopsied (e.g., fluid, soft tissue, bone, etc.)
- **The anatomic** location of the tumor (e.g., cutaneous nodule or lesion within the liver parenchyma)
- **The biopsy approach.** This should be thoughtful so as not to unnecessarily contaminate surrounding normal tissues with cancer cells. Remember that the entire biopsy tract should be included in the surgical excision of the tumor or the radiation field. A poorly planned biopsy could compromise the success of the definitive procedure by enlarging the area that needs to be treated.
- **The risk of anesthesia** if immobilization is required to obtain the biopsy

Cytology

- Cytology is the examination of individual cells or small groups of cells that have been recovered from tumor masses or from neoplastic effusions. The morphology of the cells is assessed. Malignant tumors, particularly those of epithelial or hemolymphatic origin, commonly exfoliate cells that may be recovered for cytological identification.
- Indications:
  - To identify the presence of neoplastic disease.
- Advantages:
  - Cytology specimens are usually easily recovered with minimal requirements for instrumentation (e.g., hypodermic needles for fine needle aspirates).
  - Specimens can be recovered with little disruption of the tumor and the surrounding tissues.
  - Risk of hemorrhage is minimal in most cases.
  - Multiple sites within the tumor can readily be sampled during a single biopsy procedure.
  - Preparations can be rapidly prepared and stained on microscope slides without the need for specialized processing equipment.
  - Anesthesia is usually not required.
- Disadvantages
  - Some tumors do not readily exfoliate cells. This can result in a nondiagnostic sample or a misdiagnosis (e.g., many mesenchymal tumors).
  - The cells in cytological preparations often bear no relationship to their original arrangement within the tumor or to its architecture.

Procedures in Cytology

Fine Needle Aspiration (FNA)

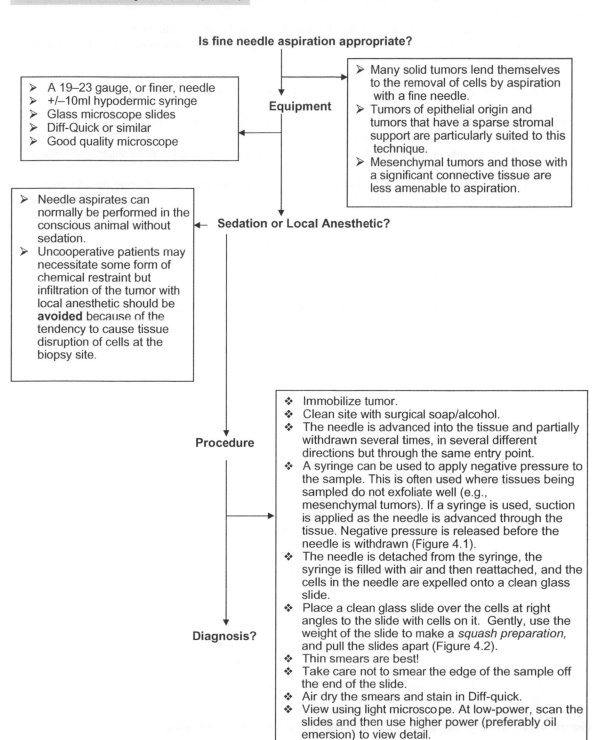

Is fine needle aspiration appropriate?

> A 19–23 gauge, or finer, needle
> +/–10ml hypodermic syringe
> Glass microscope slides
> Diff-Quick or similar
> Good quality microscope

Equipment

> Many solid tumors lend themselves to the removal of cells by aspiration with a fine needle.
> Tumors of epithelial origin and tumors that have a sparse stromal support are particularly suited to this technique.
> Mesenchymal tumors and those with a significant connective tissue are less amenable to aspiration.

> Needle aspirates can normally be performed in the conscious animal without sedation.
> Uncooperative patients may necessitate some form of chemical restraint but infiltration of the tumor with local anesthetic should be **avoided** because of the tendency to cause tissue disruption of cells at the biopsy site.

Sedation or Local Anesthetic?

Procedure

❖ Immobilize tumor.
❖ Clean site with surgical soap/alcohol.
❖ The needle is advanced into the tissue and partially withdrawn several times, in several different directions but through the same entry point.
❖ A syringe can be used to apply negative pressure to the sample. This is often used where tissues being sampled do not exfoliate well (e.g., mesenchymal tumors). If a syringe is used, suction is applied as the needle is advanced through the tissue. Negative pressure is released before the needle is withdrawn (Figure 4.1).
❖ The needle is detached from the syringe, the syringe is filled with air and then reattached, and the cells in the needle are expelled onto a clean glass slide.
❖ Place a clean glass slide over the cells at right angles to the slide with cells on it. Gently, use the weight of the slide to make a *squash preparation*, and pull the slides apart (Figure 4.2).
❖ Thin smears are best!
❖ Take care not to smear the edge of the sample off the end of the slide.
❖ Air dry the smears and stain in Diff-quick.
❖ View using light microscope. At low-power, scan the slides and then use higher power (preferably oil emersion) to view detail.

Diagnosis?

Fluid Aspirates and Exfoliative Cytology (Figure 4.1)

- One of the simplest techniques for recovery of exfoliated cells is to disturb the surface of the tumor by irrigation with saline (e.g., prostatic washing, nasal flushing, tracheobronchial washing).
- Alternatively, tumors that develop within body cavities are often accompanied by a fluid effusion that may contain neoplastic cells.
- The technique for recovery of these fluids will be dictated by the location of the body cavity (e.g., thoracocentesis, abdominocentesis, joint tap, cerebrospinal tap, bone marrow aspirate, pericardiocentesis, urinalysis).
- Irrespective of the method of recovery, several ml of the fluid should ideally be collected into an EDTA container. A total nucleated cell count (standard white blood cell count procedure) should then be used to determine the concentration of cells in the sample.
- Samples in which the cell count is normally expected to be high (e.g., bone marrow) need not be counted and preparations can be made directly from the fluid.
- Samples with cell counts of more than 10,000 cells/uL can be smeared directly onto a microscope slide (Figures 4.2, 4.3).
- Samples with cell counts of less than 10,000 cells/uL should be centrifuged at 2,000rpm for 35 minutes. The smear is then made from the sediment.

Abdominocentesis

- Indicated when there is any free fluid in the abdominal cavity.
- Equipment: as for FNA.
- Performed 3–5 cm caudal to the umbilicus and to the right of midline (avoiding the spleen).

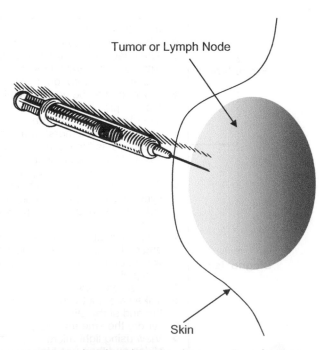

Tumor or Lymph Node

Skin

Figure 4.1. Taking an aspirate from a lymph node using a basic needle and syringe.

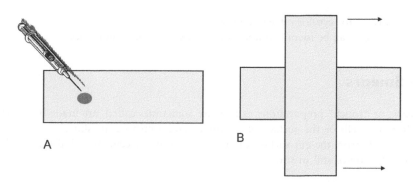

Figure 4.2.   Making a squash smear: Cells are expelled onto one slide (A). A second slide is placed flat on top of the first slide at right angles to it. This needs to be performed gently to prevent the cells being damaged. The second slide is then slid quickly and smoothly across slide 1 so that the smear to be examined is on the underside of slide 2 (B).

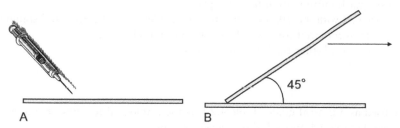

Figure 4.3.   Where aspirates are more fluid or diluted, a blood smear technique can be employed. The sample is expelled onto the slide (A). A second spreader slide is then used (a normal slide that has had one corner broken off to avoid smearing cells over the edge of the slide) to smear cells. The spreader slide is placed at a 45° angle in front of the sample and slid backward until it comes into contact with the sample drop. The spreader slide is advanced forward (B) to create a smear with a feathered edge.

- Area is clipped and cleaned as for surgery.
- 2 ml of air are drawn into the syringe and the needle is slowly advanced into the abdominal cavity.
- If no fluid is acquired after applying negative pressure, 0.5 ml of air is injected into the cavity to free the syringe of blockages.
- The procedure is repeated at different positions and depths. Fluid localized in pockets can be identified and sampled by ultrasound guidance.

Thoracocentesis

- Indicated for any free fluid in the thoracic cavity.
- Equipment as for FNA, and 3-way stopcock.
- Animal should be standing and quiet.
- Area should be clipped and cleaned as for surgery.
- Location can vary, but usually 7th or 8th intercostal space.
- The bevel of the needle should face the pleural lining. The needle (with syringe and stopcock attached) is advanced just cranially to the near rib to prevent hitting the intercostal artery.
- Negative pressure is applied.
- The 3-way stopcock is used to prevent air leaking into the chest as fluid is collected.

- Collect samples in EDTA for cytology ± bacteriology.
- Fluid localized in pockets can be identified and sampled by ultrasound guidance.

Impression Smears

- Impression smears, or "touch" preparations as they are sometimes called, are made by direct contact between the exfoliating cells on the surface of the tumor and a microscope slide.
- The smear can be made from the cut surface of an excised tumor specimen and also from the friable or ulcerating surface of a tumor still in situ.

Practical Cytological Interpretation

- Detailed cytological interpretation requires an experienced clinical pathologist. For a general practitioner, the key skills to be acquired are the following:
  - Being able to tell whether the sample/smear is of sufficient quality for a clinical pathologist to interpret
  - Being able to distinguish inflammation from neoplasia
- Samples are first reviewed with the 10× objective to ensure adequate cellularity and staining.
- Selected sections are then reviewed using the 100× oil emersion objective.
- Key things to interpret are whether the lesion represents
  - Inflammation
  - Hyperplasia
  - Neoplasia
  Table 4.1 can be used as a general guide. Table 4.2 lists the cytological features of epithelial, mesenchymal, and round cell tumors. Figures 4.4 and 4.5 show smear examples.

Table 4.1. Inflammation versus neoplasia

Inflammation	Benign Neoplasia	Malignant Neoplasia*
Acute: >70% neutrophils that may be hypersegmented, or toxic Chronic Active: 30–50% monocytes and plasma cells, significant numbers of neutrophils Chronic Granulomatous: Macrophages dominate the cell population	Uniform population of cells Lack of criteria of malignancy	Pleomorphic cell population with mitoses Anisocytosis Poor degree of differentiation (anaplasia) Large nuclear:cytoplasmic ratio Nuclear pleomorphism Multiple nuclei, hyperchromatic nuclei, and prominent and multiple nucleoli Irregular chromatin size and shape

*Some cancerous tumors are characterized by an absence of these criteria of malignancy. Examples include anal sac adenocarcinoma and thyroid carcinoma.

Table 4.2. Cytological features of epithelial, mesenchymal, and round cell tumors

Cell of Origin	Cytological Features
Epithelial tumors	Cells are round, quite large, and have a round/oval nucleus with abundant cytoplasm. Cells exfoliate in clumps, which appear adherent. Cells derived from glandular origin tend to have a vacuolated, foamy cytoplasm and are arranged in an acinus. Cells from squamous epithelium tend to resemble normal squamous cells, with abundant, pale-staining cytoplasm.
Mesenchymal tumors	Small- to medium-sized elongated (or spindle-shaped) cells. Elongated oval nucleus. Cells are often single or in dense clumps, reflecting their reluctance to exfoliate.
Melanoma	Cells can be either round or fusiform. Cytoplasm contains green/black granules. Benign and malignant lesions can have granules.
Round cell tumors	Includes lymphoma, mast cell tumor, plasma cell tumor, histiocytoma, and transmissible venereal tumor. Cells readily exfoliate and can appear as discrete cells, or as sheets of cells, if the smear is very cellular. **Lymphoma** • Often sheets of large lymphoblasts (>50%). • Large N:C ratio. • Mitotic figures often present. **Plasma cell tumor** • Abundant basophilic cytoplasm. • Nucleus positioned to one side of the cell with characteristic clumped chromatin. **Mast cell tumors:** • Pink/purple granules in the cytoplasm. • In higher grade tumors there may be fewer granules, and an increase in the number and size of nucleoli. **Histiocytoma** • Poorly exfoliative. • Abundant cytoplasm with small vacuoles. • Round nucleus, coarse chromatin, and 1–2 nucleoli • Occasional binucleate cells.

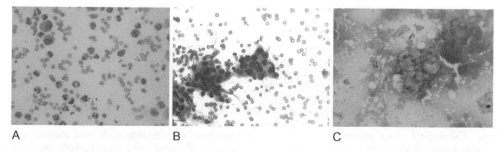

A   B   C

Figure 4.4. Cytology smear preparations demonstrating superficial inflammation (A) (a mixture of inflammatory cells with no criteria of malignancy); malignancy (B) (nasal carcinoma showing poor degree of differentiation, large nuclear: cytoplasmic ratio, nuclear pleomorphism, multiple nuclei,) and a benign tumor (C) (anal adenoma demonstrating no criteria for malignancy).

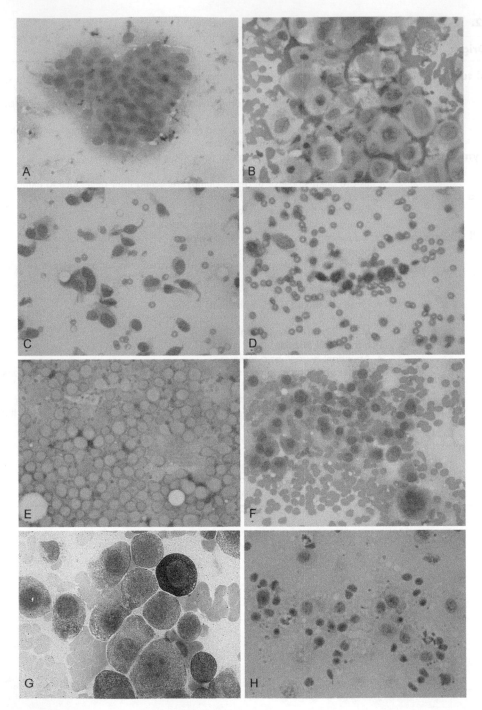

Figure 4.5. Cytological smear preparations of epithelial tumors (anal sac carcinoma, A, and squamous carcinoma, B); mesenchymal tumor (fibrosarcoma, C); melanoma, D; and a series of round cell tumors (lymphoma, E, plasma cell tumor, F, mast cell tumor, G, and canine cutaneous histiocytoma, H).

Needle Biopsy (Figure 4.6)

- Used to remove small cores of tumor tissue from solid lesions, e.g., Tru-cut needle biopsy (14 to 22 gauge).
- Used when it is important to recover sufficient tissue to establish tumor type ± architecture:
  - Recovery of tissue from tumors of internal organs without surgical procedures
  - Recovery of tissue from bone lesions (e.g., using Jamshidi needle)
- Advantages:
  - Substantially more tissue can be recovered than with needle aspirates.
  - Recovered tissue retains much of its architecture and is suitable for routine histological processing techniques.
  - Comparatively inaccessible sites (e.g., prostate, lung, etc.) may be biopsied without need for a surgical procedure.
  - Multiple samples may be removed through a single approach.
- Disadvantages:
  - Needle biopsies may result in a greater incidence of post biopsy complications (e.g., hemorrhage, swelling) than fine needle aspirates.
  - For this reason, caution should be exercised when the technique is used to biopsy potentially vascular tumors in inaccessible locations (e.g., liver, kidney).

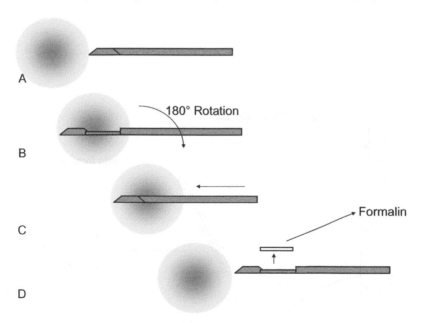

Figure 4.6.   Tru-Cut biopsy. This can be performed using either general anesthetic or sedation, and infiltration with local anesthetic. The area over the biopsy site is prepared and a small incision is made through the skin to accommodate the introduction of the needle. The needle is introduced through the skin with the central obturator and recessed biopsy groove withdrawn into the outer cannula (A). Once in the tumor tissue, the central obturator is advanced to expose the biopsy groove. The needle may be rotated through 180° at this point to ensure that the biopsy groove is adequately filled with tissue (B). The outer cannula is then advanced forward smartly to amputate the tissue within the groove (C). The unit is withdrawn and the cannula retracted to expose the biopsied tissue in the groove of the obturator (D). The tissue is recovered by gently flushing it with saline into the fixative so as to avoid damaging it by manipulation.

Skin Punch Biopsy (Figure 4.7)

- Excellent for skin and superficial soft-tissue tumors.
- Substantially more tissue can be recovered than with needle aspirates.
- Recovered tissue retains much of its architecture and is suitable for routine histological processing techniques.
- Multiple samples may be removed through a single approach.

Incisional Biopsy (Figure 4.8)

- This is the surgical removal of a solid piece of tissue from a tumor for histopathological examination.
- This is used where a substantial amount of tumor tissue is required to enable histopathological typing and grading.
- Incisional biopsy provides an **opportunity for exposure** of the biopsy site allowing accurate selection of the site for tumor sampling and reducing the risks of postbiopsy complications.
- Advantages:
  - An adequate amount of tissue can be recovered to allow a variety of histological processing techniques to be performed.
- Disadvantages:
  - Incisional biopsy normally requires general anesthesia of the patient.
  - Surgical procedures are generally more time consuming than needle techniques.
- If future treatment is not to be compromised, a few general principles of biopsy should be borne in mind:
  i.   The biopsy site should be positioned within the probable surgical or radiation field.

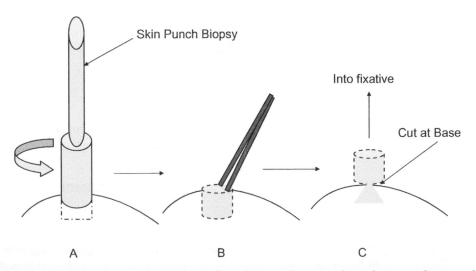

Figure 4.7. Punch biopsy technique. This can be performed using either general anesthetic or sedation, and infiltration with local anesthetic. The area over the biopsy site is prepared. The biopsy punch is placed at right angles to the surface to be biopsied (A). The punch is rotated in one direction at the same time as a firm downward pressure is applied until the punch reaches the level of the subcutis (A). The core of tissue is gently elevated with forceps or the point of a needle (B), and then finally the base of the biopsy is severed with scissors (C). The defect is closed using simple sutures.

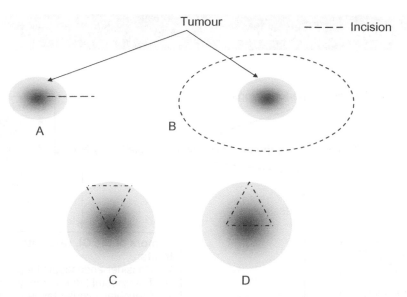

Figure 4.8.   Incisional (A) and excisional (B) biopsy. For incisional biopsy a wedge biopsy can be taken (C) to include some normal tissue. Where closure may be a problem, an inverted wedge can be removed (D).

ii.   The biopsy incision should be as small as is required, and orientated so as not to unnecessarily increase the size of the subsequent treatment area (e.g., on limbs, biopsy incisions should be orientated parallel to the long axis of the limb).

iii.   Specimens should be handled carefully and multiple samples obtained if possible. Electrocautery should not be used to obtain the sample as this will distort the architecture and make it unreadable by the pathologist. Electrocautery may be used afterward for hemostasis.

iv.   Samples should be taken from different areas of the lesion.

v.   The biopsy should result in minimal risk of local dissemination of the neoplastic disease. Uninvolved anatomic planes and compartments should not be breached and fresh instrumentation should be used for each site biopsied.

vi.   An adequate exposure should be made for both incisional and excisional biopsies to ensure that there is minimal disruption of the tumor and the adjacent uninvolved anatomic planes.

Excisional Biopsy (Figure 4.8)

- The complete surgical extirpation of a tumor, following which tissue samples are removed for histopathological examination.
- Histopathological examination should ideally be performed on **all** excised specimens in order to arrive at a definitive histopathological diagnosis.
- If a margin or normal tissue is removed with the tumor, surgical margins should be tagged to allow for histologic assessment of completeness of excision.
- Excisional biopsy should also be performed for tumors where pretreatment histopathology was not performed because
  - Of reasons of accessibility (e.g., tumors of the GI tract).
  - The proposed treatment was not influenced by the histological information (e.g., mammary tumors).

Choosing Biopsy Procedures

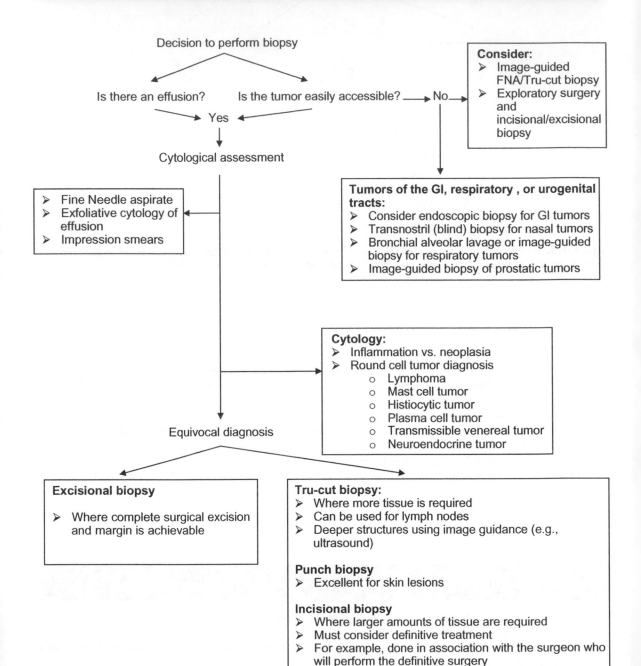

Decision to perform biopsy

Is there an effusion?   Is the tumor easily accessible? ⟶ No ⟶

Consider:
- Image-guided FNA/Tru-cut biopsy
- Exploratory surgery and incisional/excisional biopsy

Yes

Cytological assessment

- Fine Needle aspirate
- Exfoliative cytology of effusion
- Impression smears

Tumors of the GI, respiratory , or urogenital tracts:
- Consider endoscopic biopsy for GI tumors
- Transnostril (blind) biopsy for nasal tumors
- Bronchial alveolar lavage or image-guided biopsy for respiratory tumors
- Image-guided biopsy of prostatic tumors

Cytology:
- Inflammation vs. neoplasia
- Round cell tumor diagnosis
  - Lymphoma
  - Mast cell tumor
  - Histiocytic tumor
  - Plasma cell tumor
  - Transmissible venereal tumor
  - Neuroendocrine tumor

Equivocal diagnosis

Excisional biopsy
- Where complete surgical excision and margin is achievable

Tru-cut biopsy:
- Where more tissue is required
- Can be used for lymph nodes
- Deeper structures using image guidance (e.g., ultrasound)

Punch biopsy
- Excellent for skin lesions

Incisional biopsy
- Where larger amounts of tissue are required
- Must consider definitive treatment
- For example, done in association with the surgeon who will perform the definitive surgery
- Must not compromise the success of the definitive procedure

Bone Marrow Biopsy

- Bone marrow biopsy is often indicated in the diagnosis of conditions affecting the lymphoid and myeloid systems. The biopsy may take the form of an aspirate or a core biopsy.
- Indications for bone marrow biopsy
  - Nonregenerative anemia of undetermined cause
  - Investigation for secondary immune-mediated hemolytic anemia
  - Staging and/or diagnosis of hematopoeitic tumors

Bone Marrow Biopsy Procedure

Requirements for Bone Marrow Biopsy (Figure 4.9)

- Jamshidi needle (Figure 4.9A)
- Scalpel blade
- Glass microscope slides
- 10ml syringe
- EDTA blood tubes (to store excess marrow)
- Diff-Quick or similar

Technique (Figure 4.10)

- One can use the humerus, femur, or iliac crest.
- The patient is placed in sternal recumbency for an iliac crest sample and in lateral recumbency for humerus sample (Figure 4.10A).
- The animal is anesthetized or sedated for immobilization and the site is clipped and scrubbed as for a surgical procedure.
- A stab incision is made in the skin over the biopsy site.
- The bone marrow needle with stylet in place is advanced into the site and then introduced into the bone in a corkscrew fashion (Figure 4.10B).

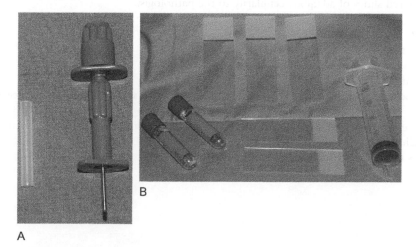

A   B

Figure 4.9. Bone marrow biopsy: materials.

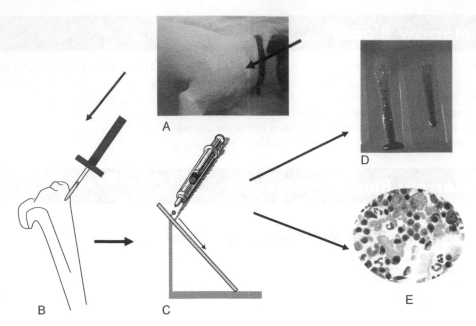

Figure 4.10. Bone marrow biopsy: technique.

- The needle should be firmly in the marrow space with no apparent wobble. The stylet is removed and a 10ml syringe attached to the needle.
- Bone marrow is aspirated.
- Marrow clots quickly; working fast is essential.
- Once marrow is aspirated, the whole needle and syringe is removed from the patient and drops of the marrow are placed on inclined slides (Figure 4.10C).
- Smears are made as for blood smears (Figure (4.10D).
- Before the animal is recovered, one of the smears is stained with Diff-Quick to ensure adequate cellularity (Figure 4.10E).
- Submit all prepared slides of adequate cellularity to the pathologist.

Bone marrow core sample
- A *Jamshidi needle* is employed.
- The procedure above is carried out, but after the aspirate has been retrieved, the needle is advanced to obtain a core sample.
- The needle is rocked forward and backward after advancement to sever the bone in the needle from its base.
- When the needle is removed, a smaller wire obturator is used to retrograde the biopsy material out of the top of the needle.
- This material is then fixed in formalin for histopathology.

Tissue Preparation and Handling After Biopsy

Key Points

The biopsy site and method will depend on the individual case. However, in general:

- The pathologist likes to see the junction between normal and abnormal tissue for accurate diagnosis. Where possible this should be achieved. One exception to this is bone neoplasia, where the biopsy is taken from the center of the lesion.
- Avoid electrocautery, surgical lasers, and crushing the artifact with forceps as these may deform tissues.
- Where possible, it is desirable that the whole tissue specimen be submitted. However, there is an absolute requirement for adequate fixation of tissue (ideally a formalin:tissue ratio of 10:1). If only part of a tissue is being submitted:
  - Avoid areas of necrosis and hemorrhage.
  - Send representative samples and margins.
  - Tissue should not be >1 cm thick or it will not fix properly.
- Where there is a requirement to evaluate surgical margins for completeness of excision:
  - Draw a diagram on the submission form representing where the lesion was removed.
  - Use surgical ink, or different colored sutures to tag appropriate margins.
  - Or, submit marginal tissue from the remaining tissue bed, separately from the main tumor mass.
- Submit:
  - Appropriately fixed material
  - The appropriate forms with diagrams
  - A clear history and clinical diagnosis
- Establish a good working relationship with your pathologist.

Interpretation of Histopathology Reports

- Read the report thoroughly.
- If the biopsy report does not correlate with the clinical scenario, you are obliged to
  - Speak to the pathologist directly and discuss any potential errors.
  - Request a second opinion.
  - Request further diagnostic immunohistochemistry.
  - Perform a second biopsy for a more representative sample.
- **It has been demonstrated that 5–10% of biopsy results may be inaccurate.**
- When a pathologist reports that the surgical margins are free from cancer cells, remember that this represents only the small fraction of slides he/she has examined from that particular tumor. For most malignant tumors, excision is considered complete (i.e., low risk of residual microscopic disease) if the histologic margin of normal tissue is 0.5–1 cm or greater. For mesenchymal tumors such as soft tissue sarcoma, a histologic margin of 1 cm or greater is preferred because these tumors commonly have long "tendrils" of microscopic cancer calls that extend beyond the detectable edges of the tumor.

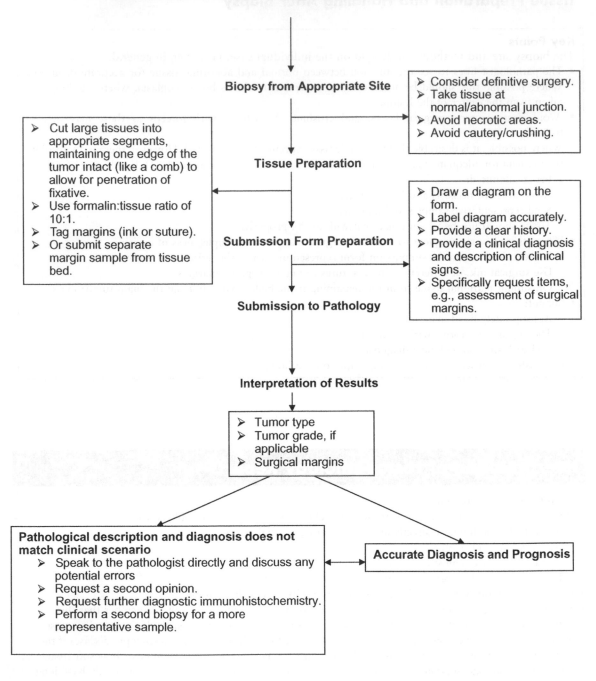

The Pathology Submission Checklist Incisional/Excisional Biopsy

Biopsy from Appropriate Site

> Consider definitive surgery.
> Take tissue at normal/abnormal junction.
> Avoid necrotic areas.
> Avoid cautery/crushing.

> Cut large tissues into appropriate segments, maintaining one edge of the tumor intact (like a comb) to allow for penetration of fixative.
> Use formalin:tissue ratio of 10:1.
> Tag margins (ink or suture).
> Or submit separate margin sample from tissue bed.

Tissue Preparation

Submission Form Preparation

> Draw a diagram on the form.
> Label diagram accurately.
> Provide a clear history.
> Provide a clinical diagnosis and description of clinical signs.
> Specifically request items, e.g., assessment of surgical margins.

Submission to Pathology

Interpretation of Results

> Tumor type
> Tumor grade, if applicable
> Surgical margins

Pathological description and diagnosis does not match clinical scenario
> Speak to the pathologist directly and discuss any potential errors
> Request a second opinion.
> Request further diagnostic immunohistochemistry.
> Perform a second biopsy for a more representative sample.

Accurate Diagnosis and Prognosis

Immunohistochemistry and Tumor-specific Histologic Dyes

- Immunohistochemistry (IHC) involves the use of labeled antibodies as reagents to localize antigens and proteins in cells to help identify the cell type.
- The use of IHC or special histologic dyes is indicated when a diagnosis is difficult using standard H/E sections.
- Typical routine stains include those shown in Table 4.3.

Table 4.3.   Tumor types and routine stains

Tumor Type	Specific Stain
Carcinoma	Cytokeratin
Mesenchymal	Vimentin
Lymphoid neoplasia	CD3, CD79a
Histiocytic tumor	CD18 / MHC II
Melanoma	S100, Melan A
Mast cell tumor	Toludine Blue*, Giemsa*

*Histologic dyes.

5
CANCER TREATMENT MODALITIES

David J. Argyle, Malcolm J. Brearley, Michelle M. Turek, and Linda Roberts

Part 1: Choosing an Appropriate Treatment Modality

Key Points

- Veterinary oncology is a fast-moving field. New drugs and other treatment modalities are continually being developed for use in the human medical field and then being applied to companion animal medicine. Occasionally, an innovative treatment modality is first investigated in companion animal patients.
- Many antineoplastic treatment options are highly involved, expensive, and potentially toxic. There is a dearth of lucid, practical, readily available written information for veterinary practitioners who feel responsible to "first do no harm" to their patients. Not surprisingly, then, antineoplastic therapy, particularly chemotherapy, is viewed with trepidation by many conscientious veterinarians.
- Yet with improvements in companion animal nutrition and preventative health care, we are dealing with an aging population of pets. In the future, we can anticipate that cancer will become an increasingly important cause of morbidity and mortality in the pet populations under our care.
- While there will always be clients who request euthanasia the moment they hear mention of the word cancer, more and more clients wish to explore and discuss treatment options for their pet.
- Sometimes euthanasia is, indeed, the most appropriate option; but more often there are alternatives that can provide a period of good quality life. Of course, some tumors can be cured surgically. This is less often true for the other treatment modalities.
- The purpose of this section is to go some way toward "demystifying" veterinary oncology. After reading this material, it is hoped that readers will feel better informed about the current "state of the art" and more willing to recommend and advise clients on treatment of the more common canine and feline tumors seen in their practices.

Key Steps in Choosing the Right Treatment Options for Animals with a Malignant Tumor (Figure 5.1)

- When presented with an animal with a neoplastic mass, some pertinent questions are worth being asked. The answers to these questions will be helpful in formulating a definitive plan for treatment.
  1. Is it in the animal's interest to remove/treat the mass?
  2. Are we going to improve the quality of life?

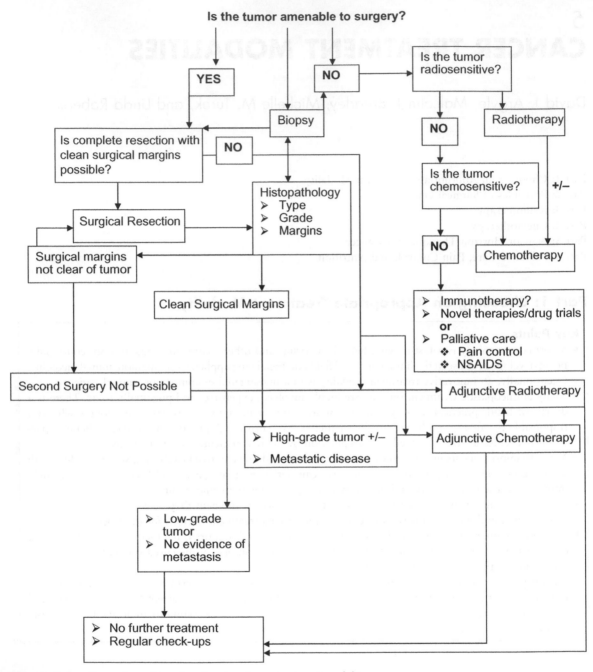

Figure 5.1. General considerations for choosing a treatment modality.

3. Are we going to prolong the animal's life with quality?
4. What investigations are needed to deliver the information needed?
5. Do we have the equipment and expertise to assist in the surgical resection of the mass?
6. What are we trying to achieve with therapy?
- The danger of not considering these questions is that one may start a surgical procedure, realize that the mass is inoperable, and then have to wonder how to close a nonclosable wound.

Is It in the Animal's Interest to Remove the Mass?

- In cases of advanced disease where organ function, cosmesis, or closure would be compromised, it may not be in the best interest of the pet to remove the mass.
- An example is a large and invasive lingual carcinoma. The tongue is critical to the swallowing mechanism and surgical resection should not be performed if the animal's ability to eat and drink would be compromised, especially since there is no way to reconstruct the tongue.

Are We Going to Improve the Quality of Life?

- A typical example is osteosarcoma.
- While amputation as the sole therapy does not influence survival, because development of metastasis is likely, removal of the painful mass dramatically improves the quality of life.

Are We Going to Prolong the Animal's Life with Quality?

- The progression of many tumors can be halted or delayed by excising the tumor, thereby extending the patient's life expectancy. If removal of the tumor will not affect the course of the disease, surgical excision may not be advisable unless it will provide palliation.

What Investigations Are Needed to Deliver the Information Needed?

- Appropriate clinical tumor staging and investigation of any concurrent disease should be performed prior to treatment consideration.

Do We Have the Equipment and Expertise?

- There are many advanced surgical procedures that should be attempted only by a board certified or experienced surgeon.
- Although chemotherapy can be performed in practice there is an absolute requirement for
  - Appropriate safety considerations
  - Knowledge of the drugs
  - Ability to cope with potential side effects
  - Adherence to National Health and Safety regulations, e.g., **COSHH (U.K.) and OSHA (U.S.)**
- Radiotherapy requires specialized equipment. The practitioner needs to know when radiotherapy is an appropriate treatment course so that a referral can be arranged.

What Are We Trying to Achieve with Therapy?

- Durable remission with good quality of life (i.e., curative intent)?
- Short-term palliation with good quality of life?

Part 2: Principles of Surgical Oncology

> **Key Points**
> - Oncological surgery involves aspects of soft-tissue surgery, orthopedic surgery and neurological surgery, and requires a comprehensive knowledge of anatomy and reconstructive procedures for tissue deficits.
> - Surgical oncology requires careful attention to surgical technique to avoid contamination of surrounding normal tissues with cancer cells.
> - Most malignant tumors have "extensions" of microscopic cancer cells that extend beyond the clinically detectable tumor. One of the objectives of surgery is to excise these microscopic cells along with the bulky tumor in order to minimize the risk of local tumor recurrence.
> - Complete surgical excision of localized tumors that have a low risk of metastasis often results in long-term tumor control.
> - Surgery is often combined with other treatment modalities including radiotherapy and chemotherapy to optimize the probability of tumor control.

What Is the Goal of Surgery?

- Diagnosis: as part of a biopsy procedure
- For curative intent: when complete surgical excision (clear surgical margins) can be achieved
- As part of a multimodality strategy to treat a tumor: e.g., cytoreduction to microscopic disease, followed by radiotherapy
- For palliation: e.g., amputation alone for dog with appendicular osteosarcoma
- For prevention of tumor development: e.g., spaying to prevent mammary tumor development
  For all of the above, the pet owner must be made fully aware of what the surgery is aiming to achieve.

General Considerations in Oncological Surgery

- Decisions about a surgical procedure must be made in association with all available data from tumor staging procedures.
- When a decision to use surgery for therapy has been made, the best possible outcome will be achieved the first time – second surgeries are less successful. This is especially important when the objective of surgery is curative-intent.
- For curative intent surgery, the best results are obtained with the first surgery
- Full consideration must be given to the potential requirement for tissue reconstruction.
- Preoperative planning of the anesthetic and analgesic regimen and the postoperative care will minimize postoperative morbidity.
- If both surgery and radiotherapy are planned or anticipated, the surgeon and the radiation oncologist should consult with one another to ensure that the therapy is optimally planned and that treatment with one modality will not compromise success of the other.

Types of Oncological Surgery

1. **Surgery for a Biopsy Procedure**
   - This is covered in Chapter 4.
2. **Prophylactic Surgery**
   - A prophylactic oncological surgery can be defined as one that results in a reduction of either the anticipated incidence rate of a particular tumor type or the risk of progression of a noncancerous lesion to a malignant one, e.g.:
     - ○ Mammary tumors in the bitch
     - ○ Benign vaginal tumors in the bitch
     - ○ Testicular tumors in the dog
     - ○ Premalignant lesions of squamous cell carcinoma in the cat

3. **Cytoreductive Surgery**
   - In some circumstances, definitive excisional curative surgery for solid tumors is not possible.
   - Certain tumor types or grades are associated with significant rates of local recurrence even after radical surgery, and resection of such tumors should always be regarded as incomplete.
   - Cytoreductive surgery reduces the numbers of tumor cells present.
   - Cytoreductive surgery is combined with other treatment modalities such as radiotherapy or local or systemic chemotherapy to try to achieve long-term remission.
   - Cytoreductive surgery improves the efficiency of these adjunctive therapies by reducing the numbers of malignant cells to be treated.
   - Examples include
     - Mast cell tumor resection to microscopic disease followed by adjunctive radiotherapy
     - Hemangiosarcoma removal followed by adjunctive chemotherapy
4. **Palliative Surgery**
   - A surgery performed to improve quality of life when progression of the cancer is expected despite surgical intervention
   - Examples of this include
     - Limb amputation for osteosarcoma causing lameness
     - Removal of large ulcerated painful mammary carcinomas
     - Placement of a permanent cystostomy catheter to relieve urine outflow obstruction in dogs with transitional cell carcinoma
5. **Definitive Surgical Excision (Figures 5.2, 5.3)**
   - This refers to the use of surgery as the sole treatment, without adjunctive radiotherapy or chemotherapy, to achieve long-term tumor control.
   - The incision, the surgical exposure, and the surgical margin are the most important aspects of a definitive surgery.
   - The incision should take into account the need to resect any scars that are a result of previous surgery or sites of biopsy. Such scars should be afforded the same margins as the bulk of the tumor because surgical scars will be contaminated by tumor cells from the primary mass.
   - The incision should also allow adequate access to the tumor to avoid rough handling and fragmentation of the neoplastic tissue.
   - The choice of the margin at surgery will profoundly affect the success of the surgery as a curative procedure.
- Definitive surgical procedures include:
  - Local excision
  - Wide local excision
  - Radical excision

Key Points: Wide Local Excision
- This surgery involves removing a significant predetermined margin of surrounding normal tissue together with the primary mass.
- To plan this surgery properly, knowledge of the tumor type and, if relevant, the tumor grade is essential.
- Anatomic considerations dictate whether a complete resection of the mass with an appropriate margin is possible.
- In certain circumstances (e.g., on limbs) appropriate depth of surgical margin cannot be achieved. However, a collagen-rich fascial plane (e.g., a muscle sheath or aponeurosis) may act as a natural boundary to tumor spread.
- In general, gross normal tissue margins of 2–3 cm should be obtained for most malignant tumors. Exceptions include
  - CNS tumors where it is not desirable to exceed the bounds of the tumor.
  - Mast cell tumors in cats where a smaller margin of normal tissue usually suffices to remove microscopic disease.
  - Soft tissue sarcomas may require >3 cm margins due to their invasiveness into surrounding tissue.

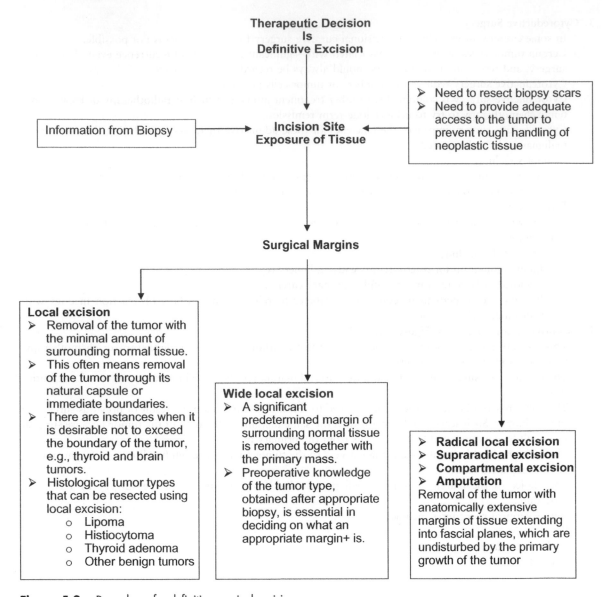

Figure 5.2. Procedures for definitive surgical excision.

Presurgical Biopsy and Complete Staging

Dissection

> Use a scalpel for the skin incision and incisions into hollow viscera as it is the least traumatic form of tissue separation.
> Scissors and swabs should be used for the separation of fascial planes, the separation of adhesions and in the body
> Blood vessels should be identified and ligated or cauterized prior to transaction.
> Tissues should be placed under moderate tension as the dissection is carried out to facilitate the identification of fascial planes and tumor margins.

Reduction of Tumor Cell Contamination of the Surgical Field

> Surgically induced tumor seeding has been identified.
> The pseudocapsule around many tumors, especially sarcomas, has viable tumor cells on its surface.
> Manipulation of and surgical exposure of the pseudocapsule promotes tumor spread via exfoliated cells.
> Solid neoplastic tissue should be manipulated using stay sutures rather than crushing forceps.
> In body cavities, neoplasms should be isolated from surrounding viscera by large laparotomy pads to minimize contamination of normal tissue.
> Lavage is recommended to effect removal of blood clots, foreign material, necrotic tissue fragments and potentially the removal of unattached tumor cells.
> Gloves, instruments, and drapes should also be changed after tumor excision and lavage.

Wound Complications

> The development of hematomas, seromas, and sepsis will all interfere with local cellular defense mechanisms and should all be avoided.
> Hemostasis, effective closure of dead space, and appropriate use of drains and perioperative antibiotics are key.

Vascular Occlusion

> Vascular supply to the tumor and venous and lymphatic drainage from it should be ligated as early as possible during surgery.
> The benefits of temporary occlusion of vascular supply to an area that includes the tumor to be resected remain unproven, and the main reason for occluding the vascular supply as soon as possible in the dissection is for the benefit that is gained from improved hemostasis.

Lymph Node Management

> The practice of routinely removing the "sentinel" or regional lymph nodes in both man and animals in order to prophylactically excise micrometastatic deposits is a matter of considerable controversy.
> Local lymph node metastasis is common for malignant melanomas and most carcinomas; intermediate for sarcomas, respiratory tumors, cutaneous carcinomas, and mast cell tumors; and rare for nervous system tumors, skeletal tumors, nasal tumors, and most endocrine tumors (e.g., insulinomas).
> Current recommendations are
  o The nondestructive biopsy of grossly normal local nodes
  o Removal of the node when
    ▪ It is histologically proven to contain tumor cells.
    ▪ It appears grossly abnormal at surgery.
    ▪ It is intimately associated with the tissue being removed and surgical margins dictate its removal.
    ▪ One case where local lymph node removal is probably beneficial is the removal of the medial iliac lymph nodes in patients with metastatic apocrine or sebaceous gland adenocarcinomas of the perineum.

Successful Tissue Closure

Reconstruction of the Resulting Tissue Deficit

Figure 5.3. Successful definitive excisional surgery.

Key Points: Radical Local Excision, Supraradical Excision, Compartmental Excision, and Amputation

- This form of surgery is required for tumors that extend along fascial planes rather than through them (e.g., sarcomas).
- This pattern of growth dictates removal of the entire anatomic compartment rather than simply wide margins of tissue.
- For example, an area is resected back to clean fascial planes on all sides with removal of all blood vessels, nerves, and lymphatics that lie within the affected compartment.
- Examples of supraradical excision/compartmental excision:
  - In the limbs, muscles with their associated fascial capsules comprise individual compartments
  - Removal of the whole pinna and vertical ear canal for resection of squamous cell carcinoma of the pinna
  - Mandibulectomy and its muscle attachments for treatment of oral tumors
  - Amputation of a limb for appendicular osteosarcoma
  - Hemipelvectomy for high hindlimb tumors
- Examples of radical resections:
  - Excision of the eyelids and orbital contents for removal of invasive squamous cell carcinomas of the eyelid
  - Total or partial orbitectomy for the treatment of periorbital tumors
  - Radical chest wall resection or abdominal wall resection for the removal of sarcomas
- If a margin of 3 cm is required, with a depth of excision to include two muscle or fascial planes, the surgery often involves resection of large compartments of tissue such as amputation. Tumor types requiring this include
  - Grade III (high grade) mast cell tumors
  - Grade II and III soft-tissue sarcomas (spindle cell sarcomas)
  - Feline vaccine-associated sarcomas

Preoperative Preparation

- The patient should be widely clipped.
- Gently clean using effective skin preparations (e.g., chlorhexidine/alcohol mixture
- Avoid vigorous palpation of tumors prior to surgery.
- The infection rates following oncological surgery have been shown to be significantly higher than for other surgical procedures.
- Use prophylactic antibiosis during surgery and in the perioperative period.
- The best results are seen when antibiotic therapy begins not more than 2 hours before the surgical procedure and continues for no more than 24 hours after the surgical procedure.
- **Primary Skin Closure**
  - The coaptation of the wound edges at the time of the initial surgery without the need for extensive skin releasing techniques.
  - Indicated for small skin deficits or where there is a lot of loose skin.
  - Tension-releasing techniques are sometimes required.
  - The wound should have no tension.
- **Secondary Skin Healing**
  - The closure of the wound by secondary intention.
  - Particularly suited to contaminated wounds or where the reconstruction of the wound is prohibited by the lack of surrounding skin.

- Specialized Reconstruction Techniques
  - Pedicle flap closure of the skin
    - ○ Closure of wounds using sliding flaps of skin, e.g., advancement flaps, rotation flaps and transposition flaps.
    - ○ It also includes the use of axial or island flaps. Such techniques can be used immediately after the excisional surgery.
  - Free skin grafts
    - ○ Particularly suited to the closure of skin deficits over the distal limbs.
    - ○ These techniques have to be delayed until after the excisional surgery to allow for the establishment of a good recipient granulation bed.
  - Local tissue augmentation
    - ○ e.g., the use of omental flaps.
  - Mesh implants
    - ○ Provide a scaffold for reconstruction of the thoracic and abdominal wall. Cutaneous reconstruction techniques are then used to close the skin.

Postoperative Care

- Effective analgesia must be provided if the secondary adverse effects of postoperative pain such as increased levels of catabolic hormones, prolonged recovery, and increased skeletal and smooth muscle tone, as well as the suffering caused by the pain itself, are to be avoided.
- The prevention of postoperative pain should start preoperatively with effective doses of multiple injectable analgesics, as well as local nerve blocks and epidurals as indicated. Postoperative local infiltration of analgesics such as lidocaine using a "soaker catheter" provides effective local analgesia. This should be avoided if complete surgical excision of cancer is not certain because the infused medication could result in seeding of cancer cells. This technique works well for limb amputations where the tumor is distal to the incision site.
- If elective surgery for a painful neoplastic lesion is planned, it is probably beneficial to provide effective analgesic therapy for several days prior to surgical intervention in order to minimize central sensitization. This could easily be provided with NSAID therapy after the animal begins taking in food.
- As the surgery planned becomes more extensive, the doses of opioids used (e.g., buprenorphine, morphine) should increase, and pre- or postoperative NSAID therapy be used.
- Careful monitoring must be used to allow the provision of effective fluid therapy in the immediate postoperative period and the instigation of oral or enteral nutrition.

Part 3: Radiotherapy

Key Points
- Radiotherapy is the use of ionizing radiation for the treatment of neoplasia. It is an effective local treatment for many solid tumors in dogs and cats.
- Radiation causes damage to the genetic material (DNA) of cells within the irradiated tissue, which leads to cellular death. This biological effect is expressed when the damaged cells attempt to divide.
- Radiation is a local therapy with no systemic effects. Side effects are limited to the tissues within the radiation field. Cancer cells outside of the radiation field will not be affected by the radiation.
- Theoretically, there is a dose of radiation that would sterilize any tumor. The most important factor that limits the dose that can be safely administered to a tumor is the tolerance of the surrounding normal tissues to radiation. The goal of radiation planning is to deliver the maximum dose to the tumor while maintaining the dose to surrounding normal tissues below their tolerance level.

- Radiation-induced side effects are predictable based on the proliferation rate of the tissue being irradiated and the dose of radiation being administered. Tissues with a rapid rate of cellular turnover are called acutely responding tissues. Radiation effects that affect these tissues develop in the immediate postradiation period and are self-limiting. Tissues with a slow rate of cellular turnover are called late-responding tissues. Late effects develop years to months after radiotherapy and are irreversible. It is paramount that radiation protocols be designed to minimize the risk of late effects.
- External beam radiation (Figure 5.4) is the most common form of radiation delivery in veterinary medicine. Linear accelerators and cobalt-60 units are devices used to deliver external beam radiation. General anesthesia is required for patient immobilization during the treatment.
- In general, the probability of local tumor control is highest when radiation is combined with surgical excision of a tumor. In this situation, detectable disease is surgically resected and peripheral microscopic cancer cells are targeted by radiation. Radiation can be delivered pre- or postoperatively.
- Radiotherapy can also be used for palliation of tumor-related clinical signs when factors such as metastatic disease or advanced local disease are likely to lead to early demise. Unlike definitive (curative-intent) protocols that call for multiple weeks of daily radiation treatments, palliative protocols involve fewer and less frequent radiation treatments, thereby minimizing the risk of clinically significant side effects.
- Optimal care of veterinary cancer patients often requires a multidisciplinary approach that combines surgery, radiotherapy, and chemotherapy. Consultation with a radiation oncologist or an oncology specialist is advisable for any case that may benefit from radiotherapy. These specialists can help formulate the best plan of action to optimize the efficacy of radiation in conjunction with the other treatment modalities that are available.

Goal of Therapy

- In general, the goal of radiotherapy is either long-term tumor control (definitive therapy, or curative intent) or short-term palliation of tumor-related clinical signs in cases of advanced disease when long-term prognosis is poor (palliative therapy) (Table 5.1).

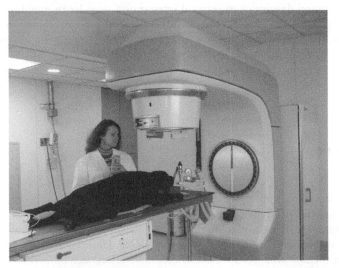

Figure 5.4. External beam radiotherapy involves the use of radiation beams whose source is located externally to the patient. External beam radiation most commonly involves use of a linear accelerator or a cobalt-60 unit. A 4 MeV linear accelerator is shown here. The beam comes out of a part of the accelerator called the *gantry,* which rotates 360° around the patient. The patient lies on a movable treatment couch and lasers are used to make sure the patient is in the proper position. Radiation can be delivered to the tumor from any angle by rotating the gantry and moving the treatment couch.

Table 5.1. Goals of radiotherapy

	Definitive RT	Palliative RT
Synonym	Curative intent Full-course	Coarse fraction
Objective	Tumor control. Life expectancy is extended because progression of the cancer is suspended.	Palliation: short-term improvement of tumor-related clinical signs resulting in improved quality of life as the disease process progresses. Tumor control is not expected. Life expectancy may not be longer than with no therapy.
When to offer it	For tumors without distant metastasis where progression of the cancer can be positively impacted (significantly delayed or even cured) with therapy. Often combined with surgery for best chance of long-term tumor control. Radiation can be used pre- or postoperatively.	For tumors that are associated with clinical signs such as pain, hemorrhage, or obstruction that are expected to lead to early demise. • Large, advanced, incurable tumors • Tumors associated with distant metastatic disease For tumors that are associated with clinical signs for which the owner does not wish to pursue definitive therapy for practical reasons, such as cost and time commitment required.
Side effects[†]	Acute effects are expected. Risk of late effects ≤5%.	Minimal to no acute effects. Risk of late effects is high but since the patient's life expectancy is limited due to the extent or nature of the cancer, late effects will not have the opportunity to develop.
Dose per fraction	Low 2–4 Gy	High 6–15 Gy
Number of fractions	10–20	1–6
Treatment schedule	Daily: Monday–Friday	Weekly or biweekly or as needed
Clinical implications	Treatment is delivered daily. Treatment is expensive. Self-limiting side effects are expected.	Less time-intensive. Less expensive. Few to no clinically significant side effects.

[†] Acute effects are side effects that affect normal tissues within the radiation field that have a rapid turnover rate, such as skin and oral mucosa. They develop in the immediate postradiation period and are self-limiting. Late effects affect tissues with a slow turnover rate, such as bone and nervous tissue. They take several months to years to develop and are irreversible. See "Normal Tissue Reactions and Radiation-Induced Side Effects" for more information.
RT = radiotherapy.

Decision Making for the Radiation Treatment Approach (Figure 5.5)

- When considering how best to use radiotherapy for treatment of a tumor, factors to consider include the owner's wishes, the stage of the cancer, the probability of tumor control, and the patient's general health as it relates to concurrent diseases and the risk of frequent anesthesia.
- Chemotherapy should be considered if it has antitumor activity against the cancer being treated, especially if the tumor is likely to metastasize.
- The radiation oncologist or oncology specialist should be consulted at the time of tumor diagnosis so that the use of radiation can be optimized in conjunction with the other treatment modalities available.

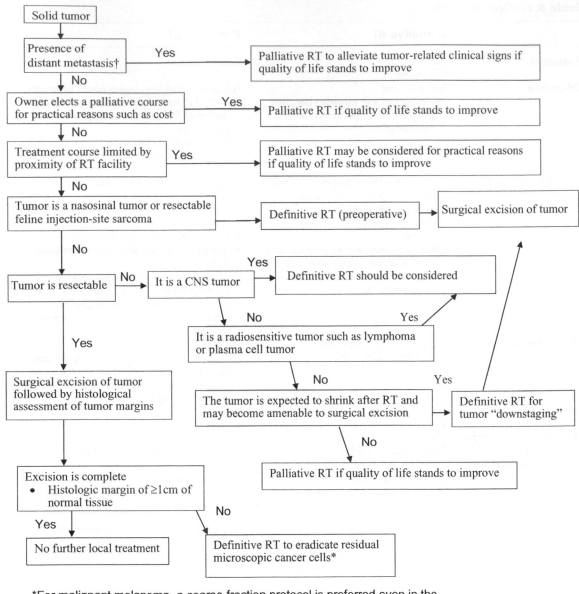

*For malignant melanoma, a coarse-fraction protocol is preferred even in the microscopic setting.
RT = radiotherapy.

Figure 5.5. Radiation treatment decision tree.

Tumors Commonly Treated with Radiotherapy (see specific chapters for further discussion of tumor types)

- Nasosinal tumors
- CNS tumors including brain or spinal tumors
  - Pituitary tumors
  - Meningioma
  - Glioma
- Oral tumors
  - Malignant melanoma
  - Squamous cell carcinoma
  - Fibrosarcoma
  - Acanthomatous epulis
- Cutaneous mast cell tumor in dogs
- Soft-tissue sarcoma
- Histiocytic tumors, in particular the cutaneous form
- Cutaneous hemangiosarcoma
- Feline injection-site sarcoma
- Ceruminous gland carcinoma
- Anal sac adenocarcinoma
- Thyroid carcinoma
- Thymoma
- Lymphoma
  - Focal disease
  - Multicentric disease in dogs (half-body irradiation)
- Primary and metastatic bone tumors (palliation)

The Biological Basis of Radiotherapy

- Radiotherapy is the treatment of cancer using ionizing radiation.
- When absorbed by tissue, ionizing radiation causes damage to genetic material (DNA) inside cells. When DNA damage is irreparable by the cellular repair mechanisms, the cell cannot survive and cellular death ensues. Both tumor cells and normal cells in the radiation field are affected. This results in tumor shrinkage and normal tissue side effects within the radiation field.
- In general, cellular death from radiation occurs during mitosis when a cell is preparing to divide. Hence, the timing of tumor shrinkage and the development of side effects is a function of the proliferation rate of the tumor or the normal tissue in question, respectively.
- Radiation-induced side effects are grouped into two categories. Those that affect tissues with a rapid rate of proliferation (acutely responding tissues) are called acute effects. Those that affect tissues with a slow rate of proliferation (late-responding tissues) are called late effects. See the section "Normal Tissue Reactions and Radiation-Induced Side Effects" for a more detailed discussion of side effects.
- Lymphoid tissue, including lymphoid neoplasia, is highly radiosensitive and is an exception to the rule that cellular death occurs at the time of cellular division. Cellular death in lymphoid tissues occurs within hours after irradiation. This is why half-body irradiation is being investigated as an adjuvant to chemotherapy for multicentric lymphoma in dogs.
- In general, radiation is most effective at eradicating cancer when there are fewer target cancer cells to kill. It follows that the probability of local tumor control is highest when radiation is used in combination with surgery. Surgery is used to excise gross (detectable) disease, and radiation is used to eradicate residual microscopic cancer cells that extend from the periphery of the tumor. This is true for two reasons:

- The oxygen effect: The presence of oxygen inside a cell is critical for maximal radiation-induced DNA damage. Large tumors that contain hypoxic cells due to limited oxygen diffusion are less sensitive to the effects of radiation. It follows that radiation is more effective at controlling cancer when tumors are small or subclinical (microscopic), as after an incomplete excision.
  - Radiation-induced cellular death follows exponential kinetics. This means that each time a tumor is exposed to radiation, a constant fraction of cells is killed, rather than a constant number. Therefore, tumor control will be best when fewer cells are required to be killed, as is the case for small or subclinical tumors.
- When radiotherapy and surgery are used in combination, the most common approach is to resect the tumor first and follow with adjuvant radiation if the excision was incomplete and subclinical (microscopic) disease remains at the surgical site. However, some tumors are best managed using preoperative irradiation. Examples include feline injection-site site sarcomas, nasosinal tumors, and some tumors that are initially nonresectable where radiation is expected to decrease tumor size and render surgical excision possible. The latter approach is called downstaging and is indicated for nonresectable thyroid carcinomas and thymomas.

Radiation Dose and Fractionation

- Radiation dose is measured in units called *gray (Gy)*.
- 1 gray represents 1 joule (J) of energy absorbed by 1 kilogram (kg)of tissue.
- In radiotherapy, the total dose of radiation is fractionated or spread out over multiple treatments.
- One radiation treatment is called a *fraction*.
- Radiation prescriptions include the dose per fraction and the number of fractions.
  - For example, 3 Gy × 19 fractions = 57 Gy total dose
- Fractionation of the total dose over a period of time capitalizes on the following biological principles:
  - Repair of normal cells. Dividing the total dose into a number of small doses allows normal cells to repair radiation-induced DNA damage between fractions. Unlike normal cells, cancer cells have a limited ability to repair DNA, which works to our advantage.
  - Reoxygenation of cancer cells. As discussed earlier, the presence of oxygen inside a cancer cell is necessary for maximal radiation-induced DNA damage that leads to cell death. Tumors contain both oxygenated and hypo-oxygenated cells. As well-oxygenated cancer cells die off during radiotherapy, oxygen is able to diffuse to hypo-oxygenated cells, making them more susceptible to radiation-induced DNA damage.
  - Redistribution of cancer cells in the cell cycle. Cells in the G2-M phase of the cell cycle are most susceptible to cell death by radiation. As radiotherapy progresses, cancer cells in the less sensitive phases of the cell cycle progress into the more sensitive phases.
- The radiation prescription for tumors varies based on the tumor type, the tolerance to radiation of the surrounding normal tissues, and the goal of treatment (i.e., definitive or palliative therapy). For example:
  - Sarcomas require a total dose of 50–60 Gy for tumor control, whereas lymphoid tumors require 30–48 Gy.
  - The ocular lens tolerates total doses up to 5–10 Gy before irreversible damage occurs, resulting in cataract formation. The skin tolerates total doses up to 60+ Gy before irreversible damage such as fibrosis develops.
  - The probability of late, irreversible side effects to normal tissues is greater when a high dose/fraction is used. When life expectancy is expected to be long, smaller doses/fractions are used to minimize the risk of late effects.
- Definitive protocols with curative intent involve daily radiation treatments for 2–4+ weeks. The objective is to deliver the required tumoricidal dose in as short a period as possible without delivering too high a daily dose to do irreversible damage to normal tissues. In contrast, palliative protocols usually call for weekly (or biweekly) treatments. The total dose of these protocols is lower and is delivered in fewer fractions to minimize side effects. For example, a commonly used palliative protocol for osteosarcoma is 8 Gy × 4 weekly fractions. The long interval between fractions allows normal tissues to repair and minimizes or eliminates the risk of acute side effects.

Normal Tissue Reactions and Radiation-Induced Side Effects

- The interactions between radiation and tissue, as well as the clinical side effects that ensue, are predictable and expected.
- The nature, severity, onset, and duration of side effects depend on the type and volume of tissues that are irradiated and on the treatment itself (total dose, dose/fraction, treatment schedule).
- The response of normal tissue depends on the proliferation rate of the cells that compose it.
- In general, acute (or early) toxicities affect rapidly proliferating tissues, and chronic (or late) toxicities affect slowly proliferating tissues.
- Rapidly proliferating tissues include skin, oral and nasal mucosa, GI tract, cornea, and conjunctiva. These are usually epithelial tissues.
- Slowly proliferating tissues include bone, nervous tissue, muscle, connective tissue, lens, and retina. These are usually mesenchymal tissues.
- Since radiation-induced cell death occurs at the time of mitosis, it follows that side effects affecting rapidly proliferating tissues (acute effects) begin to develop during therapy and resolve within 2–4 weeks after treatment. These effects are transient due to cellular renewal. They are unavoidable when definitive radiation protocols are used. Severity of acute effects correlates directly with the total dose and the duration of treatment. Examples of acute radiation effects include
  - Moist desquamation of the skin including ulceration and edema (Figure 5.6)
  - Rhinitis or oral mucositis (Figures 5.7, 5.8)
  - Corneal ulceration
  - Conjunctivitis
  - Colitis and diarrhea
- Treatment of acute effects amounts to supportive care during the healing process:
  - Prevention of self-trauma that would delay healing (e-collar, T-shirt)
  - Antibiotics to prevent secondary infection
  - Pain medication to control discomfort (narcotics, gabapentin) and inflammation (NSAIDs)
  - Occasionally, steroids to alleviate effects

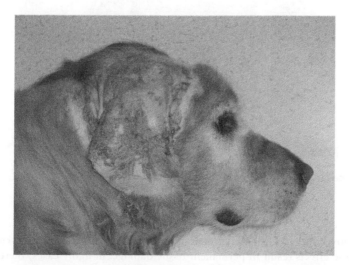

Figure 5.6. Moist desquamation is shown. Radiation damage to the skin results in sloughing of the basal cell layer and loss of integrity of the epithelial barrier. Skin changes range from erythema to inflammation to dry desquamation (flaking) to moist (exudative) desquamation. Radiation damage to hair follicles causes epilation. Cutaneous side effects are self-limiting and resolution occurs over 1–3 weeks after radiation.

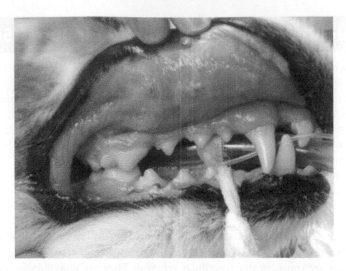

Figure 5.7. Oral mucositis is inflammation of the mucosa of the oral cavity secondary to radiation. It ranges from redness to ulceration. The whitish material shown here on the inner aspect of the upper lip represents dead epithelial cells. Due to the rapid proliferation of the oral mucosa, tissue damage is repaired within 1–2 weeks after radiation.

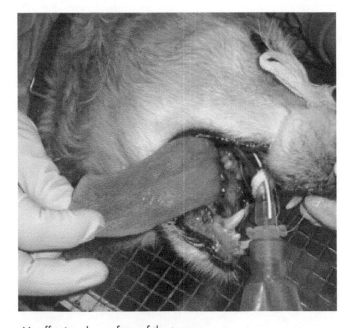

Figure 5.8. Oral mucositis affecting the surface of the tongue

- Due to the slow turnover of late-responding tissues, late effects develop months to years after treatment and do not heal. These effects result in permanent tissue damage. In many cases, there is no treatment. Hence, the primary dose-limiting factor in radiotherapy is the tolerance of late-responding tissues in the radiation field. Examples of late radiation effects include
  - Myelomalacia
  - Muscular fibrosis

- Cataract formation (Figure 5.9)
- Retinal hemorrhage and degeneration
- Radiation-induced tumor formation
- Osteomyelitis and bone necrosis (Figure 5.10A)
- Leukotrichia (Figure 5.10B)
- The probability of late toxicity is minimized in definitive protocols by appropriate treatment planning, including the use of smaller doses/fraction. Palliative protocols employ few, large-dose fractions delivered at long intervals (usually weekly). When palliative protocols are used, the implication to the normal tissues is a low risk of acute effects (due to the long interval between fractions) but a high risk of late effects (due to the large dose per fraction). This risk of late effects is accepted because the life expectancy of the patients undergoing palliative protocols is limited. The patients are not expected to be living months to years later when late effects develop.
- There is species variation. Cats appear to be more resistant to radiation side effects than dogs or people.

Types of Radiation

- Radiation is classified based on the method of delivery. The different methods relate to the position of the radiation source. See Table 5.2.
  - External beam radiation (or teletherapy)
  - Interstitial radiation (or brachytherapy)
  - Systemic radiation therapy
- External beam radiation is the most common method of radiation delivery in veterinary medicine.
- Most veterinary radiation facilities use a linear accelerator or a cobalt unit to deliver external beam radiation. These are high-energy (megavoltage) radiation devices.
- Linear accelerators and cobalt units differ in how the radiation beam is generated. In linear accelerators, radiation is generated in the form of a photon beam (called an x-ray beam) by the physical interaction between a beam of fast-moving electrons and the atoms of a solid metal target, usually tungsten. This interaction occurs within the linear accelerator when it is set to treatment mode and it results in emission of the photon beam through the collimator. In contrast, cobalt units employ a radioactive isotope of cobalt, cobalt-60, that emits a photon beam (called a gamma ray) as it decays. The radioactive cobalt source is stored within a shielded compartment of the unit when the unit is off. When it is set to treatment mode, the cobalt source is positioned at the level of the collimator and the photon beam is emitted. See Table 5.3.

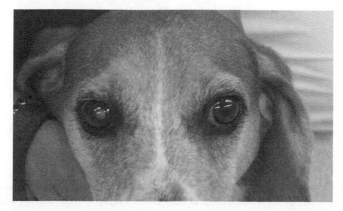

Figure 5.9. A radiation-induced cataract has developed in the left eye 10 months following radiotherapy for a nasal tumor. Damaged cells of the lens are not replaced naturally; therefore, a cataract forms as damaged cells become opaque. The lens is a late-responding tissue; hence, development of a cataract occurs several months after treatment.

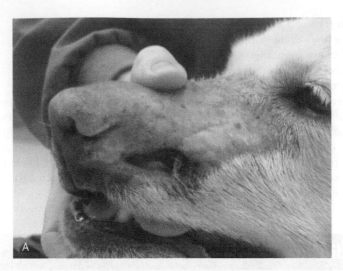

Figure 5.10A. Osteomyelitis leading to osteonecrosis is a rare late complication of radiotherapy. In the case shown here, the root of the left maxillary canine is visible through the defect in the maxilla. This lesion is not expected to heal and surgical intervention is not likely to be effective. With appropriate treatment planning and by taking into account normal tissue tolerance, the risk of development of osteomyelitis and osteonecrosis is less than 5%.

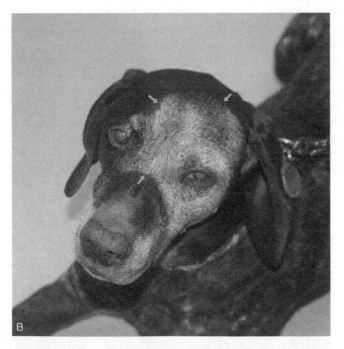

Figure 5.10B. Leukotrichia (whiteness of hair shown by the arrows) is a late effect of radiotherapy. This is an irreversible, aesthetic change with no significant clinical implications.

- The penetrability in tissue of a radiation beam is a function of its energy. Linear accelerators emit higher energy radiation with greater penetrability than cobalt units. Higher-energy beams are useful for deep-seeded tumors in large patients.
- In veterinary patients, many tumors treatable with radiation involve the skin or subcutaneous tissues. Examples include mast cell tumors, soft-tissue sarcomas, and feline injection-site sarcomas. For these

Table 5.2. Radiation classification based on the method of delivery

	External Beam Radiation	**Interstitial Radiation**	**Systemic Radiation**
Synonym	Teletherapy	Brachytherapy	–
Radiation source	Radiation is emitted from a machine that is external to the body.	Implanted directly into the body within or close to the tumor	Injected into the body
Equipment	Linear accelerator Cobalt-60 unit	Sealed radioactive material in the form of wires, tubes, ribbons, or "seeds"	Unsealed radioactive materials such as I^{131}
Clinical implications	The patient is not radioactive.	The patient is radioactive until the implants are removed. Isolation is required to minimize exposure of hospital personnel and the pet owner.	The patient is radioactive. Isolation is required to minimize exposure of hospital personnel and the pet owner. Radioactivity will leave the body through saliva and urine making these fluids radioactive.
Use in veterinary medicine	Common for treatment of cancer	Rarely used Limited availability	Common for treatment of hyperthyroidism in cats (I^{131})

superficial tumors, deep-penetrating radiation beams are not necessary and low-penetrating beams are preferred in order to avoid irradiation of underlying structures. Electron beams are particularly useful for these cases because radiation deposited by high-energy electrons penetrates only a short distance into tissues. Electron beams are available on linear accelerators of ≥ 6 MeV.

Radiation Treatment Planning

- The challenge of radiotherapy is to deliver a tumoricidal dose of radiation to a tumor while sparing critical normal tissues to minimize side effects. Radiation planning is a critical part of the treatment process.
- Radiation planning refers to the process of ensuring that the radiation dose delivered to the tumor is adequate and that critical normal tissues are maximally spared. The process includes optimization of beam orientation, beam shaping, and calculations of dose distribution in tumor and normal tissues.
- As with surgery, effective radiotherapy requires knowledge of the extent of the disease. With the use of advanced imaging, including computed tomography and MRI, we are now able to delineate precisely the extent of detectable disease (Figure 5.11) allowing for greater accuracy in treatment planning and greater probability of tumor control. Not all tumors require advanced imaging for effective treatment planning.
- When radiation treatments are planned, a margin of normal tissue around the tumor is included in the radiation field to include nondetectable microscopic cancer cells and to allow for slight variations in day-to-day patient positioning.
- The radiation fields may also include the regional draining lymph nodes if there is thought to be risk of subclinical malignant spread.
- Conventional radiation portals are rectangular due to the shape of the collimator on the linear accelerator or cobalt unit. The beam may be shaped by placing blocks between the collimator portal and the patient to block normal tissues (Figures 5.12, 5.13) The use of more modern and sophisticated computerized collimator devices called *multileaf collimators* is becoming more common in veterinary medicine. Multileaf colliators are made up of dozens of individual metal "leaves" that can move independently in and out of the path of the radiation beam in order to block tissue. They facilitate radiation delivery, thereby allowing for more complex and conformal treatments.
- Computerized treatment planning software is used to optimize radiation treatment by ensuring adequate dose to the tumor and maintaining the dose to surrounding normal tissues below their tolerance level.

Table 5.3. Megavoltage external beam radiation devices

	Linear Accelerator	**Cobalt-60 Unit**
Radiation source	X-rays[†] are generated when fast moving electrons interact with a metal target, usually tungsten.	Gamma rays[†] are emitted by a radioactive isotope of cobalt (cobalt-60).
Photon beam energy	4–15 + MeV[*]	1.25 MeV[*]
Electron beam capability	Yes	No
Penetration of the radiation beam in tissue	Photon beam: • Deep tissue penetration (greater with higher energy machines) Electron beam: • Superficial tissue penetration	There is deep tissue penetration but less than with a linear accelerator.
Clinical implications	Photon beams from higher energy units allow treatment of deep seeded tumors in very large patients. Electron beams are useful for superficial cancers located on the skin or in the subcutaneous tissues. Tissues underlying the cancer are not irradiated when an electron beam is used.	Penetration of photon beam in tissue is adequate for most veterinary patients.
Radiation exposure of personnel	No radiation exposure when the linear accelerator is in beam-off mode.	The radioactive source is housed in a shielded compartment when the machine is in beam-off mode. There is a constant, detectable, albeit very low level of radiation surrounding the unit in beam-off mode.
Use in veterinary medicine	Common	Less common than linear accelerators; many facilities are replacing cobalt units with modern linear accelerators.

[†]X-ray and gamma ray beams are both photon beams. The terminology is different to represent the different source of the photons. Gamma rays represent radiation that is emitted by decaying radioactive isotopes such as cobalt-60. X-rays are "man-made" in that they are generated as a result of a human intervention (i.e., an intentional collision between fast-moving electrons and a metal target).
[*]The energy of a radiation beam is described in units called electron volts (eV) (1 KeV = 1000 eV, 1 MeV = 1,000,000 eV).
For comparison, the energy of an x-ray beam used in diagnostic radiography is in the range of 100 KeV. Therapeutic radiation from a linear accelerator or a cobalt-60 unit is in the megavoltage (MeV) range and is at least 1000× more energetic than radiation emitted from a diagnostic x-ray machine. Therapeutic radiation is more likely to cause DNA damage resulting in cellular death.

These computerized treatment-planning systems use CT images of the patient in treatment position and calculate the radiation dose distribution in the tissue. They are essentially "radiation calculators" that allow the radiation oncologist to evaluate how the radiation will interact with the patient and to modify the beams to optimize the dose distribution (Figure 5.14).

- Although computerized treatment planning is not required for all tumors (dose calculations for simple beam arrangements can be done manually), it is especially useful for tumors in close proximity to critical normal structures, such as the eyes, CNS, heart, lungs, liver, GI tract, and kidneys.
- Accuracy of beam placement relative to the tumor is critical for effective therapy and is a function of patient positioning at the time of treatment. Patient positioning and beam placement is verified at the beginning of therapy and at regular intervals thereafter using portal images. These are radiographic images of the patient using the actual treatment beam. Visualization of the treatment field and surrounding anatomy allows assessment of the positioning of the beam (Figure 5.15 and 5.16).

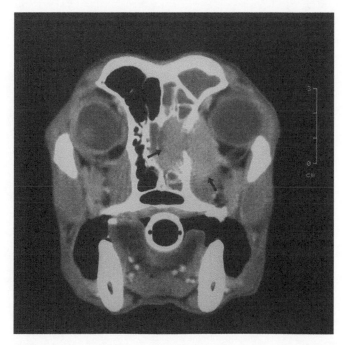

Figure 5.11. Contrast-enhanced CT image of a dog with nasosinal cancer. The tumor has eroded the frontal bone as well as the cribiform plate. There is tumor extension into the retro-orbital space and the calvarium. Advanced imaging is necessary to delineate the extent of the tumor in this patient and ensure optimized irradiation.

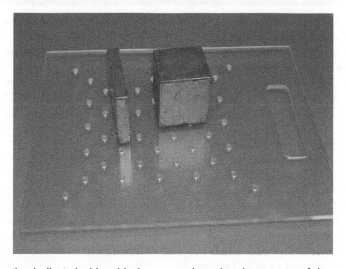

Figure 5.12. Metallic (lead alloy) shielding blocks are used to alter the intensity of the radiation treatment beam. They serve to block selected anatomical structures from the beam. Two shielding blocks are shown fastened to a tray that will be mounted on the linear accelerator.

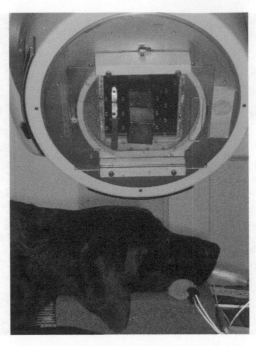

Figure 5.13. The shielding blocks are placed in the path of the radiation beam to spare selected tissues from exposure to radiation.

Multimodality Treatment

- Although radiotherapy can be used as the primary therapy for some tumors, it is more effectively used in combination with surgery and/or chemotherapy.
- Radiation is commonly combined with surgery when surgical excision alone is not adequate for eradication of microscopic or subclinical disease at the periphery of the tumor.
  - As discussed earlier, radiotherapy is most effective when there are fewer target cancer cells to kill. This is due to the fact that the presence of oxygen in cells maximizes radiation-induced DNA damage, as well as to the exponential kinetics of radiation-induced cell death. (See "The Biological Basis of Radiotherapy.")
  - It follows that for many tumors, it is advantageous to resect gross disease surgically and follow with postoperative radiation to target residual cancer cells.
  - Preoperative radiotherapy is considered when postoperative radiotherapy would not be feasible for reasons such as the position of the incision. This is often the case for feline injection-site sarcomas. Excision of these tumors results in a long incision that is difficult to irradiate effectively due to the close proximity of critical organs (CNS, lung, abdominal organs). In these cases, it is preferred to irradiate the tumor bed preoperatively (the radiation field is smaller) to sterilize the microscopic disease that is expected to remain after subsequent surgical excision. Preoperative radiation is also considered for tumors that are not initially resectable, where a decrease in tumor size is expected following radiation making surgical excision potentially feasible. This is referred to as *downstaging*.
- Chemotherapy is used in conjunction with radiotherapy to improve local control of chemosensitive tumors and for tumors that are likely to metastasize.
- Some chemotherapy drugs are considered to be radiation sensitizers. These drugs make the cancer cells more sensitive to the effects of radiation.
  - Platinum drugs (cisplatin, carboplatin)
  - Doxorubicin
  - Gemcitabine

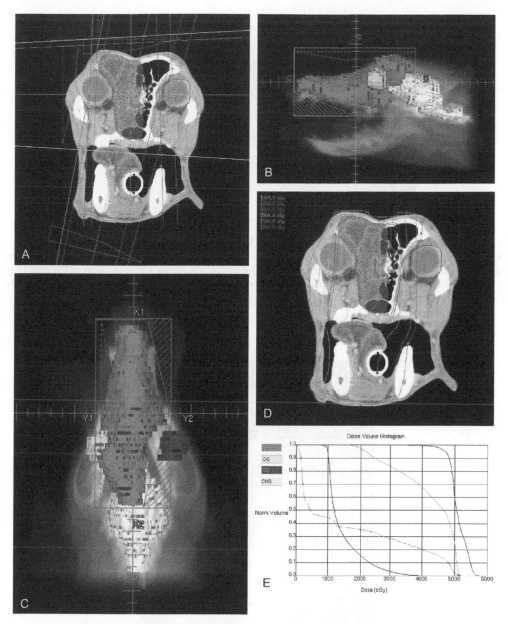

Figure 5.14. Computerized planning allows different treatment approaches to be virtually tested using a CT image of the patient to optimize radiation delivery. Image A shows a three-beam treatment plan using wedges. Wedges are metallic beam modifiers that are placed in the path of the beam to alter the spatial distribution of the radiation intensity. Radiation dose accumulates at the intersection of the beams in the tissue. The target tumor volume is highlighted in red. Critical normal structures are outlined. Images B and C show the beam's eye view for the lateral and dorsal beams, respectively. The hatched lines represent shielding blocks that are placed in the path of the beam to protect normal tissues. Image D shows the radiation dose distribution in the patient. Note that the tumor volume receives the target radiation dose of 4800 cGy (48 Gy) and that the right eye is spared from high dose-radiation to prevent blindness. Image E is a dose-volume histogram that shows the radiation dose delivered per percentage volume of critical normal tissues.

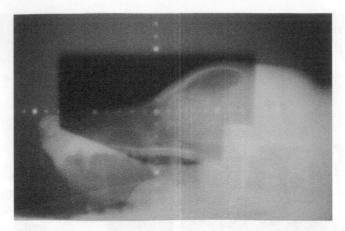

Figure 5.15. A portal film of the lateral beam in Figure 5.14. A double exposure is performed. The first exposure is of the actual treatment field with shielding blocks in place. During the second exposure, the collimator of the linear accelerator is fully opened to expose the normal anatomy. The portal film allows for verification of the placement of the beam and the shielding blocks relative to the patient's position on the treatment couch. Note the placement of the blocks over the CNS and the cranioventral maxilla, as shown in Figure 5.14B.

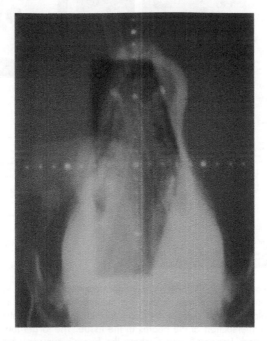

Figure 5.16. A portal film of the dorsal beam in Figure 5.14. Note the placement of the blocks on the right side of the beam to shield the right eye, a portion of the right side of the brain, and the right lip, as shown in Figure 5.14C.

- Consultation with a radiation oncologist or an oncology specialist is advisable at the time of tumor diagnosis for any case that may benefit from radiotherapy. These specialists can help formulate the best plan of action to optimize the use of radiation in conjunction with the other treatment modalities available.

Part 4: Chemotherapy

The Biological Basis of Chemotherapy

Key Points
- At the turn of the century cancer was regarded as a disease that began locally, and only at a very late stage spread to distant sites. Thus, initial attempts at disease control were confined to radical local excision or radiotherapy.
- Over time it became clear that many tumors metastasize early and patients may still die despite the primary tumor site remaining clear. It was therefore necessary to develop some form of systemic therapy.
- Many of the cancer chemotherapy drugs used today stem from seminal experiments conducted during the 1940s onward.
- **Alkylating agents** originated from research into chemical warfare and the **antimetabolite** class of drugs were born from research into nutrition and nucleic acid metabolism.

Why Do Cancer Chemotherapy Drugs Work?

- In many branches of pharmacology the aim is to treat a disease with a drug that is specific for the disease or the diseased tissue.
- In cancer patients, this specificity is, in part, provided by the rapidly dividing cells of the tumor as compared to the rest of the animal's normal tissues.
- This is because most chemotherapy or "cytotoxic" drugs act upon the process of **cell division.**
- To understand how these drugs work, and kill cancer cells, we must first consider the basic biology of cancer cells and how tumors grow.

The Cellular Targets for Chemotherapy Drugs

- Most chemotherapy or "cytotoxic" drugs act upon the process of **cell growth** and **division.**
- The cytotoxic drugs used in cancer chemotherapy can be broadly divided into the following six classes on the basis of their mode of action:
  - Alkylating agents
  - Antimetabolites
  - Antitumor antibiotics
  - Mitotic Spindle Inhibitors
  - Glucocorticoids
  - Miscellaneous agents
- Their cellular targets are depicted in Figure 5.17.

Cancer Cell Cycle Dynamics

- Like any other dividing cell, the cancer cell undergoes a cycle of activity (the cell cycle) which allows the genetic material to be doubled, and the cell to divide. The phases of the cell cycle are shown in Figure 5.18.
- Essentially, the cells in a tumor will either be dividing (in various stages of the cell cycle, from G_1 to M), or nondividing (G_0).
- Once a cell has acquired the necessary genotypic and phenotypic characteristics of a cancer cell, in general there is an exponential growth of a tumor, with very few cells in G_0.

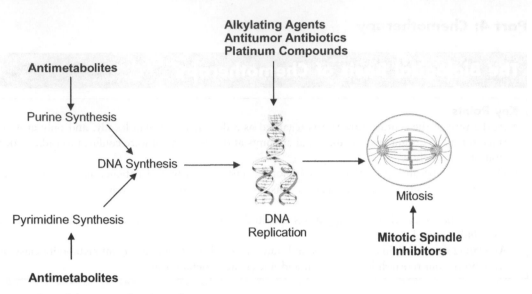

Figure 5.17. The cellular targets for chemotherapy.

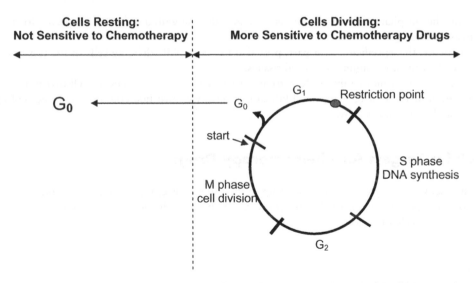

Figure 5.18. Cell division is a cyclical process whereby a cell "programmed" to divide will progress through several stages involving growth and DNA replication, ultimately leading to mitotic division. Cells, which are not dividing, are said to be in G_0 or the *resting phase* but can be recruited into the *cell cycle* in response to stimuli.

- However, this growth soon slows through many factors including the outgrowth of nutrient supply.
- These classical growth characteristics of tumors are referred to as *gompertzian growth* (Figure 5.19).

What Are the Consequences of These Growth Characteristics?

- Tumor growth kinetics is such that there is an initial rapid growth curve, which then flattens as the growth rate slows.
- The actual growth rate of a tumor is described in terms of **mass doubling time (MDT),** or the time taken for a tumor to double in size.

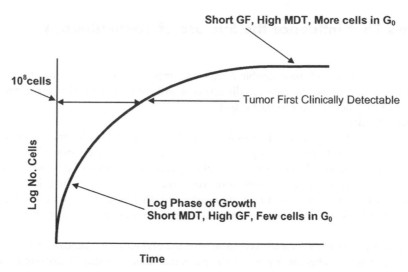

Figure 5.19. The gompertzian growth of tumors.

- As described earlier, tumor growth is considered to be gompertzian, which means that mass doubling times are much shorter during the early stages of tumor growth.
- It follows that MDT is a function of
  - The number of cells that are actively dividing, or the **growth fraction (GF)**
  - The cell cycle time
  - The number of cells being lost by cell death
- Tumors with a high growth fraction have a short MDT.
- Because most chemotherapeutic agents act upon the process of cell division, it follows that chemotherapy is likely to be more successful where tumors have a **high GF** and a **low MDT**.
- Cells in G_0 are relatively resistant to the action of cytotoxic drugs.
- Some cytotoxic drugs are termed **cell cycle specific**, in that they are active only on cells at a certain stage of cell division (e.g., vincristine during the M phase). Other drugs such as cyclophosphamide are not cell cycle specific and act on all dividing cells.
- Small tumors with a high growth fraction and short MDT will be more susceptible to the action of cytotoxic drugs.
- Many tumors are not clinically detected (palpation/imaging) until they are in the slower phases of growth (10^8–10^9 cells). Consequently, chemotherapy is less effective in large bulky disease.
- Initially, metastatic lesions have a higher GF and shorter MDT than the primary tumor from which they arose, and they are potentially more susceptible to chemotherapy drugs.

The Effects of Cytoreductive Surgery

- Consider the gompertzian growth curve for a tumor.
- A tumor is excised (cytoreductive surgery) when the tumor is in the plateau phase of growth.
- There is microscopic disease in the tissue bed.
- The cells left behind move into a phase of cell division and adopt a higher GF and shorter MDT than the removed mass. This is known as **recruitment**.
- This is when the cells are most sensitive to the effects of chemotherapy drugs.
- Consequently, adjunctive chemotherapy is given a short time after surgery, a balance between allowing enough time for healing, but hitting as many dividing cancer cells as possible.

Other Factors That Influence the Success of Chemotherapy

- Tumor Cell Type
  - While the growth fraction and mass doubling time are important in determining the success of chemotherapy, even some tumor types that are rapidly growing will not respond well to cytotoxic drugs by virtue of their inherent resistance to antineoplastic agents.
- Tumor Cell Heterogeneity
  - In addition to changes in growth rate, a naturally occurring tumor will evolve and accumulate other mutations, which can alter their biological properties (e.g., their ability to expel cytotoxic drugs or their ability to metastasize). Consequently, despite similar morphology, the population of cells within a tumor are considered heterogeneous with respect to many properties, including drug handling. If there is a small subpopulation of cells within a population that are resistant to a particular cytotoxic drug, continued use of that drug can lead to selection for the resistant cells, eventually leading to treatment failure.
- Drug Resistance
  - Drug resistance is the ability of a tumor cell to survive the actions of an anticancer agent.
  - Drug resistance can be an **inherent** feature of the particular tumor or can be **acquired resistance**, arising through genetic mutations within the tumor.
  - There are several mechanisms that may confer resistance to anticancer agents. Drugs that share similar chemistry often share resistance mechanisms, and this allows us to choose sensible rescue drugs.
  - Relapsing tumors can acquire resistance to drugs that have not been used to treat the tumor initially (**multidrug resistance, MDR**). In practice, drug resistance is the most common form of treatment failure.:
    - Avoid any treatment prior to induction.
    - Treat early and aggressively to achieve good first remission.
    - Avoid rescue drugs with a similar mode of action.

Summary: The Biological Basis for Chemotherapy

The major factors, in terms of tumor growth, that determine the success or failure of chemotherapy are
- Tumor growth fraction
- Mass doubling time
- Tumor cell type
- Tumor cell heterogeneity
- The development of drug resistance

The Practicalities of Cytotoxic Drug Administration

Key Points
- The theoretical basis of cytotoxic drug administration and scheduling has been determined through clinical research and extrapolation from human clinical trials.
- Despite this, it is still the art of administering highly toxic compounds, at doses being calculated by means of enlightened empiricism.
- Work carried out in the 1960s on a rat model of leukemia established one of the most important basic principles of anticancer chemotherapy.
- It was found that cytotoxic drugs kill tumor cells according to first-order kinetics, i.e., a given dose of a cytotoxic agent kills a fixed percentage of the total mass of cells in a tumor rather than a fixed number of cells; this is known as the **tumor cell kill hypothesis**.
- This is a theoretical model only and assumes that the tumor is homogeneous in terms of chemosensitivity, and drug distribution is even.
- However, this hypothesis has aided in the development of the following guidelines for cytotoxic drug administration:

- In all cases the maximum tolerated dose should be used and as often as possible.
- Because a cytotoxic drug kills tumor cells according to first-order kinetics, a single dose of an agent is unlikely to eradicate an entire tumor population.
- Chemotherapy is likely to be most effective when the tumor burden is at its lowest and is unlikely to be effective in extensive or advanced disease.

Applying These Principles to the Clinical Case

How do we dose patients?

- Because of the high likelihood of toxic effects in cases of overdose and the serious risk of tumor recurrence if the patient is underdosed, it is important that dosing of chemotherapeutic drugs be as accurate as possible.
- When dosing toxic drugs on the basis of weight there is a tendency to overdose large animals and underdose small ones.
- For this reason, it has become common practice for veterinary oncologists to dose many chemotherapeutic drugs according to the calculated body surface area (BSA) of the patient rather than the body weight.
- BSA is used in preference to weight because, for a variety of species, the maximum tolerable dose of a variety of toxic drugs has been shown to correlate much better with BSA than with weight.
- Overall, use of this system has certainly helped to decrease drug toxicity in large-breed dogs receiving chemotherapy. However, through extensive experience it has recently become clear that BSA-based dosing *increases toxicosis in small dogs.* The practical consequence of all this is that many veterinary oncologists now dose their small-breed canine patients on a mg/kg body weight basis, especially with the more toxic drugs like doxorubicin. Alternatively, they use a lower mg/m^2 dose rate for small dogs than for large dogs. For example, a dose of 30 mg/m^2 for dogs $\geq$15 kg, 25 mg/m^2 for dogs $\leq$15 kg, and 1 mg/kg for toy breed dogs has been suggested for doxorubicin.
- For animals of 15 kg body weight and less, we recommend that veterinarians calculate the dose both ways and err on the side of caution, i.e., tend to dose on the low side for the first treatment until tolerance is established.
- Because cats have their own separate BSA-based dose rates for chemotherapeutic drugs (often lower than those for dogs), and because cats tend to vary in weight much less than do dogs; there is no clear evidence that small cats are experiencing increased toxicosis when dosed according to the same formulae as large cats.
- Notwithstanding these problems and complications with BSA-based dosing, it remains an effective system for avoiding overdose of heavier animals. Table 5.10 (at the end of the drugs section) provides a convenient conversion table from body weight to BSA for use in dogs. Table 5.11 provides the same information for cats.

Body weight is used to calculate the surface area by the following formula:

$$\text{Surface area}(m^2) = \frac{k \times \text{body wt}(kg)^{0.66}}{10^4}$$

$$k = 101.1 \text{ for dogs}, \quad k = 10 \text{ for cats}$$

Timing and intervals between doses of drugs

- The dose of drugs to be administered is limited by the toxicity to normal tissues, the most common form of toxicity being myelosuppression and gastrointestinal toxicity.
- These tissues have enormous capacity for repair compared to the tumor and therefore a drug schedule is developed that allows the drug to be administered at intervals rather than continuous treatment.
- The intervals are carefully timed such that the normal tissue has time to repair without expansion of the residual tumor population.

The ideal situation is demonstrated in Figure 5.20. The dosing schedule is such that normal tissue has time to recover, but the tumor does not recover completely.

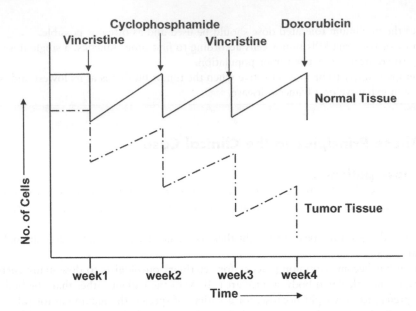

Figure 5.20. The ideal dosing schedule allows for tumor reduction over time, but recovery of normal tissue.

Combination versus single-agent chemotherapy
- In the previous section we described how tumor cell heterogeneity may contribute to chemotherapy failure. Exposure of a tumor cell population to just one drug may allow for the selection of a resistant population of cells.
- For this reason, where chemotherapy is being used as the sole treatment modality, a combination of drugs is used to treat a tumor rather than a single agent.
- Drug combinations are used that
  - Affect various stages of cell division
  - Have different modes of action
  - Have no overlapping toxicity
  - Do not interfere with each other's actions

When should we consider using chemotherapy?
The four main scenarios for using chemotherapy in small animal practice are
- A single modality to cure a cancerous condition:
  - This is a rare indication in veterinary medicine.
  - Quality of life is more important than quantity and very often we are not trying to cure the cancer but give the patient a good quality of life for a reasonable amount of time.
  - Because quality of life is a balance between toxicity and efficacy, a cure is rarely attained.
- As a single modality to attain long-term remission:
  - Most frequently used for the treatment of
    - Lymphoma
    - Leukemia
    - Myeloma
    - Multifocal histiocytic disease
- As a single modality for disease palliation:
  - This is sometimes applied when long-term remission is unattainable but short-term, good quality of life is required, e.g., the use of corticosteroids as a single agent in lymphoma.
- As part of multimodality therapy for cancer:
  - This could be in the adjuvant setting (following a primary modality, such as surgery) or neoadjuvant (just prior to primary therapy).

- Examples include
  - The use of an adjuvant platinum drug to treat osteosarcoma in dogs following amputation
  - The neoadjuvant use of chemotherapy to downstage (shrink) a thymoma prior to surgery

In general:

- The usefulness of chemotherapy is often limited to very few tumor types, which is also true in human medicine.
- Doses are usually a compromise between efficacy and toxicity, and the potential toxic side effects of the drugs must be fully explained.
- The owner must be counseled thoroughly and must be committed to the treatment.

The flow chart in Figure 5.21 illustrates the stages and types of treatment a tumor-bearing patient might undergo (e.g., a dog with multicentric lymphoma).

Chemotherapy Drugs (Figure 5.22)

- Details of dosages and indications for the chemotherapy drugs can be found in the section "Tables of Specific Drug Classes," later in this chapter.
- Chemotherapeutic drugs may be divided into a number of categories, each of which work by different mechanisms and at different stages in the cell growth cycle:
  - **Alkylating agents:** substitute an alkyl group for an H+ ion in DNA causing cross-linking and breaking of DNA molecules; thus, DNA strands are unable to separate during DNA replication and RNA transcription. Examples are cyclophosphamide, CCNU, ifosfamide, chlorambucil, dacarbazine, and melphalan. Cisplatin also behaves in many respects like an alkylating agent.
  - **Mitotic spindle inhibitors:** bind to cytoplasmic microtubular proteins and arrest mitosis in metaphase. Examples are the vinca alkaloids, including vincristine, vinblastine, and vinorelbine, as well as the taxanes, including paclitaxel and docetaxel.
  - **Antimetabolites:** mimic normal substrates needed for nucleic acid synthesis. They inhibit cellular enzymes or lead to the production of nonfunctional molecules so that DNA synthesis is prevented. Examples are methotrexate, cytarabine (*syn.* cytosine arabinoside), 5-flurouracil, and gemcitabine.
  - **Antitumor antibiotics:** use a variety of mechanisms to prevent DNA and RNA synthesis, including breaking of DNA strands, cross-linking of base pairs, free radical production, and inhibition of topoisomerase II. Examples are doxorubicin, mitozantrone, and dactinomycin.
  - **Glucocorticoids:** are cytolytic for lymphoid tissues and are therefore useful in the treatment of some lymphoid malignancies. Their mechanism of antitumor action is unclear.
  - **Miscellaneous:** Other agents with a variety of mechanisms of action are used in chemotherapy. These include the platinum compounds (cisplatin, carboplatin, and L-asparaginase).

Alkylating Agents

- **Cyclophosphamide** (Cytoxan™, Bristol-Myers Squibb)
  - This alkylating agent can be **given orally or intravenously.**
  - This is a pro-drug requiring hepatic activation.
  - The drug undergoes activation to alkylating metabolites by the mixed function microsomal oxidase systems in the liver.
  - Cyclophosphamide is useful in a wide range of companion animal neoplasms.
  - Toxic effects seen in some animals are gastrointestinal signs (anorexia, nausea, vomiting) and myelosuppression.
  - The sterile hemorrhagic cystitis that sometimes occurs in dogs and people is less of a problem in cats.
  - Sterile hemorrhagic cystitis is a consequence of formation of a toxic metabolite called *acrolein* that is excreted in the urine and is irritating to the bladder wall.
  - In dogs, the incidence of sterile hemorrhagic cystitis is dramatically reduced when furosemide is used at a dose of 1–2 mg/kg IV 30 minutes prior to IV injection of cyclophosphamide. The use of prednisolone in many chemotherapeutic protocols may similarly reduce the risk of cystitis.

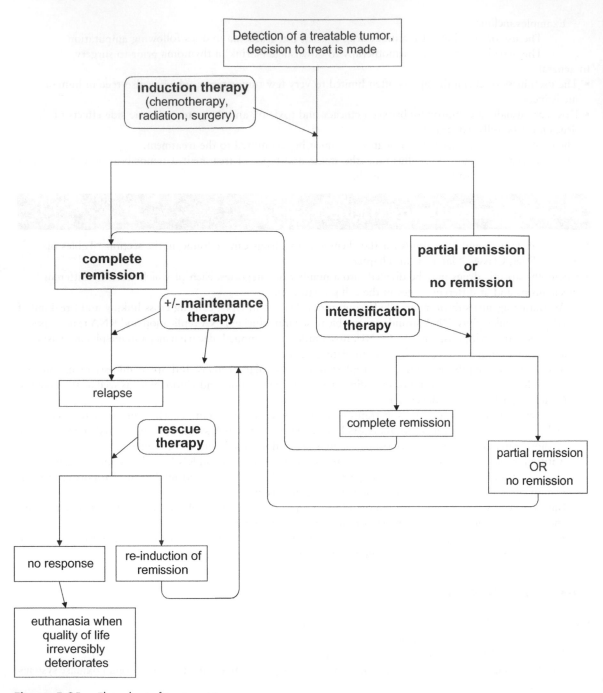

Figure 5.21. Flow chart of treatment types.

- CCNU (Lomustine™, Bristol-Myers Squibb)
  - It is given orally.
  - Activity against lymphoma, including cutaneous lymphoma, mast cell tumors, histiocytic disease, and brain tumors.
  - It crosses the blood-brain barrier.

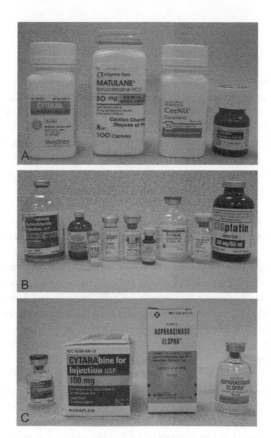

Figure 5.22. Chemotherapy drugs for oral (A), intravenous (B), and subcutaneous (C) use.

- Common toxicities include myelosuppression and gastrointestinal effects such as vomiting, diarrhea, and anorexia.
- Myelosuppression can be prolonged (4–6 weeks) in cats.
- Myleosuppression can result in cumulative thrombocytopenia.
- Hepatotoxicity can develop in a cumulative and dose-related manner. It is characterized by a marked elevation of liver enzyme activity and nonspecific histologic findings. It can be subclinical and can result in liver failure if treatment is not discontinued. Liver enzyme activity should be monitored in dogs that receive CCNU.
- Renal toxicity can occur but is rare.
- **Chlorambucil** (Leukeran™, GlaxoSmithKline)
  - It is given orally.
  - It has been used to replace cyclophosphamide in patients that develop, or are considered at high risk to develop, sterile hemorrhagic cystitis.
  - It is used for treatment of small-cell, epitheliotropic lymphoma in cats.
- **Melphalan** (Alkeran™, GlaxoSmithKline)
  - It is given orally.
  - It is used with prednisolone to treat plasma cell neoplasms, including multiple myeloma.
- **Busulphan** (Myleran™, GlaxoSmithKline)
  - It is given orally.
  - It is used to treat chronic myelogenous leukemia (CML) and polycythemia rubra vera.

Antimetabolites

- Methotrexate
  - Methotrexate is an antimetabolite and an analogue of folic acid.
  - It enters the cells via an active transport system for reduced folates and, due to relatively irreversible binding, exerts its cytotoxic effect by competitively inhibiting the enzyme dihydrofolate reductase, which catalyzes the conversion of folic acid to tetrahydrofolate.
  - This interferes with the synthesis of thymidylic acid and purines which in turn inhibits DNA synthesis and cell reproduction and, to a lesser extent, protein and RNA synthesis.
  - The affinity of dihydrofolate reductase for methotrexate is far greater than its affinity for folic or dihydrofolic acid and, therefore, even very large amounts of folic acid given simultaneously will not reverse the effects of methotrexate.
  - Methotrexate seems also to cause an increase in intracellular deoxyadenosine triphosphate, which is thought to inhibit ribonucleotide reduction and polynucleotide ligase, an enzyme concerned in DNA synthesis and repair.
  - It is rarely used as part of the treatment of lymphoma and leukemia in some protocols.
  - Myelosuppression and intestinal epithelial damage are the major toxic effects.
- Cytarabine (also called *cytosine arabinoside*, Cytosar-U™ Pharmacia and Upjohn Co.)
  - This synthetic antimetabolite is converted intracellularly to form the metabolite cytarabine triphosphate. It is a pyrimidine analog that inhibits DNA synthesis.
  - The precise mechanism of action is unknown, but cytarabine triphosphate is thought to competitively inhibit DNA polymerase, which results in inhibition of DNA synthesis.
  - Cytarabine has no effect on nonproliferating cells nor on proliferating cells unless in the DNA synthesis (S) phase, and thus is a classic example of a cell cycle phase–specific antineoplastic agent.
  - The drug may be given subcutaneously, intravenously (often as a slow infusion over several hours to days), and even intrathecally.
  - It is part of some protocols used in the treatment of lymphoma and some leukemias.
  - It crosses the blood-brain barrier, and therefore is used as part of protocols to treat lymphoma in the brain.
- 5-fluorouracil
  - **THIS ANTINEOPLASTIC DRUG IS CONTRAINDICATED FOR USE IN CATS (see below).** It causes a fatal neurotoxicity in this species.
  - It can be administered intralesionally, intracavitarily, and topically as well as intravenously.
  - As an aside, companion animals are sometimes fatally poisoned by ingesting tubes of 5-FU–containing ointment intended for treatment of human skin diseases.
  - Fluorouracil is an analogue of uracil, a component of ribonucleic acid. The drug is believed to function as an antimetabolite.
  - After intracellular conversion to the active deoxynucleotide, it interferes with the synthesis of DNA by blocking the conversion of deoxyuridylic acid to thymidylic acid by the cellular enzyme thymidylate synthetase. Fluorouracil may also interfere with RNA synthesis.
  - In addition to myelosuppression and gastrointestinal effects, it can be neurotoxic in dogs. 5-FU neurotoxicity is fatal in cats.

Mitotic Spindle Inhibitors

- Vincristine (Oncovin™, Eli Lily)
  - This mitotic spindle inhibitor is an alkaloid derived from the periwinkle plant (*Vinca rosea* L.).
  - It must be given intravenously, and causes irritation if it is inadvertently administered perivascularly (see the later section "Managing Complications of Chemotherapy").
  - Vincristine is only modestly myelosuppressive.
  - Gastrointestinal toxicity is common.

- A rare complication of its use is peripheral neuropathy, manifesting as pelvic limb weakness or as constipation when the pelvic limbs and gastrointestinal tract are affected, respectively.
  - Vincristine is relatively inexpensive.
  - The recommended formulation is a 1 mg/ml aqueous solution that has a good shelf life.
- **Vinblastine (Velban™, Eli Lily)**
  - This is a close relative of vincristine.
  - It is more myelosuppressive than vincristine, but may be more effective in treatment of some tumors, including mast cell tumors.
  - Similarly to vincristine, it is an irritant if inadvertently extravasated during IV injection.
- **Vinorelbine (Navelbine™, GlaxoSmithKline)**
  - Like the other drugs in its class, this semisynthetic vinca alkaloid inhibits mitosis at metaphase by interfering with microtubule assembly.
  - In dogs, it has clinical activity against primary pulmonary carcinoma.
  - Myelosuppression causing neutropenia is the dose-limiting toxicity.
  - It is an irritant if inadvertently extravasated during IV injection.
- **Taxanes**
  - The taxanes are relatively new anticancer cytotoxics that stabilize cellular microtubules preventing cellular division.
  - The two taxanes in clinical use in people are paclitaxel (Taxol™, Bristol-Myers Squibb) and docetaxel (Taxotere™, Aventis).
  - Both drugs bind to the beta-subunit of tubulin, resulting in the formation of stable, nonfunctional microtubule bundles and thus interfering with mitosis.
  - Paclitaxel acts at the G2/M-phase junction, whereas docetaxel is primarily active in the S-phase of the cell growth cycle.
  - The taxanes can also induce apoptosis and have antiangiogenic (i.e., antimetastatic) properties.
  - These agents are widely accepted to be effective components of therapy for advanced breast, lung, and ovarian carcinomas in people.
  - Paclitaxel is being used in dogs and cats.
  - Administration to dogs and cats is involved, because the Cremophor carrier is so prone to induce mast cell degranulation and consequent anaphylaxis.
  - Patients must be pretreated with steroids, and then given cimetidine, diphenhydramine, and dexamethasone on the day of infusion.
  - Even with these precautions, anaphylaxis is possible and the infusion may have to be slowed or stopped.
  - Seek advice if you are considering use of paclitaxel in one of your patients.
  - A new veterinary formulation is being developed and may be available after this book goes to press.

Antitumor Antibiotics

- **Doxorubicin HCl (Adriamycin™, Pharmacia and Upjohn Co.; also hydroxydaunorubicin)**
  - This anthracycline antibiotic is a potent, expensive drug with many uses.
  - Over the last decade it has become the cornerstone of most effective veterinary chemotherapeutic protocols.
  - It is red in color.
  - Common toxicities include myelosuppression and gastrointestinal toxicities in dogs. Myelosuppression can be severe. Rarely, hemorrhagic colitis can develop.
  - Doxorubicin can be nephrotoxic in cats. It should be used with caution in cats with renal insufficiency.
  - Doxorubicin must be given intravenously. It is a vesicant, which means that perivascular injection is calamitous, often resulting in a severe tissue necrosis that does not heal.
  - The drug is delivered as a 5 to 20 minute IV infusion through a "one-stick" peripheral venous catheter in a controlled setting.
  - In case of extravasation, dexrazoxane (Zinecard™), a free radical scavenger, may be administered IV within hours at a dose of 10:1 to the dose of doxorubicin.

- If doxorubicin is given by rapid infusion, it can cause acute cardiac toxicity with dysrhythmias.
- Doxorubicin can cause a rare hypersensitivity-like reaction caused by degranulation of mast cells. Patients can exhibit head-shaking, pinnae and lip swelling, hives, and vomiting. Intravenous dexamethasone is used if these signs develop during infusion of doxorubicin.
- In dogs and man, dilated cardiomyopathy is a potential, cumulative, dose-dependent toxic effect of doxorubicin. The mechanism involves damage to cardiomyocytes by doxorubicin-induced free radicals.
- To reduce the risk of development of cardiomyopathy in dogs, it is suggested that a total lifetime cumulative dose of 180 mg/m^2 is not exceeded.
- Dogs with decreased cardiac contractility should not receive doxorubicin.
- Dexrazoxane (Zinecard™), a free radical scavenger, is used in people as a cardioprotectant in patients at risk of dilated cardiomyopathy. Its efficacy in dogs for this purpose has not been investigated.
- Cardiomyopathy has not been reported as a clinical complication of therapy in the cat, but cardiac lesions similar to those found in other species have been found in cats after treatment.
- Mitozantrone HCl (Novantrone™, Immunex Corporation)
  - Mitozantrone (or mitoxantrone) is an expensive anthracycline derivative similar to doxorubicin, but is considered less cardiotoxic.
  - It is blue in color.
  - It can be used instead of doxorubicin in dogs with decreased cardiac contractility, in dogs that have reached the maximum recommended dose of doxorubicin, or in cats with renal dysfunction.
- Glucocorticoids
- Prednisolone
  - Not often thought of as a chemotherapeutic agent, prednisolone is, nevertheless, cytotoxic for lymphoid tissues and therefore useful in the treatment of lymphoma and some leukemias.
  - Prednisolone is not myelosuppressive and its side effects are familiar and mostly benign (polydipsia, polyuria, and polyphagia).
  - The doses used in chemotherapy are often immunosuppressive, but most of these patients are, in any case, immunocompromised by their disease. Treatment does not usually make matters worse.
  - Prednisolone penetrates the central nervous system and enters cerebrospinal fluid. Unfortunately, most tumors rapidly become resistant to glucocorticoids.

Miscellaneous Cancer Chemotherapeutics

- Cisplatin
  - **CISPLATIN IS ABSOLUTELY CONTRAINDICATED FOR USE IN CATS** because of often-fatal acute pulmonary toxicity.
  - Cisplatin is a potent antineoplastic agent with biochemical properties similar to those of alkylating agents.
  - The drug inhibits DNA synthesis by producing intrastrand and interstrand cross-links in DNA.
  - Protein and RNA synthesis are also inhibited to a lesser extent.
  - Cisplatin does not appear to be cell cycle specific.
  - This drug has been used to treat a wide range of canine tumors, including osteosarcoma, a variety of carcinomas, and mesothelioma.
  - In dogs, it is most commonly delivered as an intravenous infusion. On occasion, it is mixed with a medical-grade sesame oil or collagen matrix for injection directly into tumors. It can also be administered into body cavities.
  - Nephrotoxicity is a potential problem in treated dogs. There is a therefore a relative contraindication for use of cisplatin in tumor-bearing dogs with concurrent, preexisting renal insufficiency or failure.
  - A standardized 6-hour saline diuresis is administered along with the drug to minimize the risk of nephrotoxicity,
  - Due to the large volume of IV fluids used for diuresis, advanced heart disease where there is a risk of congestive heart failure is also a relative contraindication to treatment with cisplatin.
  - Cisplatin causes nausea and vomiting at administration. This is prevented with pretreatment use of potent antiemetics.

- Saline diuresis is administered along with the drug, so advanced heart failure is also a relative contraindication.
- Avoid use of aluminum needles with this drug, as aluminum can react with cisplatin leading to drug inactivation and precipitate formation.
- The use of cisplatin has largely been superceded with carboplatin. Carboplatin has similar efficacy, fewer toxicities, and is less labor-intensive to administer and handle.
- Carboplatin
  - This is a second-generation platinum drug.
  - It is less toxic than cisplatin, without loss of antitumor efficacy.
  - It can be used in cats and is appropriate for dogs that have mild to moderate preexisting renal insufficiency or cannot withstand the relatively intense diuresis required to administer cisplatin.
  - Carboplatin has been used for a wide range of canine and feline tumors, such as osteosarcoma, melanoma, various other sarcomas, and carcinomas, both as a sole agent and as part of adjuvant or combination therapy.
  - It is given intravenously over about 15 minutes or, like cisplatin, it is sometimes injected directly into tumors or body cavities.
  - Both cisplatin and carboplatin can react with aluminum, so it is recommended that aluminum needles are not used for reconstitution or administration of these drugs.
  - Common toxicities include myelosuppression and gastrointestinal effects.
  - The neutrophil nadir associated with carboplatin use in cats can occur twice in one cycle: at 7–10 days, and then a second nadir at 21 days. For this reason, Carboplatin protocols in cats often have a four week interval.
- Hydroxyurea
  - This works by inhibiting the enzyme ribonucleoside diphosphate reductase. It is given orally and has been used successfully to treat refractory chronic myelogenous leukemia and is useful as a first-line drug for polycythemia rubra vera.
- L-Asparaginase (Elspar™, Merck & Co.)
  - This enzyme derived from bacteria, *E. coli*, breaks down extracellular asparagine, an amino acid, to L-aspartic acid and ammonia.
  - Lymphoma cells cannot synthesize asparagine and require the extracellular supply for protein synthesis. They die when it is absent.
  - Normal cells synthesize their own asparagine and are unaffected by the extracellular depletion of this amino acid by L-asparaginase.
  - Subcutaneous injection is the preferred and most convenient route of administration.
  - Some administer this drug intramuscularly.
  - L-asparaginase is a foreign protein, and may provoke an anaphylactic reaction after repeated injections.
  - The clinician should be ready to deal with this complication, should it occur. For prevention, the patient may be pretreated with an antihistamine 15–30 minutes prior to administration of L-asparaginase. Dogs should be monitored for at least 15 minutes after the treatment.
  - Tumors may become rapidly resistant to L-asparaginase. The drug is expensive, and some formulations are thought to have a very short shelf life once reconstituted.
  - L-asparaginase is available only in aliquots of 10,000 units. The shelf life of an opened, reconstituted vial is about 8 hours.

Chemotherapeutic Agents Specifically *Contraindicated* in Cats

- Cats have gained a reputation for being metabolically incompetent. Perhaps this is because they have difficulty with hepatic glucuronidation of phenolic compounds.
- The clinician should recognize that cats *are* different from dogs and some drugs affect them adversely. Below are two antineoplastic drugs useful in dogs and humans, which are absolutely contraindicated in cats.
- **5-Fluorouracil**

- This antimetabolite causes severe neurotoxicity in the cat, characterized by acute blindness, ataxia, and hyperexcitability followed by opisthotonus, convulsions, dyspnea, and death.
- Cisplatin
  - This agent, which has a similar mechanism of action to the alkylating agents, is very useful for a wide range of tumors in dogs and man. Unfortunately, even low doses cause pulmonary edema in the cat as a result of damage to the pulmonary microvasculature. It should not be used in this species. Fortunately, carboplatin can be used to treat feline tumors instead.

Figure 5.23 outlines a decision tree for cytotoxic drugs.

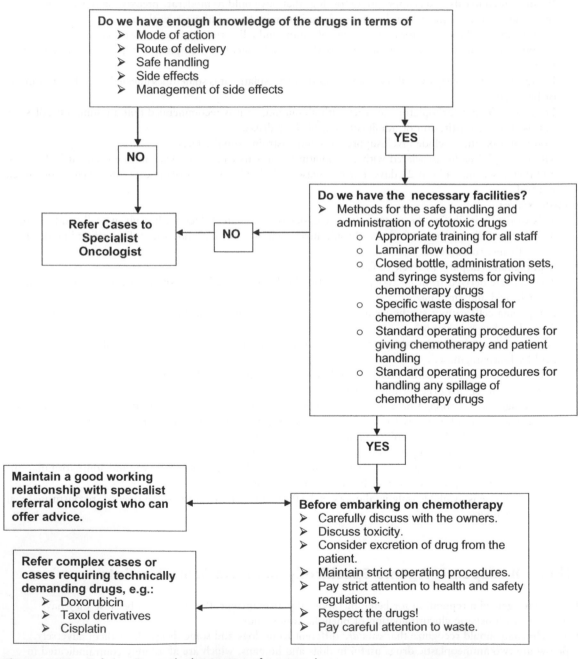

Figure 5.23. Safe handling and administration of cytotoxic drugs.

Advice to Clients Prior to Starting Chemotherapy

In addition to a detailed discussion with the clients regarding the goals and expectations of treatment with cancer chemotherapeutics, it is also essential that clients are made absolutely aware of the nature and danger of cytotoxic drugs:

- Drug may be metabolized and excreted in their active form in saliva, urine, and feces.
- Dogs and cats on current corticosteroid therapy may produce more urine or have urine "accidents" in the house.
- Particular care should be taken in explaining these issues if the client has young children in the house, or they themselves have a clinical condition that makes them immunosuppressed.
- Many specialist oncology referral centers provide detailed written information prior to beginning therapy or as part of the consent form. It is advisable for general practices to consult with local cancer specialists to obtain any client information sheets that may be available.

Handling Cytotoxic Drugs

Key Points

These are only guidelines. The practitioner should always, in addition, follow the safety regulations laid down by the individual country.

- Many cytotoxic drugs have been shown themselves to be carcinogenic, mutagenic, or teratogenic.
- They can also be extremely irritant, producing harmful effects if they come into contact with the skin or the eyes. They should therefore be used with extreme care and respect.
- The toxic effects of therapeutic doses of chemotherapeutics are well known, but the effects of long-term occupational exposure are not clearly established. Personnel exposure should therefore be minimized through safety awareness and safe handling techniques.
- The major risks are as follows:
  - Absorption via the skin or mucous membranes
  - Aerosol formation when removing liquid chemotherapy
  - Inhalation of aerosols or dust
  - Self-inoculation when administering injectable agents
- The author recommends the use of a vertical laminar airflow hood for all drug handling (Figure 5.24).
- However, the access to these facilities is often limited to the major veterinary hospitals and so the following are guidelines for the safe handling of tablets and injectable agents in veterinary practice.

Handling and administration of tablets or capsules

- Pill-counting equipment designated for chemotherapy use only should be used.
- Tablets or capsules should never be divided, broken, or crushed.
- Disposable gloves should always be worn when handling or administering the drug.
- If tablets are provided in "blister packs," they should be dispensed in this form.
- Staff and owners should receive clear instruction on administration.
- Staff and owners should wash hands after administering drugs.
- Excess or unwanted drugs should be incinerated in a chemical incinerator.

Handling and administration of injectable agents

- All injectable drugs should be prepared in a vertical flow laminar hood (Figure 5.25).
- Closed bottle systems (e.g., PhaSeal by Carmel Pharma, Inc.) are available and should be used where possible. This includes a system of bottles, drip sets, and injection ports that offer a completely closed system (Figure 5.26).

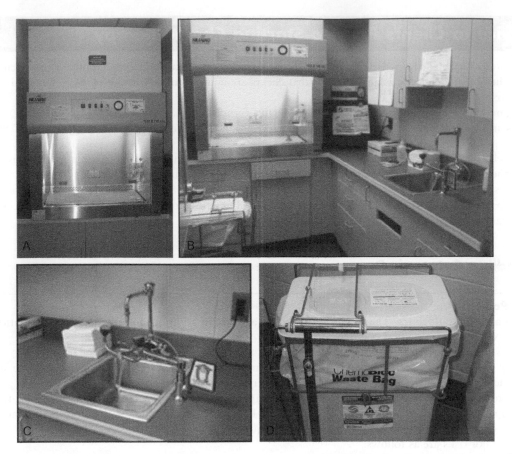

Figure 5.24. Laminar flow hood for chemotherapy drug preparation (A). Typical well-ordered room for chemotherapy preparation (B), containing a sink specifically designated for chemotherapy (C) and specialist waste disposal (D).

- Note that surgical or filter masks are not protective against inhalation of aerosols or dust.
- Most injectable cytotoxic drugs are administered via the intravenous route and an intravenous catheter should always be used for this purpose (Figure 5.27).
- Locking syringe fittings are preferable to push connections.
- Plastic-backed absorbable pads should be used on work surfaces during chemotherapy handling and administration.
- Patients should be adequately restrained, and some may need to be sedated.
- Protective clothing, including a nonabsorbent diposable gown, protective eye wear, powder-free latex gloves, and mask, should be worn at all times. Gloves should be thick, or doubled up if using standard examination/surgical gloves (see Figure 5.27).
- Low-transit areas with minimal draft should be used for drug handling and administration.
- No food, drink, chewing gum, or application of cosmetics should be allowed in the chemotherapy area.
- Pregnant woman should avoid the chemotherapy area.

Waste disposal
- Sharps should be placed in an impenetrable container, specific for chemotherapy, and then sent for incineration when full.
- Solid waste should be placed in polyethylene bags and incinerated.
- Practices must comply with National Health and Safety regulations. Chemotherapy waste needs to be treated differently from general hospital waste. The company employed to remove waste from practices should be made aware of specific chemotherapy waste bins.

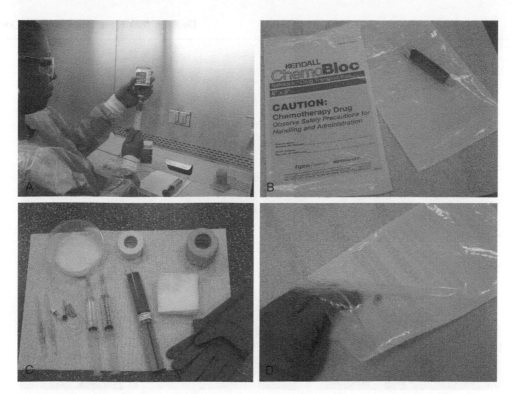

Figure 5.25. Chemotherapy drugs are prepared in a laminar flow hood and wearing appropriate protective clothing (A). Drugs can then be labeled (patient, drug, dosage, and dose) and placed in a ziplock bag for later use (B). All required materials for administration are laid out in advance (C). When the cap of the chemotherapy syringe is removed for application of a needle or connector, this is done within the ziplock bag (D).

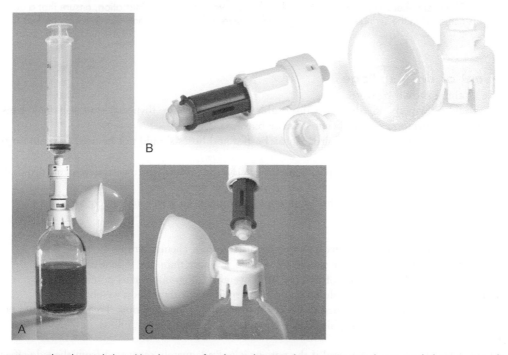

Figure 5.26. The PhaSeal closed bottle system for chemotherapy drug preparation by Carmel Pharma, Inc. The system allows for a closed preparation and administration of drug (A). The sealed airtight chamber captures aerosols and vapors while maintaining equal pressure in the vial during drug preparation (B). The injector provides a sealed transfer and "locks" into safe mode when procedures are complete to prevent exposure and contact. It also allows the operator to retrieve all of the drug from the vial (C). Images courtesy of Carmel Pharma, Inc.

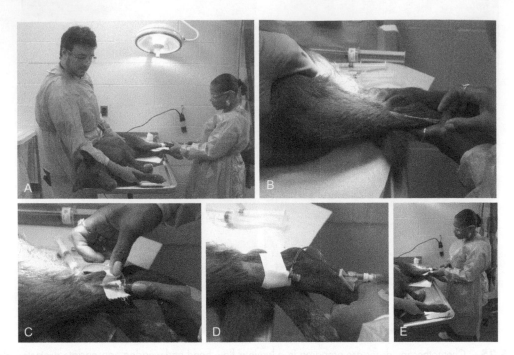

Figure 5.27. Safe administration of intravenous chemotherapy. The patient is adequately restrained by a second operator (A), and both operators are clothed in protective gowns, face masks, and latex gloves. Intravenous catheter placement is performed under sterile conditions and only a "first stick" placement is used (B). The catheter is securely taped and the line flushed with saline (C). Avoid heparin with drugs such as doxorubicin as it may cause some precipitation of the drug. The chemotherapy syringe is attached to the catheter. Prior to administration, ensure that a good drawback of blood is achieved in the syringe (D). The drug is administered slowly, and blood drawback is checked at intervals (E).

In the event of drug spillage

- Protective clothing should be worn.
- The spill should be wiped with absorbent disposable towels, which are then sealed in polythene bags and disposed of in the chemotherapy designated waste bins.
- To avoid aerosolization of the spilled drug, spray bottles and hoses should not be used to clean up the spill.
- Spill kits containing the necessary supplies (protective clothing, absorbent towels, detergent, disposal bags, etc.) are commercially available for ease of use should a spill occur.
- Contaminated surfaces should be washed with copious amounts of water and detergent.

Patient safety

- The patient's identity should be verified before administration of chemotherapy.
- Calculation of the chemotherapy dose should be verified by more than one individual to avoid mathematical errors or incorrect use of units of body weight (kilograms versus pounds)
- Chemotherapy dose calculations should be based on current (same day) body weight
- Adequate cell counts must be confirmed prior to chemotherapy administration. Treatment should be delayed if treatment-induced neutrophil or platelet counts are lower than 1,500/uL or 75,000/uL, respectively.
- A treatment delay should be considered if the patient is not adequately recovered from the side effects of the previous chemotherapy treatment.
- Patients should be adequately restrained, and some may need to be sedated to ensure safe chemotherapy administration and to reduce the risk of drug extravasation.
- A "single-attempt" IV catheter should be used for all intravenous chemotherapy administration.

- This is especially important for irritant and vesicant drugs such as the vinca alkaloids, doxorubicin, dactinomycin, and mechlorethamine.

Managing Complications of Chemotherapy

The major dose-limiting factor in chemotherapy protocols is drug toxicity, which can be broadly divided into the categories discussed in the following sections.

Gastrointestinal Effects (Figure 5.28)

Gastrointestinal effects

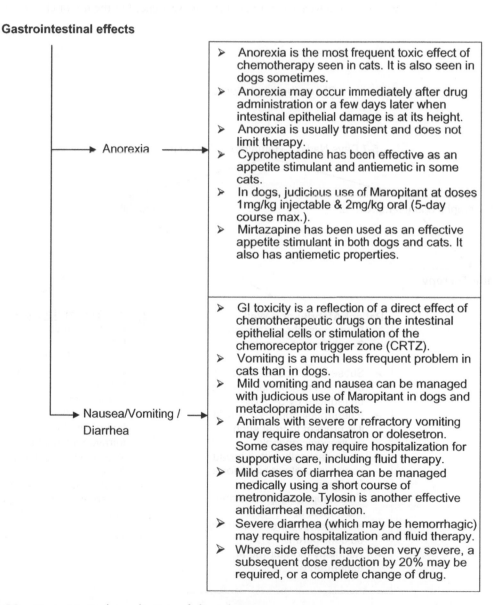

Anorexia
- Anorexia is the most frequent toxic effect of chemotherapy seen in cats. It is also seen in dogs sometimes.
- Anorexia may occur immediately after drug administration or a few days later when intestinal epithelial damage is at its height.
- Anorexia is usually transient and does not limit therapy.
- Cyproheptadine has been effective as an appetite stimulant and antiemetic in some cats.
- In dogs, judicious use of Maropitant at doses 1mg/kg injectable & 2mg/kg oral (5-day course max.).
- Mirtazapine has been used as an effective appetite stimulant in both dogs and cats. It also has antiemetic properties.

Nausea/Vomiting / Diarrhea
- GI toxicity is a reflection of a direct effect of chemotherapeutic drugs on the intestinal epithelial cells or stimulation of the chemoreceptor trigger zone (CRTZ).
- Vomiting is a much less frequent problem in cats than in dogs.
- Mild vomiting and nausea can be managed with judicious use of Maropitant in dogs and metaclopramide in cats.
- Animals with severe or refractory vomiting may require ondansatron or dolesetron. Some cases may require hospitalization for supportive care, including fluid therapy.
- Mild cases of diarrhea can be managed medically using a short course of metronidazole. Tylosin is another effective antidiarrheal medication.
- Severe diarrhea (which may be hemorrhagic) may require hospitalization and fluid therapy.
- Where side effects have been very severe, a subsequent dose reduction by 20% may be required, or a complete change of drug.

Figure 5.28. Gastrointestinal complications of chemotherapy.

Myelosuppression/Sepsis (Figure 5.29)

- Fast-dividing bone marrow stem cells are killed by most chemotherapeutic agents. As a consequence, peripheral blood cytopenias occur, with the lowest point, or nadir, usually occurring 5–10 days after drug administration, though sometimes earlier or later.
- Neutropenia and thrombocytopenia are the most frequent cytopenias because of the relatively short half-lives of these cells in the peripheral blood (6–8 hours for neutrophils and 5–7 days for platelets).
- Cell counts usually return to normal 2–3 days after the nadir. Marked neutropenia can result in sepsis, which is a serious complication that requires aggressive medical management including intravenous fluid therapy and antibiotics. Bleeding as a consequence of chemotherapy-induced thrombocytopenia is rare.
- In a "new" chemotherapy patient, hemotology should be about a week (7–10 days) after giving each myelosuppressive drug for the first time. If the neutrophil count is below 1.5×10^9/L, or the platelet count below 75×10^9/L, it is wise to seek advice from a veterinarian experienced in the use of chemotherapy.

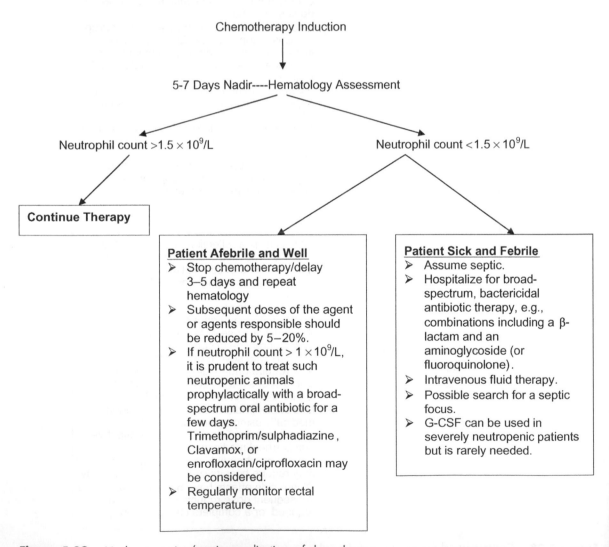

Figure 5.29. Myelosuppression/sepsis complications of chemotherapy.

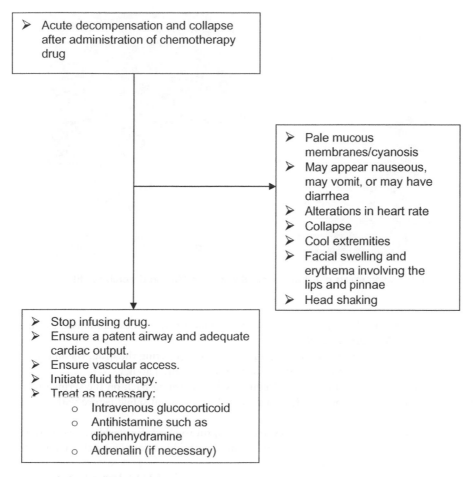

Figure 5.30. Anaphylaxis/allergic reactions from chemotherapy.

Anaphylaxis/Allergic Reactions (Figure 5.30)

- These can occur after injections with L-asparginase (foreign protein), doxorubicin infusions and as a reaction to cremaphor carrier in taxol derivatives.
- Prevention is better than dealing with the problem:
  - Avoid intravenous injections with L-asparaginase.
  - Premedication with antihistamines is advisable if risk is considered high.
  - Taxol derivatives should be administered by specialist oncologists only and adhering to strict pretreatment protocols with corticosteroids.

Drug Extravasation (Figure 5.31)

- Drugs that cause soft tissue damage following inadvertent perivascular injection are called *irritants* or *vesicants,* depending on the severity of tissue damage that they cause.
- The vinca alkaloids (vincristine, vinblastine, vinorelbine) are considered irritants.
- Extravasation results in self-limiting inflammation, erythema, and discomfort.
- Doxorubicin, mechlorethamine, and dactinomycin are vesicants because they cause catastrophic, progressive soft tissue necrosis at the extravasation site.

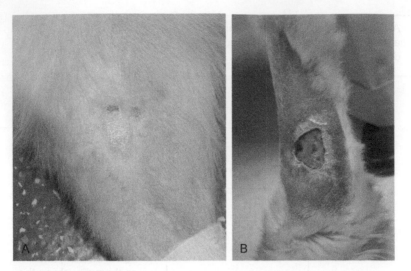

Figure 5.31. Skin damaging effects of extravasation of vincristine (A) and doxorubicin (B).

- Clearly, prevention is better than cure. Doxorubicin and vincristine are best administered through a well-secured, *"single-stick" intravenous catheter.*
- The patient should be well-restrained for venipuncture. Before injecting the drug, the line should be flushed with about 5 ml normal saline and checked for flashback to ensure patency.
- During injection, patency should be checked frequently by aspirating back on the syringe plunger. After injection, the line should be thoroughly flushed with 5–10 ml normal saline before withdrawal of the needle or catheter.
- During this final flushing stage, it is not necessary or helpful to check for flashback as there is a small chance that the flush solution may become contaminated with blood containing the irritant drug.
- In the event of perivascular injection:
  - If an irritant or vesicant is inadvertently injected perivascularly, **STOP** drug administration immediately. The needle or catheter should be left in place and attempts made to withdraw as much of the drug as possible by suction.
  - Once this has been done, the needle or catheter is withdrawn, and a 25- or 26-gauge needle and syringe is used to withdraw any more of the visible subcutaneous bleb.
  - **For vinca alkaloid extravasation:**
    - Infiltrate the site with sterile water.
    - Apply *warm* compresses for 15–20 minutes QID for 24–48 hours to promote vasodilation and increase blood flow. The reaction seen with extravasation of vincristine is often rather mild to moderate and is due in part to excessive licking and self-trauma following extravasation. An ulcer or large eschar may occur at the site. If this happens, it is unlikely that the vein will ever be patent in the future.
  - **If doxorubicin is extravasated:**
    - Immediately try to remove as much of the drug as possible, as above.
    - Apply *cold* packs for 15–20 minutes QID for 72 hours to promote vasoconstriction to restrict spread of the drug.
    - You can give 5 ml of sodium bicarbonate 8.4% IV, ±DMSO solution 50–99%, applied topically 2–4 times daily for 2–14 days.
    - Dexrazoxane (Zinecard®), a free radical scavenger, prevents doxorubicin-induced skin necrosis in experimental laboratory animals. Experience in companion animals is limited but anecdotal evidence suggests it may be effective in dogs and cats. The dose is 10:1 that of doxorubicin given IV within 3 hours of extravasation and repeated daily for 2 additional days.
    - Contact a veterinarian experienced in administration of chemotherapy **AS SOON AS POSSIBLE** if extravasation of doxorubicin is suspected.

- ○ Immediate surgical excision of surrounding tissue may be advised if the extravasation area is limited to resectable tissue. If a large quantity of the drug is known to have been extravasated, future limb amputation may be necessary.
- ○ Tell the owner to expect frequent follow-up visits for the first few weeks, and the probability that future surgical debridement of the site may be required. The full extent of the injury may not be evident for up to 2 weeks.

Cardiotoxicity

- Doxorubicin causes dose-dependent cardiotoxicity in the form of dilated cardiomyopathy. For this reason, it is recommended not to exceed a total cumulative dose of 180 mg/m^2 in dogs.
- Cats are more resistant to this form of toxicity, but total doses exceeding 150–200 mg/m^2 can have clinical consequences. Given that each individual dose is typically 20–25 mg/m^2 in cats and 30 mg/m^2 in dogs, no more than a total of 6 doses is recommended without serious consideration of risks versus benefits.
- Echocardiography and ECG should be done prior to initiation of doxorubicin treatment in any canine patient with a heart murmur and after 120 mg/m^2 and 180 mg/m^2 total dose. Physical examinations should be done at every visit. In subclinical cardiotoxicity a new murmur, gallop, sound or dysrhythmia may be auscultated. A wide range of ECG abnormalities are possible: bundle branch blocks, supraventricular or ventricular dysrhythmias, and changes in R wave amplitude. On echocardiography, subclinical cardiotoxicity may be associated with poor cardiac contractility (i.e., reduced shortening fraction) and other changes. When overt clinical signs develop, the patient will show signs typical of congestive heart failure.

Nephrotoxicity and Sterile Hemorrhagic Cystitis

- Doxorubicin in cats and cisplatin in dogs are the drugs most likely to cause nephrotoxicity. Methotrexate (dogs) and carboplatin (dogs and cats) can also do it, though less commonly.
- Cyclophosphamide and the newer alkylating agent ifosfamide are oxazophosphorines that can cause sterile, hemorrhagic cystitis in dogs. Acrolein, a metabolite of these drugs that is excreted in the urine, is an irritant for the bladder wall. Cats are much less likely to be affected. Affected animals show hematuria (often severe), pollakiuria, stranguria, and dysuria. Signs can take weeks to months to resolve.
- Prevention is easier than trying to manage this condition. Concurrent administration of furosemide (1– 2 mg/kg IV) 30 minutes prior to intravenous cyclophosphamide administration has markedly reduced the incidence of this condition.
- If sterile cystitis does occur, no universally effective treatment exists. Clinical signs may be minimized by intravesicular infusion of 20 ml of 25% DMSO solution. Sedation is advised to prevent immediate micturition after infusion. Treatment can be repeated in 7 days if needed. Unfortunately, DMSO is not always effective. Oxybutynin, an antichoninergic medication, is often used to decrease muscle spasms associated with sterile hemorrhagic cystitis. It is dosed at 0.2 mg/kg PO BID, with most dogs receiving 1.25–5 mg total dose BID. The bladder mucosa sometimes has to be cauterized to minimize blood loss.
- Cyclophosphamide should then be discontinued and chlorambucil substituted.

The Effect of Chemotherapy on Wound Healing

- Cytotoxic drugs affect rapidly dividing cells and therefore theoretically can have a deleterious effect on wound healing when chemotherapy is being combined with surgery or following a major biopsy procedure.
- However, in practice most cytotoxic drugs can be used in the perioperative procedure where there is an indication to do so.

- Major problems can arise if the patient is extremely leukopenic and there is the possibility of wound infection, or if the patient is severely cachectic. In cases where wound healing may be a problem, the administration of vitamin A may reduce the effects of cytotoxic drugs on wound healing.

Other Complications of Chemotherapy

- In certain conditions such as the lymphoproliferative or myeloproliferative diseases, the administration of cytotoxic drugs at the start of therapy may lead to rapid lysis of the tumor.
- This can cause a severe metabolic disturbance resulting in hyperkalemia, hyperphosphatemia, and hypocalcemia, the end result being renal and/or cardiac failure.
- This condition is termed *tumor lysis syndrome* and is relatively rare.

Appendix A: Tables of Specific Drug Classes

Alkylating Agents

The drugs in Table 5.4 are cell cycle nonspecific and act by interfering with DNA replication and RNA transcription, this being directly related to their ability to alkylate DNA.

Table 5.4. Alkylating agents

Drugs	Indications	Dose	Potential Toxicity
Cyclophosphamide (Cytoxan®)	Lymphoma Various sarcomas Resistant multiple myeloma	50 mg/m^2 PO daily for the first 4 days of each week OR 250 mg/m^2 IV weekly	Myelosuppression GI effects Sterile hemorrhagic cystitis
Chlorambucil (Leukeran®)	Chronic lymphocytic leukemia Feline epitheliotropic GI lymphoma Instead of cyclophosphamide in cases of sterile hemorrhagic cystitis	2 mg/m^2 PO daily, reducing to every other day in CLL OR 1.4 mg/kg IV weekly OR 20 mg/m2 PO q 2 weeks in cats	Bone marrow suppression, but this is rare
Busulphan (Busilvex®, Myleran®)	Chronic granulocytic leukemia	Initially 2–6 mg/m^2, then reduced according to response	Bone marrow suppression Long term can lead to chronic pulmonary fibrosis
Melphalan (Alkeran®)	Multiple myeloma	0.1 mg/kg PO daily for 10 days, then 0.05 mg/kg PO daily	Myelosuppression including cumulative, chronic thrombocytopenia GI effects
CCNU (Lomustine®)	Lymphoma Mast cell tumor Brain tumors	Dogs: 60–90 mg/m^2 PO q 3 weeks Cats: 55–65 mg/m^2 PO q 3–5 weeks	Myelosuppression including cumulative, chronic thrombocytopenia GI effects Hepatotoxicity Renal toxicity (rare)

Antimetabolites

These are a class of drugs that interfere with normal cell metabolism. They can be broadly divided into the antifolates (e.g., methotrexate), the purine analogues (e.g., azathioprine), and the pyrimidine analogues (e.g., cytosine arabinoside, gemcitabine, 5-fluorouracil). They are cell cycle specific. Table 5.5 gives a brief summary of the commonly used antimetabolites in veterinary practice.

Antitumor Antibiotics

The drugs in Table 5.6 form stable complexes with DNA and thus inhibit DNA synthesis and replication. They tend not to be cell cycle specific but are more active in the s phase.

Vinca Alkaloids

The drugs in Table 5.7 are plant alkaloids derived from the periwinkle. Their mode of action is to bind to tubulin during M phase so as to inhibit the formation of the mitotic spindle. Thus they are cell cycle.

Table 5.5.   Antimetabolites

Drugs	Indications	Dose	Potential Toxicity
Cytosine Arabinoside (Cytosar®, Ara-C. cytarabine®)	Lymphoma	400–600 mg/m^2 IV as a slow infusion over 4–24 hours or divided SC over 2 days	Myelosuppression Mild diarrhea
Azathioprine	Immune-mediated disease	2 mg/kg daily or every other day	Myelosuppression rare Pancreatitis

Table 5.6.   Antitumor antibiotics

Drugs	Indications	Dose	Potential Toxicity
Doxorubicin (Adriamycin®, also called *hydroxydaunorubicin*)	Wide range of indications including • Lymphoma • Other lymphoid malignancies • Osteosarcoma • Other sarcomas • Carcinomas	Dogs: ≥15 kg: 30 mg/m^2 IV q 2–3 weeks <15 kg: 25 mg/m^2 IV q 2–3 weeks **Toy breeds: 1 mg/kg IV q 2–3 weeks** Cats: 1 mg/kg IV q 2–3 weeks	Severe tissue necrosis if extravasated Myelosuppression (can be severe) GI effects including hemorrhagic colitis Hypersensitivity-like reaction Cardiotoxicity (dose not to exceed a total of 180 mg/m^2)
Epirubicin	As above (isomer of doxorubicin)	As above	Less cardiotoxic than doxorubicin
Mitoxantrone (Novantrone®)	Lymphoma Substitute for doxorubicin when it cannot be used Carcinomas	5–5.5 mg/m^2 IV q 3 weeks	Myelosuppression GI effects Overall, toxicity is less than for doxorubicin)

Hormones

The major drug in this class is prednisolone (Table 5.8). Although this drug is reported to be lymphotoxic and thus beneficial in lymphoma patients, the major action is probably antiinflammatory, which allows tumor shrinkage by virtue of removal of the inflammatory component of the tumor.

Miscellaneous Agents

Table 5.9 lists miscellaneous agents not included in the previous tables of specific drug classes.

Tables 5.10 and 5.11 provide a convenient conversion table from body weight to BSA for use in dogs and cats, respectively.

Table 5.7. Vinca alkaloids

Drugs	Indications	Dose	Potential Toxicity
Vincristine (Oncovin®)	Lymphoma Other lymphoid malignancies Sarcoma TVT	0.5–0.75 mg/m^2 IV weekly	Soft tissue irritation if extravasated Minimally myelosuppressive GI effects Peripheral neuropathy including constipation
Vinblastine (Velban®)	Many similar indications as vincristine In particular, mast cell tumor	2–2.5 mg/m^2 IV weekly	As above, but more myelosuppressive

Table 5.8. Hormones

Drugs	Indications	Dose	Potential Toxicity
Prednisolone	Lymphoma Other lymphoid malignancies Mast cell tumor Terminal patients	0.5–2 mg/kg PO daily, tapering dose	Iatrogenic Cushing's disease Polydipsia, polyuria, polyphagiza Behavior change

Table 5.9. Miscellaneous agents

Drugs	Indications	Dose	Potential Toxicity
Cisplatin	Osteosarcoma Carcinoma Mesothelioma	50–70 mg/m^2 IV every 3 weeks. This is combined with a standardized diuresis protocol.	Nephrotoxicity (must be given with diuresis) Should NEVER be given to cats Myelosuppression GI effects Vomiting during infusion
Carboplatin	Osteosarcoma Other sarcomas Carcinomas Mesothelioma	Dog; 300 mg/mg^2 IV q 3 weeks Cat: 265 mg/m^2 IV q 3 weeks	Myelosuppression GI effects Less nephrotoxic than cisplatin Safe to use in cats
L-Asparaginase	Lymphosarcoma Other lymphoid malignancies	400 IU/kg or 10,000 IU/m^2 by SQ injection (maximum total dose of 10000 IU)	Hypersensitivity
Hydroxyurea	Polycythemia Rubera vera (primary erythrocytosis)	50 mg/kg daily per. os.	Myelosuppression

Table 5.10.   Body surface area tables: Dogs

Kg	m²	Kg	m²
1.0	0.10	26.0	0.88
2.0	0.15	27.0	0.90
3.0	0.20	28.0	0.92
4.0	0.25	29.0	0.94
5.0	0.29	30.0	0.96
6.0	0.33	31.0	0.99
7.0	0.36	32.0	1.01
8.0	0.40	33.0	1.03
9.0	0.43	34.0	1.05
10.0	0.46	35.0	1.07
11.0	0.49	36.0	1.09
12.0	0.52	37.0	1.11
13.0	0.55	38.0	1.13
14.0	0.58	39.0	1.15
15.0	0.60	40.0	1.17
16.0	0.63	41.0	1.19
17.0	0.66	42.0	1.21
18.0	0.69	43.0	1.23
19.0	0.71	44.0	1.25
20.0	0.74	45.0	1.26
21.0	0.76	46.0	1.28
22.0	0.78	47.0	1.30
23.0	0.81	48.0	1.32
24.0	0.83	49.0	1.34
25.0	0.85	50.0	1.36

Table 5.11.   Body surface area tables: Cats

Kg	m²	Kg	m²
2.0	0.159	3.6	0.235
2.2	0.169	3.8	0.244
2.4	0.179	4.0	0.252
2.6	0.189	4.2	0.260
2.8	0.199	4.4	0.269
3.0	0.208	4.6	0.277
3.2	0.217	4.8	0.285
3.4	0.226	5.0	0.292

Part 5: New or Horizon Therapies for Cancer

Both chemotherapy and radiation therapy rely on the nature of dividing cells in cancer. With an increased understanding of the mechanisms in cancer, newer drugs are being developed that target specific pathways. Table 5.12 offers an insight into drugs in development, targeting cancer pathways, and also a brief overview of some of the other modalities that may be available at specialist centers.

Table 5.12. Drugs in development

Therapeutic Modality	Description and Availability
Drugs targeting signal transduction pathways in cancer	Receptor tyrosine kinases (RTKs) are an important group of cell surface receptors that trigger cellular activation resulting in cell proliferation, differentiation, and survival when stimulated by their cognate ligands. Activation of RTKs has been shown to precipitate malignant transformation implying a key role as "gatekeepers" that control diverse cellular processes. Development of new drugs that block RTK activity by competitive inhibition of ATP binding is a fiercely contested arena in the pharmaceutical industry. The unparalleled success of the RTK inhibitor STI-571 (Imatinib mesylate) for the treatment of human chronic myelogenous leukemia, resulted in its rapid and unprecedented quick approval by the Food and Drug Administration under the commercial name Gleevec®. Unfortunately, Gleevec is toxic to dogs and cats, but new generation RTK inhibitors offer promise in the veterinary setting.
Cancer vaccines or immunotherapy	There is strong evidence that a cancer patient can mount an immune response against specific tumor antigens. For many years, there has been a range of approaches adopted to try and harness the immune response against cancer in the form of therapeutic cancer vaccines. These approaches have included • Whole cell vaccines • Peptide vaccines • Cytokine-based approaches • DNA vaccines Despite extensive research into these modalities, immunotherapy has yet to become accepted as first line clinical practice. There are many factors that contribute to the lack of efficacy of immunotherapy, including • Host factors • Difficulty in identifying tumor-specific target antigens • The role of T-regulator cells • Direct inhibition of the immune system by the tumor A therapeutic melanoma vaccine distributed by Merial has been licensed for clinical use in canine melanoma in the U.S. This vaccine is not available in Europe.
Photodynamic therapy	This form of therapy utilizes the application of a photosensitizer to a tumor. The subsequent application of light of a particular wavelength results in activation of the photosensitizer and generation of oxygen free radicals, which cause cell death within the tumor. This is available at selected specialist centers. This has been used successfully for the treatment of squamous cell carcinoma of the nasal planum in cats.

Part 6: Palliative Care, Pain Control, and Nutrition

Palliative Therapy for Cancer

Key Points
• Palliative care refers to relieving the clinical signs of a disease or disorder without effecting a cure.
• This may be achieved through several means, depending on the disease, the patient and the owners' expectations.

Nonsteroidal Antiinflammatory Drugs (NSAIDS) and Palliative Care

- Epidemiological studies in man have demonstrated a protective effect of chronic aspirin intake in the incidence of colorectal cancer. Further, the use of antiinflammatory drugs to abrogate tumor growth has shown promise in several animal model systems and clinical cancer cases.
- Active research is underway in several laboratories to identify the cellular mechanisms mediating this effect. The majority of NSAIDs inhibit the isoforms of cyclo-oxygenase (COX-1 and COX-2) to varying degrees or are selective for one isoform. The COX inhibition, antiinflammatory and antitumor effects in vivo are exerted in a parallel dose-dependent manner. However, despite clear evidence for pro-apoptotic and antiproliferative effects in tumors, the mechanism by which NSAIDs cause protective and direct antitumor effects is still to be determined.
- Induction of COX-2 expression has been reported in various canine cancers.
- Dogs with neoplastic disease treated with NSAIDs are usually selected on the basis that standard therapy has failed, is precluded on medical grounds, is declined by the owner, or does not exist.
- The nonsteroidal antiinflammatory drug **piroxicam** (Feldene™ 10 mg and 20 mg tablets, Pfizer) has activity against a variety of tumors in humans and dogs. In dogs, it has seen most use in the treatment of transitional cell carcinomas (TCC) of the urinary bladder and urethra. It has also shown benefit in treatment of some squamous cell carcinomas and mammary adenocarcinomas. The dose is 0.3 mg/kg PO every 24 hours given with food.
- Owners commonly report that patients receiving piroxicam or **meloxicam** appear to have an improved quality of life, manifested as increased activity and alertness.
- Toxicity appears to be uncommon; however, oral piroxicam has been associated with gastrointestinal ulceration and renal papillary necrosis.
- The increased COX-2 selectivity of meloxicam or other selective COX-2 inhibitors makes for an attractive alternative to piroxicam in the treatment of cancer, since it may reduce possible gastrointestinal side effects.

Pain Control

- The alleviation of pain is important from physiological and biological standpoints, but also from an ethical point of view.
- The role of the veterinarian is to alleviate suffering and maintain the welfare of the animals in his or her care.
- Recognizing pain:
  - Animals that are in pain, especially pain associated with the musculoskeletal system, do not move around as much as they did prior to the pain (more difficult to assess in cats).
  - Localized joint, bone, or soft-tissue damage or disease producing pain will result in lameness, muscle wastage, or altered gait.
  - Oral pain can result in an uneven appearance to tartar buildup on teeth, with more tartar being found on the painful side, and can also result in problems with eating, or anorexia.
  - In cats, grooming often is decreased.
  - In dogs in particular, attention is paid to painful areas, indicated by licking at such areas.
  - Both cats and dogs in pain have decreased appetites, but drinking is usually unaffected, unless the pain is severe. Psychogenic polydipsia can occur.
  - Another very good way to determine whether a cat or dog is in pain is to examine the response to analgesic therapy.

Management of Cancer Pain

- The use of drugs is the mainstay of cancer pain management (Figure 5.32), and is based on the use of the following "groups" of analgesics:
  - Nonopioid analgesics (e.g., nonsteroidal antiinflammatory drugs, acetaminophen)
  - Weak opioid drugs (e.g., codeine)
  - Strong opioid drugs (e.g., morphine)
  - Adjuvant drugs (e.g., corticosteroids, tricyclic antidepressants, anticonvulsants, NMDA antagonists)

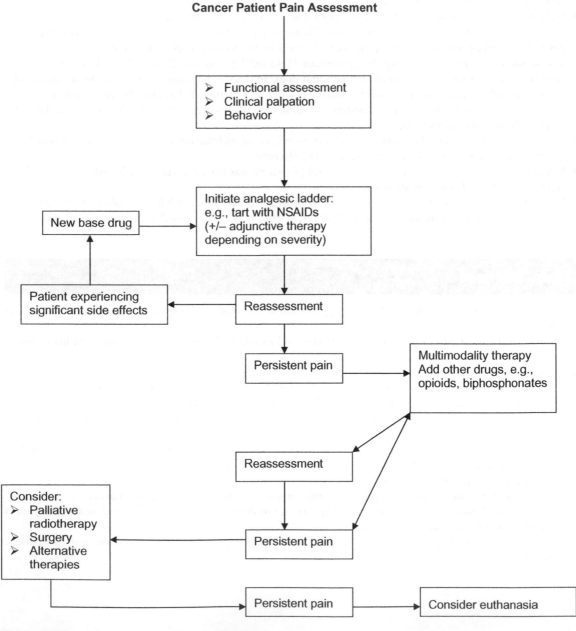

Figure 5.32. Decision tree in pain management.

- The use of these drugs follows a "ladder" in that:
  - Some types of pain will respond to nonopioid therapy alone.
  - Pain of a greater intensity may require the combination of a nonopioid and a "weak" opioid.
  - More severe pain requires the addition of a higher dose of opioid, and the use of a "strong" opioid that is titrated to the pain present (± adjuvant).
- Once pain has been present for a period of time, changes have taken place in the central nervous system that alters the way pain signals are processed. This alteration in processing (central sensitization) makes analgesics less effective, and requires that multiple classes of analgesics be used, concurrently, to minimize the pain. *This is known as multimodal pain therapy.*
- Once the pain is minimized and central changes are partially reversed, the amounts of drugs being administered, and the numbers of classes of analgesic drugs being used, can be decreased.

Drugs used for cancer pain (Table 5.13)
- Nonsteroidal antiinflammatory drugs (NSAIDs)
  - Carprofen, meloxicam and piroxicam have been found to be preferential COX-2 inhibitors, with carprofen being the most preferred. Deracoxib is a very selective COX-2 inhibitor, currently only approved for use in dogs in the U.S. Meloxicam is recommended for cats.

Table 5.13. Pain drugs and doses

Drug Class	Drug	Dog	Cat
NSAID	Piroxicam	0.3 mg/kg PO q 24 hrs with food	0.3 mg/kg PO q 48 hrs with food if renal function is normal
	Meloxicam	0.1 mg/kg PO q 24 hrs	0.1 mg/kg PO q 24 hrs daily OR q 48 to 72 hrs if using chronically
	Deramaxx	1–2 mg/kg PO q 24 hrs	–
Opioid and opioid-like drugs*	Morphine	0.3–1 mg/kg q 6–8 hrs OR 0.3–0.5 mg/kg q 12 hrs of the sustained release preparation	–
	Codeine	1–2 mg/kg PO q 6–8 hrs	0.1–1 mg/kg PO q 6–12 hrs
	Buprenorphine	Not given sublingually because transmucosal absorption has not been shown	0.02 mg/kg sublingually q 12 hrs
	Transdermal fentanyl patch	<5 kg: 12–25 mcg/hr 5–10 kg: 25 mcg/hr 10–20 kg: 50 mcg/hr 20–30 kg: 50–75 mcg/hr >30 kg: 50–100 mcg/hr	12–25 mcg/hr
	Tramadol Note that split tablets have a bitter taste	1–5 mg/kg PO q 4–12 hrs	12.5 mg q 12 hrs
Anticonvulsant	Gabapentin	4–8 mg/kg PO q 8–12; can increase to 15 + mg/kg	Consider 1–3 mg/kg q 12–24 hrs but not commonly used
Antiviral	Amantadine	3–5 mg/kg q 24 hrs	–
Tricyclic antidepressants	Amitriptyline	1 mg/kg q 12–24 hrs	0.5–1 mg/kg q 12–24 hrs
Other	Acetominophen	2–5 mg/kg q 24 hrs if liver function is normal	Do not use in cats
	Acetaminophen-codeine	Dose based on codeine dose of 1–2 mg/kg q 6–8 hrs	Do not use in cats

*For all opioids, the lowest effective dose is best.

- If the drug is effective, it should be continued. If not, therapy should be switched to another NSAID. The patient should be monitored for toxicity.
- If pain relief with NSAID therapy is inadequate, oral opioid medications, such as morphine or tramadol can be administered. Transdermal fentanyl can also be used but it is expensive. Fentanyl, morphine, or tramadol can be used for dogs that cannot be given NSAIDs. Other agents that are used to treat chronic pain include amantadine (an NMDA antagonist); anticonvulsants, such as gabapentin; and tricyclic antidepressants, such as amitriptyline. These can all be combined with NSAIDs.
- **Opioids**
  - Opioids can be a very effective part of the management of cancer pain as part of a multimodal approach (i.e., including NSAIDs, or adjunctive analgesics).
  - Side effects of opioids can include anorexia, vomiting, diarrhea, occasionally sedation or restlessness, and constipation with long-term use.
  - The drugs that appear to have been used clinically most often for the alleviation of chronic cancer pain are oral morphine, transdermal fentanyl, oral butorphanol, sublingual buprenorphine (cats only) and oral codeine.
  - None of these drugs have been fully evaluated for clinical toxicity when administered long-term or for efficacy against chronic cancer pain.
  - It is important to realize that dosing must be done on an individual basis.
  - There is currently no information on the long-term use of opioids for chronic pain in the cat.
- **Combination analgesics**
  - Tramadol (Ultram) is classified as an opioidergic/monoaminergic drug and has been found to be effective in the alleviation of pain associated with osteoarthritis in humans, as part of a multimodal approach. While it has been used successfully in the dog for alleviation of cancer-related pain, it has not been evaluated for toxicity in companion animals.
- **Corticosteroids**
  - Corticosteroids have a mild analgesic action and can also produce a state of euphoria, and they are often used for these reasons to palliate cancer and cancer pain in cats and dogs. They should not be used concurrently with NSAIDs.
- **Biphosphonates**
  - Bone pain induced by primary or metastatic bone tumors is thought to be due to, in large part, osteoclast activity and drugs that block osteoclast activity can markedly reduce bone pain.
  - Biphosphonates are a class of drug that inhibit osteoclast activity and can produce analgesia via this action.
  - Biphosphonates are analogues of pyrophosphate and are potent inhibitors of osteoclastic bone reabsorption. Their use in metastatic bone pain is becoming widely established in human oncology.
  - In the dog, injectable pamidronate and zoledronate have been used anecdotally. In human oncology these agents have been shown to impact greatly on morbidity in patients with bone lesions from multiple myeloma or breast cancer.
  - Initial studies in dogs indicate that this will be a powerful group of drugs, which will find greater prominence in the treatment of cancer patients in veterinary practice. However, large-scale clinical studies are warranted to demonstrate this conclusively.
- **Radiotherapy**
  - In cases of tumor-related pain, palliative radiotherapy to the effected area can provide relief.
  - The most common indication is bone pain caused by primary bone tumors such as osteosarcoma, metastatic bone lesions, and bony destruction caused by invasive soft-tissue tumors.
  - Tumors limited to soft tissues can also be palliated with radiotherapy when their size or location is causing discomfort to the patient.
  - See Part 3: Radiotherapy, earlier in this chapter, for further information.
- **Alternative Therapies**
  - Acupuncture is an ancient practice in which fine needles are inserted into the skin at strategic points on the body to, among other purposes, relieve pain.
  - Although there is a lack of objective clinical evidence supporting the efficacy of acupuncture for pain control in veterinary medicine, pet owners are increasingly seeking alternative modalities to treat their animal

companions, and anecdotal experience suggests that acupuncture can be effective at alleviating discomfort in some animals.

Nutrition and the Cancer Patient

Key Points
- Any cancer patient is at risk of becoming malnourished due to a lack of appetite or ability to eat.
- Cancer patients may be debilitated, in pain, or nauseous; they may be stressed by hospitalization, have obstructive tumors, or have had surgery in the head/neck/stomach area, preventing them from wanting to or being able to ingest food.
- Nutritional goals can be met by providing protein, carbohydrate, fat, and other nutrients in a form which can be utilized by the body with maximum efficiency, minimal adverse effects, and minimum discomfort.
- Increased protein breakdown occurs in response to malnutrition, illness, or injury. It can impair wound healing, as well as immune, cellular, organ, and potentially cardiac and respiratory functions, and affect the prognosis for recovery.
- When subjected to starvation, body tissue (except brain and bone) loses cell mass in varying degrees. Tumors and wounds may act as additional burdens, which further increase a patient's calorie and nutrient requirements. The degree of metabolic deviation is dependent on the severity of illness or injury and its associated tissue damage.
- When the body utilizes exogenous rather than endogenous nutrients, the breakdown of lean body mass is slowed and the patient's response to therapy optimized.
- Nutrition is often overlooked in hospitalized patients, as other matters take priority, e.g., food is often withheld in order to conduct diagnostic tests or procedures on successive days.
- Nutritional support may be inadvertently delayed until a patient reaches an advanced malnourished state or the provision nutritional support may be inadequate postoperatively.
- These patients may suffer through failure to recognize and treat increased nutritional needs due to injury or illness. When hospitalized, a patient's body weight should be recorded at least daily; food intake should be observed, measured, and recorded often, and there should be careful handovers of care, e.g., at shift changes.

In general, nutritional support is indicated when there is
- Loss, or anticipated loss, of more than 10% of body weight
- Anorexia for longer than 3 days
- Trauma or surgery
- Severe systemic infiltrative disease
- Increased nutrient loss through diarrhea
- Vomiting
- Draining wounds or burns, associated with decreased serum albumin
  Other factors that should be considered include
- Gastrointestinal tract function
- The patient's ability to tolerate tube or catheter feeding (presence of any organ failure – e.g., renal, hepatic)
- The patient's ability to tolerate physical or chemical restraint required for placement of tubes or catheters
- Venous accessibility
- Whether the patient is at risk for pulmonary aspiration (i.e., megaesophagus)
- The availability of nursing care and equipment
- The client's financial resources

Nutritional Assessment

- In order to make a nutritional assessment, a complete physical examination should be performed and a detailed history obtained from the owner.
- A full biochemistry and hematology should be performed, the patient's body weight recorded and the body condition assessed.
- Body condition scores used for healthy animals often do not apply to sick animals. When an animal is physiologically stressed, it will catabolize lean body mass as a preferred energy source, whereas healthy animals use stored body fat for energy. This will result in increased catabolism of body protein.
- A patient may present with increased amounts of body fat, yet be at serious risk of malnutrition-associated complications, associated with protein catabolism.
- Careful examination, including palpation of skeletal muscles over bony prominences, may identify muscle wasting consistent with protein catabolism.

Calculating Energy Requirements

- Calorific requirements are determined by body weight and may be calculated using the resting energy requirement (RER) for healthy adults, at rest, in environmentally comfortable cages. The functions and requirements equal those for the calculated RER amounts.
  Working calculation:
  $$\text{RER:}$$
  $$\text{dogs} = 70 + (30 \times \text{body weight [kg]})$$
  $$\text{cats} = 40 \times \text{body weight (kg)}$$
- Patients that eat more than the calculated RER should not be discouraged from doing so while recovering from surgery or trauma (the hospital is not the place to start a weight-loss program).

Implementing Feeding Orders

- Staff responsible for patient care should be given clear instructions on the type of food to be fed, as well as how much and how often. For all hospitalized patients, it is essential to record the following:
  - The amount and type of food offered
  - The time it was presented
  - The technique used to encourage the patient to eat
  - The quantity eaten (e.g., score out of 10)
  - Whether the patient showed any interest in, or aversion to, the food offered
- Such record-keeping provides the clinician with an accurate assessment of food intake and the nursing staff with successful feeding methods for individual patients (especially during shift changes).
- Meeting nutritional requirements is an important part of the care of cancer patients. Good nutrition has been shown in both people and in animals not only to improve quality of life, but also length of life by enhancing the beneficial effects of surgery, chemotherapy, and radiation therapy while at the same time reducing the side effects of these therapies. Although the ideal cancer diet for veterinary patients is not known, there are some general concepts that may be followed:
  - Provide a diet with an appetizing aroma and taste.
  - Minimize simple carbohydrates (starches and sugars). It is currently thought that dogs with certain malignant diseases have changes in carbohydrate, protein, and fat metabolism. It is believed that by using foods low in soluble carbohydrate and high in fat and high-quality protein ± supplementation with omega-3 fatty acids and arginine, the metabolic changes associated with cancer may be addressed. Enhancing levels of polyunsaturated omega-3 fatty acids may inhibit the growth and metastasis of certain tumors.
- Generally, cancer patients will be fed on a diet appropriate to their current clinical needs. These needs should be continuously reassessed (e.g., on initial presentation the patient may be anorexic and cachexic, but after 3 months of corticosteroids, it may be polyphagic and obese).

- The challenge for feeding cancer-bearing pets includes prevention and treatment of a finicky appetite. It is important not to make dramatic dietary changes at the same time as chemotherapy or other drugs are administered, especially if these drugs have the chance of causing nausea. This may result in "food aversion," – where the patient may associate the uncomfortable feeling with the food, as opposed to the treatment or hospital experience.

Hints for Increasing Oral Intake

- Make sure pain is well controlled and the patient is kept as unstressed as possible.
- Hand-feed and fuss over the patient during feeding.
- Warm the food to just below body temperature. (If microwaved, mix the food well before feeding.)
- Try adding warm water to dry foods or make a slurry from canned foods.
- Use cat food (for dogs) or human food (fish, chicken, cheese, yogurt, etc.) as a "top dressing" to the prescribed diet, to improve acceptance.
- Try various shapes and types of bowls (e.g., shallow dishes for cats and brachycephalics; plastic may have a strange smell, metal may be too noisy, etc.).
- Use foods that have a strong odor or smell (e.g., pilchards or sardines in tomato sauce).
- Offer small amounts of fresh food often; if not eaten, remove. Don't "carpet" the kennel with a buffet. Veterinary patients generally don't refuse to eat because they don't like the food offered, or you haven't selected the right flavor.
- Try feeding in different environments (e.g., most pets are not accustomed to being fed in their beds; some dogs may normally eat outside, etc.). Playing with food may stimulate a "hunting" response (mainly cats), or encourage dogs to "catch" or chase food. Ask for behaviors in exchange for food – e.g., sit for a biscuit, etc.
- Consider appetite stimulants such as cyproheptadine (cats) or mirtazapine (dogs and cats) to "jump start" the feeding process (usually ineffective over the long term).
- When oral intake is not possible (e.g., following surgery or radiotherapy), assisted tube feeding is an option to enhance both quality of life and longevity. The (permanent or temporary) placement of feeding tubes allows stress-free administration of medication, fluids, and nutrition to patients either in the hospital setting or at home. Various techniques may be employed – including placement of nasoesophageal, esophagostomy, gastrostomy, or jejunostomy tubes – depending on the patient's condition. Tube feeding should be instigated before significant weight loss/cachexia occurs.

Suggested Further Reading

Oncological Surgery

Dobson, J.M., Lascelles, B. Duncan X. 2003. BSAVA Manual of Canine and Feline Oncology (British Small Animal Veterinary Association), 2nd edition. British Small Animal Veterinary Association.

Fossum, T.W. 2006. Small Animal Surgery Textbook, 3rd edition. Mosby College Publishing, St. Louis, Missouri.

Saunders D.S. 2003. Textbook of Small Animal Surgery: 2-Volume Set, 3rd edition. W.B. Saunders, Encinitas, California.

Withrow, S.J., Vail, D.M. 2007. Small Animal Clinical Oncology, 4th edition. W.B. Saunders, Encinitas, California.

Radiotherapy

Bentel, G.C. 1995. Radiation Therapy Planning, 2nd edition. McGraw-Hill Medical, New York.

Bomford, C.K., Kunkler, I.H. 2002. Walter & Miller's Textbook of Radiotherapy: Radiation Physics, Therapy and Oncology, 6th edition. Churchill Livingstone/ Elsevier, Amsterdam.

Withrow, S.J., Vail, D.M. 2007. Small Animal Clinical Oncology, 4th edition. W.B. Saunders, Encinitas, California.

Chemotherapy

Souhami, Tannock, Hohenberger, and Horiot, editors. 2002. Oxford Textbook of Oncology, 2nd edition. Oxford University Press.

Withrow, S.J., Vail, D.M. 2007. Small Animal Clinical Oncology, 4th edition. W.B. Saunders, Encinitas, California.

Horizon Therapies, Pain Management, and Nutrition

Withrow, S.J., Vail, D.M. 2007. Small Animal Clinical Oncology, 4th edition. W.B. Saunders, Encinitas, California.

6
TUMORS OF THE SKIN AND SUBCUTIS

Valerie MacDonald, Michelle M. Turek, and David J. Argyle

Key Points
Dogs
- Most common tumor in this species
- Accounts for $1/3$ of all reported neoplasms
- Approximately 20–40% of skin tumors are malignant

Cats
- Second most common tumor overall
- Accounts for $1/4$ of all reported neoplasms
- Approximately 50–65% of skin tumors are malignant

Special Note
Occasionally tumors of the skin represent **metastatic lesions**. The best example of this is the syndrome of digital and cutaneous metastasis associated with lung cancer in cats (less commonly seen in the dog).

Classification (Table 6.1)

Generally classified according to the following:
- Tissue of origin (epithelial, mesenchymal, round, or melanotic)
- Cell of origin if possible (e.g., mast cell tumor)
- According to degree of malignancy

Frequency of Occurrence of Cutaneous Neoplasms in the Dog and Cat

The 10 Most Common Skin Tumors—Dogs

1. Mast cell tumors
2. Perianal adenoma
3. Lipoma
4. Sebaceous adenoma/hyperplasia
5. Histiocytoma
6. Squamous cell carcinoma
7. Melanoma
8. Fibrosarcoma
9. Basal cell tumor
10. Hemangiopericytoma

129

Table 6.1. Classification of cutaneous neoplasms in domestic animals

EPITHELIAL TUMORS
- Basal cell carcinoma
- Squamous cell carcinoma
- Papilloma
  - Adnexal tumors
    - ○ Sebaceous gland tumors
    - ○ *Sebaceous adenoma*
    - ○ *Sebaceous epithelioma*
  - *Sebaceous adenocarcinoma*
- Tumors of perianal glands
    - ○ *Hepatoid gland adenoma*
    - ○ *Adenocarcinoma*
- Sweat gland tumors
    - ○ *Apocrine adenoma/adenocarcinoma*
- Tumors of hair follicles
    - ○ *Pilomatricoma*
    - ○ *Trichoepithelioma*
- Intracutaneous cornifying epithelioma

MELANOCYTIC TUMORS
- Benign melanoma
- Malignant melanoma

MESENCHYMAL TUMORS (SOFT TISSUE SARCOMAS)
- Fibrous tissue
  - *Fibroma*
  - *Fibrosarcoma*
  - *Hemangiopericytoma**
- Nervous tissue
  - *Peripheral nerve sheath tumor*
  - *Neurofibrosarcoma**
- Adipose tissue
  - *Lipoma*
  - *Liposarcoma*
- Smooth muscle
  - *leiomyoma*
  - *leiomyosarcoma*
- Myxomatous tissue
  - *myxoma*
  - *myxosarcoma*

VASCULAR TUMORS
- Hemangioma
- Hemangiosarcoma

MAST CELL TUMOR
- Grade 1 (Patnaik)
- Grade 2 (Patnaik)
- Grade 3 (Patnaik)

LYMPHOMA
- Dermatropic
- Epitheliotropic (Mycosis fungoides)

HISTIOCYTIC DISEASES
- Canine cutaneous histiocytoma
- Reactive histiocytosis
- Systemic histiocytosis
- Histiocytic sarcoma
- Hemophagocytic histiocytic sarcoma

Collectively, mast cell tumors, cutaneous lymphoma, cutaneous plasma cell tumors, transmissible venereal tumors (TVT), histiocytomas, and neuroendocrine (Merkel cell) tumors are referred to as **round cell tumors.**

The 5 Most Common Skin Tumors—Cats

1. Basal cell tumor
2. Mast cell tumor
3. Fibrosarcoma
4. Squamous cell carcinoma
5. Sebaceous adenoma

Common Clinical Findings

- Owner usually discovers growth.
- Benign tumors usually present for a long period of time.
- Benign tumors are usually painless, slow growing, and movable.
- Malignant tumors may have history of rapid growth and may be fixed to underlying structures.
- Both malignant and benign tumors may be ulcerated.
- Appearance of growth varies depending on type of tumor and location.

Diagnosis (Figure 6.1)

- Detailed history and physical exam.
- Measure tumor, photograph, and identify the location of tumors on a body map.
- Lymph node examination and fine needle aspirate if possible.
- Fine needle aspirate of mass.
- Tissue biopsy (excisional versus incisional) for histologic evaluation may be indicated. Further diagnostics may be indicated depending on pathology of lesion and/or patient evaluation (i.e., thoracic radiographs, abdominal ultrasound).

Table 6.2.   Staging for canine and feline epidermal and dermal tumors (excluding mast cell tumors and lymphoma)

T	**Primary Tumor**
T_{is}	Preinvasive carcinoma (carcinoma in situ)
T_0	No evidence of tumor
T_1	Superficial tumor <2 cm maximum diameter
T_2	Tumor 2–5 cm maximum diameter, or with minimal invasion (irrespective of size)
T_3	Tumor >5 cm maximum diameter, or with invasion of subcutis (irrespective of size)
T_4	Tumor invading other structures such as fascia, bone, muscle and cartilage
	• Where there are multiple tumors arising simultaneously, these should be mapped and recorded.
	• The tumor with the highest T value is recorded and the number of tumors recorded in parentheses: e.g., $T_4(6)$.
	• Successive tumors are classified independently.
N	**Regional Lymph Node**
N_0	No evidence of lymph node metastasis
N_1	Movable ipsilateral nodes
	• N_{1a}: Nodes not considered to contain growth
	• N_{1b}: Nodes considered to contain growth
N_2	Movable contralateral nodes or bilateral nodes
	• N_{2a}: Nodes not considered to contain growth
	• N_{2b}: Nodes considered to contain growth
N_3	Fixed lymph nodes
M	**Distant Metastasis**
M_0	No evidence of distant metastasis
M_1	Distant metastasis detected

General Treatment Options for Skin Tumors (Figure 6.1 and Table 6.3)

- Complete surgical excision is standard of care.
- Cytoreductive surgery may be used for palliation of large tumors.
- Amputation for large tumors on extremities.
- Radiation therapy for incompletely excised tumors.
- Other treatment modalities may include photodynamic therapy, cryosurgery, laser ablation, and hyperthermia.

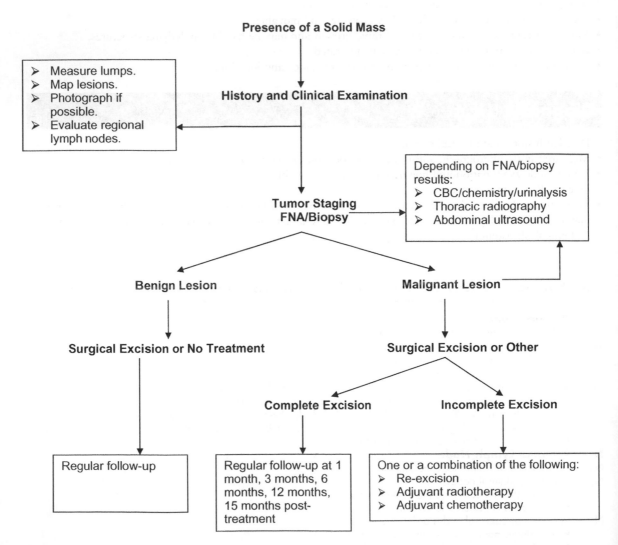

Figure 6.1. Diagnosis, staging, and treatment.

Epithelial Tumors

Table 6.3. Epithelial tumors

Tumor Type	Characteristics and Specific Management
Papilloma	This is common in dogs, rare in cats. This is associated with DNA papilloma virus. It is more common in young dogs where spontaneous resolution is common, occurring over a period of about 3 months. If treatment is necessary, surgery or cryotherapy can be used.
Squamous cell carcinoma	This accounts for 15% of feline and 5% of canine cutaneous tumors. This is often associated with poorly pigmented skin and UV exposure. In dogs, the most common area for SCC development is in the nail bed (subungual). It can also be found on the nasal planum, scrotum, flank, and abdomen. In cats, the most common areas for SCC development are the nasal planum, the eyelids and the pinnae. The tumor may be "productive," forming a papillary growth with a cauliflowerlike appearance, or "erosive," forming a shallow ulcer with raised edges. In both instances the lesion is frequently ulcerated, infected, and associated with a chronic inflammatory infiltrate. It is not uncommon for these tumors to be dismissed as infective/inflammatory lesions on initial presentation. Multifocal distribution of superficial lesions has been reported in cats. This is referred to as "multicentric SCC in situ" or **Bowen's disease**. Bowen's disease is an unusual feline skin condition of unknown origin. Recently, papillomavirus antigen has been demonstrated in 45% of the feline skin lesions using immunohistochemical methods. Unlike solar-induced SCC, Bowen's disease is found in haired, pigmented areas of the skin and is unrelated to sunlight exposure. Lesions are confined to the epithelium with no breach of the basement membrane. Lesions are crusty, easily epilated, painful, and hemorrhagic. When excision is possible, recurrence has not been reported; however, similar lesions often develop at other sites.
Basal cell tumor	Considered benign tumors. Common in cats, rarer in dogs. Surgery is the treatment of choice, and it is often curative. Rare cases of metastasis have been reported with basal cell carcinoma.
Sebaceous gland tumor	Includes • Sebaceous hyperplasia • Sebaceous epithelioma • Sebaceous adenoma • Sebaceous adenocarcinoma Surgery is the treatment of choice.
Sweat gland tumor	Apocrine gland adenoma or adenocarcinoma. Malignant tumors tend to be invasive but with low metastatic potential. Wide surgical excision is the treatment of choice.
Keratoacanthoma (intracutaneous cornifying epithelioma)	Considered a benign lesion. Can be solitary or multiple (mainly in Arctic Circle breeds such as Norwegian Elkhound and Keeshond. Solitary lesions are treated with surgery. Multiple lesions have been treated with cryosurgery, but recommend referral to a specialist oncologist.
Tumors of the hair follicles	Include trichoblastomas, trichoepitheliomas, and pilomatrixomas. Generally considered benign. Good prognosis following surgical excision.

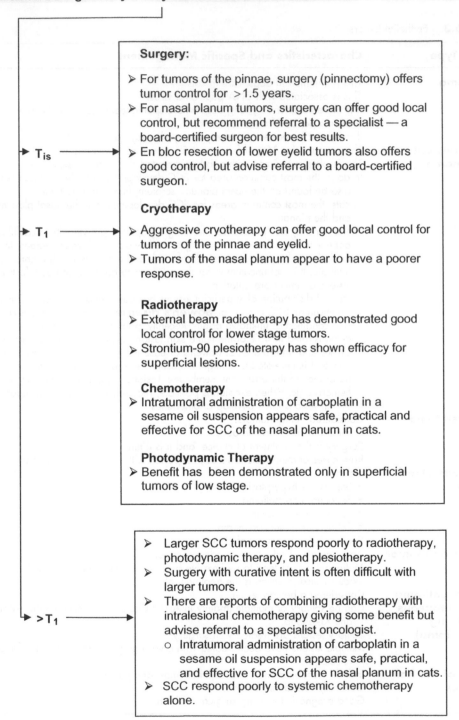

Figure 6.2. Feline squamous cell carcinoma.

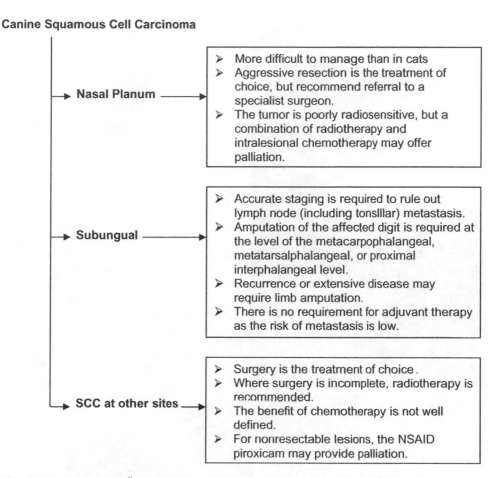

Figure 6.3. Canine squamous cell carcinoma.

Mesenchymal Tumors of the Skin (Soft-Tissue Sarcomas)

- In total, these tumors represent 9–14% of all canine skin neoplasms.
- The term *soft-tissue sarcoma* refers to a group of tumors of mesenchymal origin that develop in the subcutaneous tissues. Tumors include fibrosarcoma, peripheral nerve sheath tumors, neurofibrosarcomas, hemangiopericytomas, myxosarcomas, liposarcomas, and others.
- Irrespective of tissue type, soft-tissue sarcomas may be considered as a group since they are characterized by common morphological and behavioral features. However, these tumors do vary in their degree of malignancy and a definitive diagnosis is necessary for prognosis (Figure 6.5, 6.6; Table 6.4).
- Soft-tissue sarcomas are more common in the dog than in the cat.
- The most common soft-tissue sarcomas in the dog are peripheral nerve sheath tumors and hemagiopericytoma (may be of similar cellular origin). In the cat fibrosarcoma is the most common tumor. Feline injection-site sarcomas of cats are discussed in more detail in the musculoskeletal section.
- Soft-tissue sarcomas usually develop in older animals with a mean age of 9 years in dogs and cats. Fibrosarcomas have occasionally been found in dogs as young as 6 months of age. The distribution of soft-tissue sarcomas is widespread and sites include the head, limbs, and trunk.
- The rate of growth is variable. Most soft tissue sarcomas are slow-growing, while the anaplastic tumors often grow at an alarming rate.

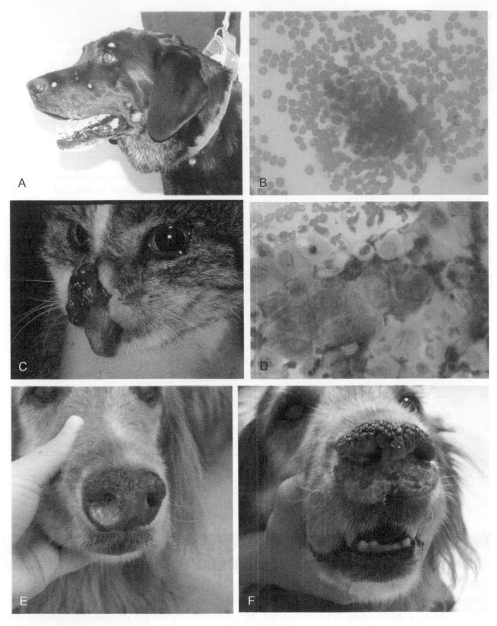

Figure 6.4. Epithelial tumors in dogs and cats: canine papillomas (A), cytology of canine basal cell tumor (B), highly aggressive and advanced feline squamous cell carcinoma affecting the nasal planum (C), and cytology of squamous cell carcinoma (D). Squamous cell carcinoma of the nasal planum in a dog at presentation (E) and at progression (F). (Images courtesy of E. Milne, M. Turek, and D. Argyle.)

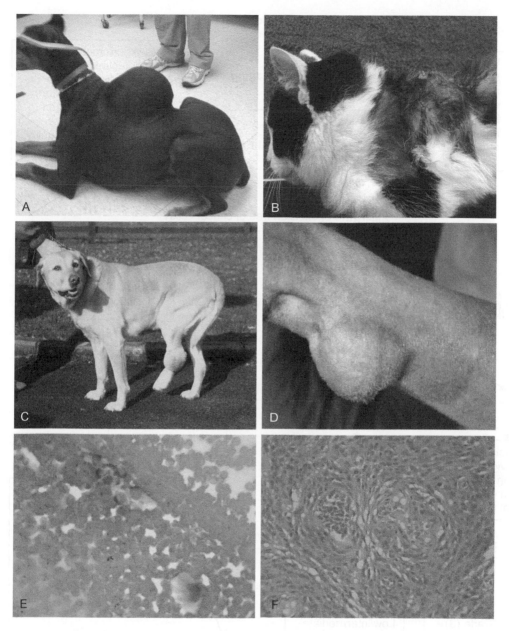

Figure 6.5. Mesenchymal tumors: large fibrosarcoma affecting the dorsum of a Doberman pinscher (A), feline injection site sarcoma (B), canine myxosarcoma (C), canine hemangiopericytoma (D) with cytology (E) and histology (F). (Images courtesy of E. Milne, M. Turek, and D. Argyle.)

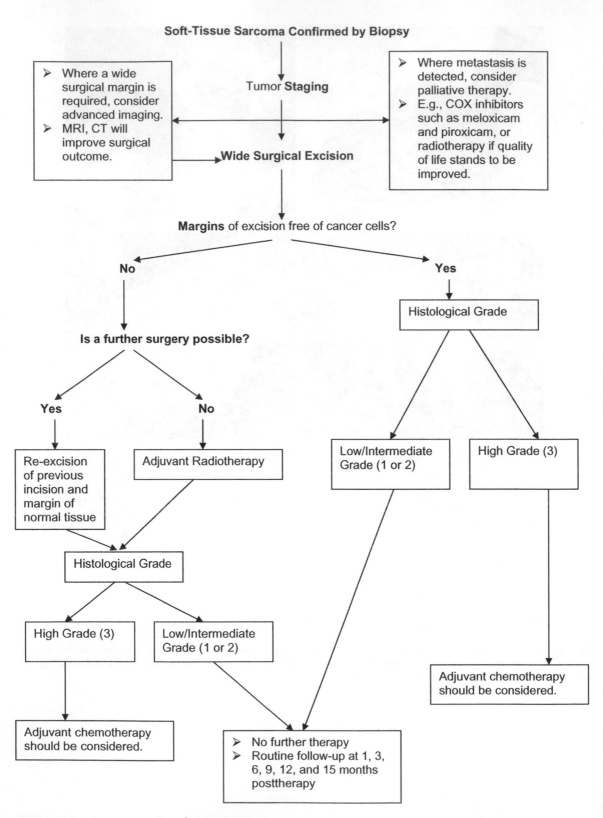

Figure 6.6. Decision tree for soft-tissue tumors.

Table 6.4. Staging system for canine soft-tissue sarcomas

Stage	T	N	M	Grade
I	Any T	N_0	M_0	I–II
II	T_{1a-1b}, T_{2a}	N_0	M_0	III
III	T_{2b}	N_0	M_0	III
IV	Any T	N_1	Any M	I–III
	Any T	Any N	M_1	I–III

T_1 = Tumor <5 cm at largest diameter.
T_{1a} = Superficial tumor.
T_{1b} = Deep tumor.
T_2 = Tumor >5 cm at largest diameter.
T_{2a} = Superficial tumor.
T_{2b} = Deep tumor.
N_0 = No lymph node metastasis.
N_1 = Lymph node metastasis.
M_0 = No distant metastasis.
M_1 = Distant metastasis.

- As a group, these tumors are characterized by
  - **An infiltrative pattern of growth.** The tumors may appear to be encapsulated due to the formation of a **pseudocapsule** composed of compressed cancer cells. The tumor invariably extends beyond this structure.
  - Regional lymph node or distant metastasis is **uncommon** except for high-grade tumors.
  - **In dogs, histopathological grade is predictive of metastasis**, and the completeness of surgical excision predicts local recurrence. Histopathological grade is determined by the degree of cellular differentiation, the percent of necrosis, and the mitotic rate of the tumor.
  - Large bulky tumors tend to have a poor response to radiotherapy and chemotherapy.
- The treatment of choice is wide surgical excision; in most cases it is necessary to resect the entire anatomic compartment if all neoplastic cells are to be eradicated.
- Failure to achieve this aim accounts for the high rate of local recurrence. It is therefore essential to identify the tumor and to carefully plan the surgical procedure prior to attempting therapy.
- The diagnostic approach for mesenchymal tumors is as for other tumors described. However, where extensive surgeries are required, **advanced imaging using either CT or MRI is highly recommended for accurate surgical planning.**
- The potential for metastatic spread is variable and correlates directly with histologic grade. In general, hemangiopericytoma has a high rate of local recurrence if not treated adequately but rarely metastasizes. Approximately 20–25% of fibrosarcomas metastasize and, although metastasis is frequently stated as being via hematogenous dissemination to the lung, in our experience lymph node involvement is quite common.
- Hemangiosarcoma is a tumor of mesenchymal origin (endothelial cells) that can affect the skin. However, its biologic behavior is distinctive from that of the tumors collectively referred to as soft-tissue sarcomas.
- Hemangiosarcoma is a particularly malignant tumor that may arise at any site, and metastatic rates as high as 90% are documented.
- In the cutaneous form, hemangiosarcoma tumors that invade the subcutis or deeper are associated with a worse prognosis, due to a higher probability of metastasis, than tumors confined to the dermis.

Key Points

Therapy for Soft-Tissue Sarcomas

- Surgery is the treatment of choice with wide surgical margins. Where surgical excision is incomplete, and no further surgery is possible, external beam radiotherapy offers excellent local tumor control and increased survival time.
- Adjuvant chemotherapy protocols tend to be restricted to
  - Patients with incomplete resections and no access to radiotherapy.
  - Patients with grade III tumors and at higher risk of metastasis.
  - Subcutaneous hemangiosarcoma.
  - Typical protocols include doxorubicin, which is administered at 25–30 mg/m^2 IV every 21 days for 4–5 cycles.
- In general, prognosis for most soft-tissue sarcomas is good if local disease can be controlled. For certain tumors with high rates of metastasis, including hemangiosarcoma, the prognosis remains poor.

Injection-Site Sarcomas in Cats

Key Points

- Injection-site sarcoma in cats is a complex disease with a poorly understood pathogenesis.
- It is considered to be a disease associated with postvaccination inflammation through both rabies and FeLV vaccination strategies.
- The term *injection-site sarcoma* is used because tumor development has been reported after administration of other injectable medications such as methyl prednisolone and certain antibiotics. However, a statistical link has only been made for FeLV or rabies vaccine administration.
- The incidence of the disease varies between countries, but has rapidly increased over the past 10 years.
- Tumors are typically mesenchymal in origin and fibrosarcoma is the most common. Other histologies include osteosarcoma, chondrosarcoma, malignant fibrous histiocytoma, undifferentiated sarcoma, and others.
- Histologically, these tumors are distinct from soft tissue sarcomas. They are more likely to have necrosis, inflammatory cell infiltrates, increased mitotic rate, and pleomorphism.
- This is a locally aggressive disease associated with a risk of metastasis of about 20%.
- The latency period of tumor development is variable, ranging from a few months to several years.

The following is a synopsis of recommendations:

1. Decision Making: Vaccination

The epidemiological evidence puts vaccination as an inciting cause for this disease. Consequently, recommendations are now in place to promote prevention of the disease, or at least early detection. These include the following:

- Avoid administering vaccinations in the interscapular space.
- Subcutaneous rather than intramuscular vaccination is preferred because tumor development can be detected more easily and earlier.
- Rabies/FeLV vaccines should be administered on the distal aspect of the right (rabies) and left (FeLV) pelvic limbs. Other vaccines should be administered in the right distal shoulder.
- Administration of any vaccine should proceed only after strong consideration of the patient's exposure risk, the zoonotic potential, and the overall medical significance.

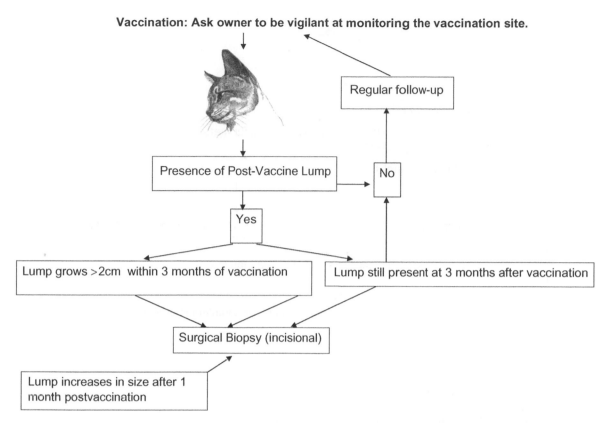

Vaccination: Ask owner to be vigilant at monitoring the vaccination site.

Figure 6.7. Decision making: Past vaccination lumps. Feline image courtesy of Romina Chirre, GraphicXperts, USA.

- The pet owner should be informed about the risk of vaccine-associated sarcoma and asked to monitor the site closely.

2. Decision Making: Postvaccination Lumps

- Some rabies and FeLV vaccinations will produce postvaccination lumps (inflammatory granulomas) in nearly 100% of cats vaccinated (Figure 6.7).
- Most of these will resolve over a 2–3 month period, and most vaccine-associated sarcomas will not occur prior to 3 months following vaccination.
- Consequently it is recommended that all postvaccination lumps be removed if still present at 3 months after vaccination, if they grow beyond 2 cm within 3 months, or if they increase in size after 1 month postvaccination.
- Surgical biopsy is recommended prior to definitive removal.

3. Decision Making: Injection-Site Sarcoma in Cats

- In light of the invasive nature of this tumor, the key to effective treatment is aggressive intervention early in the course of the disease.
- Once a vaccine-associated tumor develops, management and control can be difficult. Here is a summary of appropriate steps (Figure 6.8):
  - Presurgical tissue biopsy is highly recommended. Cytology is unreliable due to the pleomorphic appearance of fibroblasts in granulomas that cannot be easily distinguished from malignant mesenchymal cells.

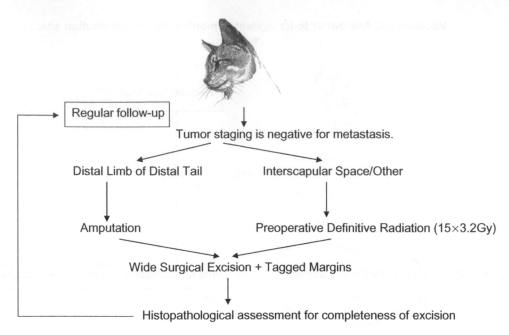

Figure 6.8. Decision making in FISS.

- Complete staging:
  - Blood count and chemistry.
  - Urinalysis.
  - Thoracic radiography to rule out pulmonary metastasis.
  - MRI or CT is highly recommended for accurate surgical assessment of the extent of disease.
- Due to the relatively low metastatic rate, treatment is aimed at achieving local tumor control.
- Due to the invasive nature of the disease, single surgical excision, even with wide margins, is rarely curative for vaccine-associated sarcoma.
- Local recurrence is common and a second surgery is always difficult. For lesions on limbs, amputation would appear to have a higher success rate than single surgeries for VAS in alternative sites.
- Radiotherapy has been shown to improve outcome over surgery alone.
- Two options are available:
  - Preoperative radiotherapy (has been shown to give local control to 23 months).
  - Postoperative radiotherapy (has been shown to give control to 12 months in 1 study).
- The aim of preoperative radiotherapy is not necessarily to reduce the size of palpable tumor, but rather to "sterilize" any residual microscopic disease that might be left after radical surgical excision. Among the advantages of this approach is the fact that the radiation treatment field is smaller than in the postoperative setting, because no surgery has been performed and no surgical scar is present. This limits the amount of normal tissue that is exposed to radiation and makes the radiation field easier to manage and treat effectively.
- For cats with tumors or incisions that are overlying vital organs such as CNS, kidney, or lung, we recommend radiotherapy using an electron beam from a linear accelerator.
- Following radiation, surgical excision is performed and margins examined for completeness of resection. At surgery, excisional margins are tagged and/or dyed with India ink.
- The most favorable clinical outcome is achieved when cats are treated at a referral institution where radical surgical excision is more common. Radical surgery often includes removal of 3–5 cm margins of normal tissue, multiple tissue planes, body wall resection, or ostectomy as indicated.
- In summary, optimal treatment of injection-site sarcoma without metastasis involves preoperative radiation followed by radical surgical excision. In some cases where amputation will result in a large margin of normal tissue, preoperative radiation may not be indicated. These cases are rare.

4. The Role of Chemotherapy

- The role of chemotherapy is poorly defined. In general, this tumor is considered poorly chemosensitive.
- For animals that do not undergo radiation, or whose margins are in doubt after radical surgery, or who have metastatic disease, chemotherapy may be offered as an adjunct.
- For patients that have had wide surgical excision following radiation, the addition of chemotherapy would appear to have little benefit.
- For cats that do not have radiation but have surgery alone (with curative intent), the addition of chemotherapy may improve the time to tumor recurrence.
- Drugs that have been used include doxorubicin, carboplatin, doxil (liposome encapsulated doxorubicin). There is no benefit of doxil over doxorubicin.

The prognosis of cats with Injection-site sarcomas remains guarded; however, prolonged local tumor control is achievable with aggressive intervention including radiotherapy and surgery early in the course of disease.

Round Cell Tumors (Figure 6.9)

- Collectively, mast cell tumors, cutaneous lymphoma, cutaneous plasma cell tumors, transmissible venereal tumors (TVT), histiocytomas, and neuroendocrine (Merkel cell) tumors are referred to as **round cell tumors** due to the morphology of the cancer cells.
- These tumor types are covered in other chapters in this book. Often the clinician is faced with a histopathological diagnosis of round cell tumor, and will require special stains or Immunohistochemistry to further identify the cell type and ascertain the appropriate diagnosis.
- Table 6.5 is intended as a guide, and an indication of the service that your pathologist should offer (i.e., a typical round cell immunohistochemical panel).

Melanocytic Tumors

Key Points
- Melanomas arise from melanocytes situated in the basal layer of the epidermis (cutaneous or dermal melanoma), the epithelium of the gingiva (oral melanoma), or the nail bed (digital melanoma).
- Cutaneous and digital melanomas are less common tumors than oral melanomas.
- Cutaneous melanomas arising from haired skin are usually benign. They are classically small (<2 cm), pigmented nodules. Instances of spontaneous regression of such lesions are documented. Mitotic rate is highly predictive of malignant behavior. A mitotic rate of <3/10 high-power fields is highly predictive of benign behavior.
- Melanomas arising from the mucocutaneous junction have a higher risk of metastasis than dermal tumors.
- Digital melanomas also have a higher risk of metastasis.
- Malignant melanomas may be pigmented, but amelanotic forms are recognized.
- Ulceration and secondary infection are common features of malignant tumors.
- Regional lymph node metastasis and widespread distant metastases frequently occur early in the course of the disease in association with malignant melanoma. It is essential that clinical staging includes a thorough physical evaluation of regional lymph nodes and radiographic evaluation of the thoracic and abdominal cavity.

Table 6.5. Typical round cell immunohistochemical panels

Stain	Results
Toluidine Blue Chymase HC Tryptase IHC	Positive = Mast cell tumor
CD3	Positive = T cell lymphoma If CD18 and MHCII are also positive, the tumor may be of histiocytic origin.
CD79a/Pax 5	Positive = B cell lymphoma **or** plasmacytoma If CD18 and MHCII are also positive, the tumor may be of histiocytic origin.
CD18 MHC II	When other stains are negative: • If CD18 is positive and MHC II is positive, the tumor may be of histiocytic origin. • If CD18 is positive and MHC II is negative, the tumor may be a mast cell tumor,

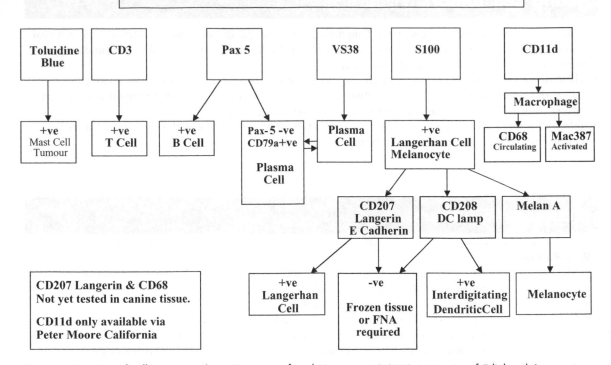

Figure 6.9. Round cell tumors markers. (Courtesy of Neil Macintyre, R(D)SVS, University of Edinburgh.)

Therapy for Melanocytic Tumors

• For benign cutaneous lesions (pigmented, located on haired skin, <2 cm in diameter, mitotic rate <3/10 HPF), surgery is curative.
• Therapy for primary malignant tumors requires radical surgical excision; surgical margins of up to 3 cm are necessary to ensure complete resection. Digital melanoma requires at least amputation of the affected digit. Limb amputation may be necessary to achieve an adequate margin.

- Alternative therapies include radiation, photodynamic therapy, local hyperthermia, and intralesional platinum-based chemotherapeutic compounds. Referral to a specialist oncologist is recommended for these modalities.
- Therapeutic melanoma vaccines have been used with varying degrees of success. Only one vaccine product (distributed by Merial) is conditionally licensed for use in the United States in dogs with oral melanoma, and it is not available in Europe.
- Efficacy of systemic chemotherapy is considered poor for malignant melanoma.
- Oral melanomas are considered in Chapter 11.

Ear Canal Tumors of Dogs and Cats

Key Points
- These are not uncommon tumors in both species, and may be associated with chronic inflammation from otitis externa.
- Clinical signs include chronic irritation, presence of a mass lesion, aural discharge, pain, and odor. In severe cases, with middle or inner involvement, patients may present with vestibular signs or Horner's syndrome.
- The most common benign tumors in both species are
  - Inflammatory polyps
  - Ceruminous adenomas
  - Papillomas
  - Basal cell tumors
- The most common malignant tumors are
  - Dogs
    - Ceruminous gland adenocarcinoma
    - Squamous cell carcinoma
    - Carcinoma of undetermined origin
  - Cats
    - Ceruminous gland adenocarcinoma
    - Squamous cell carcinoma

Therapy

- For benign lesions, conservative surgical resection in both species offers a good prognosis.
- For malignant lesions, ear canal ablation and lateral bulla osteotomy should be considered the treatment of choice:
  - Prognosis for dogs is better than for cats.
  - Local radiotherapy may be considered where incomplete resection is achieved.

7
MAST CELL TUMORS

Suzanne Murphy and Malcolm J. Brearley

Part 1: Cutaneous Mast Cell Tumors in the Dog

Key Points
- Mast cell tumors (MCTs) are common skin tumors of dogs (16–21% of all cutaneous tumors).
  - Primary MCTs can occur in other tissues: conjunctiva, connective tissue or the gastrointestinal tract. The noncutaneous MCTs are rare with a different biological behavior and will not be discussed here.
- Cutaneous MCTs occur in middle-aged dogs.
- No sex predilection reported.
- Overrepresented breeds include Boxer, Staffordshire Bull Terrier, Labrador, Golden Retriever, Weimeraner, Beagle, Schnauzer, Boston Terrier, and Shar-pei.
- The etiology is generally unknown but chronic skin inflammation may be a predisposing factor.

Pathology and Behavior

- MCTs exhibit a wide range of behavior.
- All MCTs are locally infiltrating to varying degrees.
- Approximately 30% are aggressive, rapidly metastasizing to adjacent skin, the drainage lymph node, and distant organs (in particular liver, spleen, and bone marrow).
- Mast cells have intracytoplasmic granules containing biologically active molecules (e.g., proteases, cytokines, heparin, and histamine) important in mast cell's normal role of mediating inflammation.
- These intracytoplasmic granules stain metachromatically.
- Tumor cells may degranulate, releasing these vasoactive amines spontaneously or following trauma.
- These chemicals induce an inflammatory reaction that causes the mass of the tumor to increase rapidly in size and then decrease again as the inflammation recedes.
- Some MCTs present with associated local edema, pruritus, and hemorrhage.
- Simple palpation of an MCT may induce erythema and wheal formation associated with degranulation (so-called "Darier's sign").
- Systemic absorption of histamine can also cause paraneoplastic vomiting together with gastric or duodenal ulceration leading to melena.
- Other uncommon systemic effects include hypotensive collapse and respiratory distress.

Clinical Presentation

- MCTs can mimic any other skin lesion.
- They may develop anywhere on the body.
- Well-differentiated cutaneous MCTs tend to be slow-growing, hairless, solitary lesions and may be present for months.

- Poorly differentiated MCTs tend to be rapidly growing, ulcerated, and pruritic lesions with small *satellite lesions* close by. There may be evidence of local lymphadenopathy or organomegaly on abdominal palpation.
- A significant minority of MCTs look and feel like lipomas—fine needle aspirate cytology can be used to differentiate.
- 10–15% of dogs have multiple primary MCTs either at initial presentation or as subsequent events. This clinical picture is different from regrowth or a poorly differentiated tumor with satellite metastases.

Diagnostic Investigations

- For the majority of MCTs FNA cytology gives a diagnosis (but not grade) and allows presurgical planning.
- Mast cell tumors, like most round cell tumors, readily exfoliate.
- Cytologically the cells can be distinguished from other round cells by their metachromatically staining granules, and the "spotty fried egg" appearance of the cells usually makes diagnosis easy (Figure 7.1).
- Poorly differentiated MCTs may lack these granules, necessitating more specialized staining techniques.
- FNA cytology cannot replace histopathology when it comes to predicting the tumor behavior.
- FNA cytology can be used to examine local lymph nodes, but beware—draining lymph nodes can contain significant numbers of *normal* mast cells.

Staging

- Table 7.1 shows the modified WHO Clinical Staging System for canine MCTs.
- NB: Several controversies with the current staging scheme.
- Dogs with multiple MCTs are automatically assigned to stage III.
- However, survival is dictated by the grade of each tumor rather than the fact that the dog has had a tumor before or has more than one at presentation.

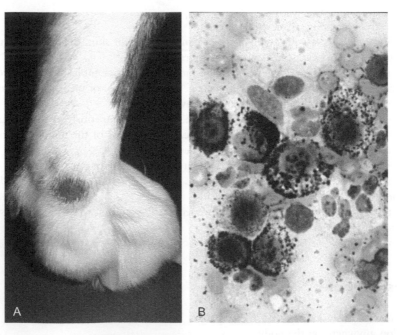

Figure 7.1. Mast cell tumors can present in many guises (A). However, cytological examination can be diagnostic (B). B demonstrates the typical cytological picture of canine mast cell disease with metochromatic granules. (Images courtesy of Suzanne Murphy.)

Table 7.1. WHO staging for canine mast cell tumors

Clinical Stage	Description
0	One tumor incompletely excised from the dermis, identified histologically, without regional lymph node involvement
I	One tumor confined to dermis without regional lymph node involvement
II	One tumor confined to the dermis with regional lymph node involvement
III	Multiple dermal tumors or large infiltrating tumor with or without regional lymph node involvement
IV	Any tumor with distant metastasis or recurrence with metastasis

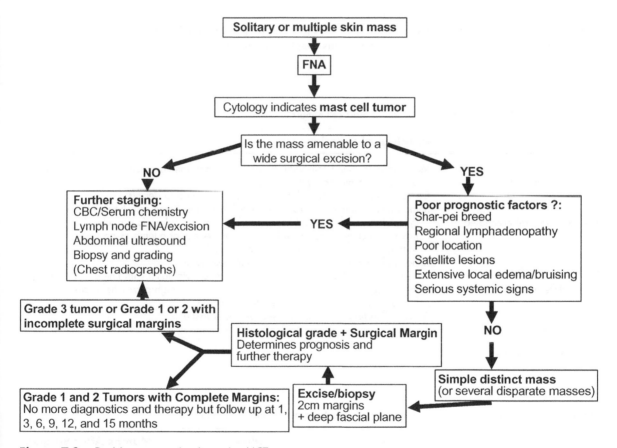

Figure 7.2. Decisions on staging in canine MCT.

- A number of breeds (Boxer, Visla, Weimeraner, Golden Retriever) seem particularly prone to multiple mast cell tumors.

The mechanics of staging
- A pragmatic approach, based on clinical judgment together with cytological evaluation, is recommended as to whether to stage the tumor before knowing the grade or resect the tumor and then stage as appropriate.
- An algorithm for MCT staging in the dog is given in Figure 7.2.

- Most dogs will have tumors that are unlikely to metastasize.
- The regional lymph node is the most common site for metastatic spread.
- A few mast cells can be normal in a lymph node, especially one draining any mast cell tumor.
- Mast cell rich buffy coat is **not** specific for mast cell tumor metastasis.
- Few dogs will have mast cells identified in bone marrow biopsies.

Prognostic Factors

- The most useful predictor of outcome for these dogs is the histological grade of mast cell tumors (Tables 7.2, 7.3):
  - The grade is based on cell morphology together with tumor invasiveness into the normal surrounding tissue.
  - Cytology alone cannot fully assess the grade.
- Well-differentiated MCTs treated by surgery alone carry a good prognosis as metastatic spread is very rare (see the section "Treatment Options," later in this chapter; see also Figure 7.3).

Table 7.2. Histological criteria for grade of mast cell tumors*

Grade	Histological Criteria
1 Well differentiated	Monomorphic round cells with distinct cytoplasm, medium-sized intracytoplasmic granules, no mitotic figures noted. Compact groups or rows of neoplastic cells *confined to dermis*.
2 Intermediately differentiated	Some pleomorphic cells – round to ovoid in shape. Some cells having less distinct cytoplasm with large and hyperchromatic intracytoplasmic granules, but others have distinct cytoplasm with fine granules. Areas of edema or necrosis are noted. Mitotic figures are 0–2 per high power field. Tumor *infiltrating lower dermis/subcutaneous tissue*.
3 Poorly differentiated	Dense sheets of pleomorphic cells with indistinct cytoplasm with fine or not obvious intracytoplasmic granules. Mitotic figures 3–6 per high-power field. Edema, hemorrhage, necrosis and ulceration common. Tumor *infiltrating lower dermis/subcutaneous tissue*.

*Patnaik et al., 1984.

Table 7.3. Grade as a predictor of survival in dogs treated with surgery alone

Study	Grade	% alive	Months After Surgery
Bostock 1973	Well	77	7
	Intermediate	45	7
	Poor	13	7
Patnaik et al. 1984	Well	93	48
	Intermediate	47	48
	Poor	6	48
Murphy et al. 2004	Well	100	18*
	Intermediate	87	18
	Poor	36	18

*Median follow-up time.

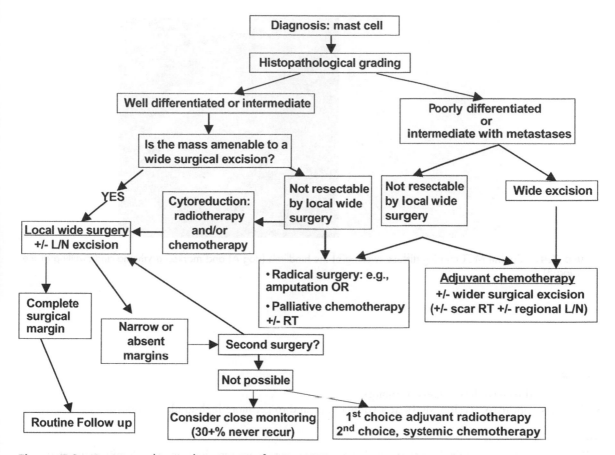

Figure 7.3. Decision making in the treatment of canine MCT.

- Intermediate-grade tumors generally have a good prognosis (85% alive at 2 years) although 10–15% will undergo metastatic spread:
  - Ki-67 and Ag-NOR counts may help define this subset.
- Poorly differentiated tumors carry a poor prognosis as 80+% will metastasize.

Predictors of Behavior at Presentation (i.e., Before the Grade Is Known)

History
- Dogs with tumors present unchanged in size or appearance for months prior to surgery are reported to do well.
- Rapidly growing tumors tend to carry a poor prognosis.
- Any paraneoplastic signs (anorexia, vomiting, melena) or widespread edema or erythema have a poorer prognosis (Figure 7.4).

Clinical stage
- Draining lymphadenopathy, enlarged liver/spleen, or a primary tumor with satellite lesions would be viewed as worrying.

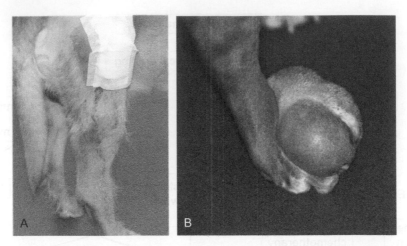

Figure 7.4. Canine MCT causing diffuse swelling of the hindlimb (dog A) and marked erythema and swelling of the foot (dog B).

Breed
- Boxers tend to have less aggressive tumors.
- Shar-peis appear to develop MCTs at a younger age and to get more high-grade tumors.

Site
- Perianal, preputial, inguinal, or subungual sites or mucocutaneous junctions are anecdotally associated with a poorer prognosis.

Treatment Options (see also Figure 7.3)

Surgery

- Pretreat with an H1 and H2 blocker prior to surgery, as necessary.
- Apply basic oncological surgical principles when the tumor is resected.
- Current recommendations for surgical margin are:
  - 2 times diameter of tumor, up to 2 cm, in each direction.
  - Include a deep fascial plane in all cases.
  - Almost certainly curative for well differentiated MCTs and majority of intermediates.
  - At least 30% of intermediate MCTs with histologically incomplete or narrow margins do not regrow.
- Submit tumor(s) for histopathological grading.
- For MCTs that are well- or intermediate-grade without evidence of metastatic disease surgery has the potential to cure.
  - *These are the majority of mast cell tumors.*
- For poorly differentiated tumors, surgery may alleviate the signs associated with the primary lesion, but these tumors are very infiltrative and are prone to wound breakdown so they should be approached with care.
- Adjuvant chemotherapy is recommended against metastatic disease.

Radiotherapy

- The major role of radiotherapy is in the adjuvant setting.
- Well- or intermediate-grade MCTs with incomplete margins in an area of a second surgery are unlikely to produce a better result (e.g., distal limbs).
  - NB: at least 30% of intermediate MCTs with histologically incomplete or narrow margins do not regrow.
- For small MCTs at difficult surgical sites, RT can be used as sole modality.
- Beware of gross degranulation of bulk tumors with severe systemic effects.

Chemotherapy

- Chemotherapy alone is rarely curative. Its main indications are
  - Palliative therapy for metastatic intermediate or high grade tumors
  - Adjuvant therapy for poorly differentiated MCTs
  - Neo-adjuvant therapy prior to a definitive surgery or radiotherapy
- Vinblastine, prednisolone, and CCNU appear to be the most active drugs.
  - Vinblastine: 2 mg/m^2 IV weekly ×4 weeks, then alternate weeks
  - Prednisolone: 1 mg/kg po b.i.d 7–14 days, reducing to once daily and then to alternate day
  - CCNU: 70 mg/m^2 p.o. q.21d or 90 mg/m^2 p.o. q.28d
- Two main combination protocols have been described:
  - Vinblastine + prednisolone (Table 7.4)
  - CCNU single agent (Table 7.5)
  - The current recommendation is to use the Vinblastine/Prednisolone protocol in the first instance.

Multiple Tumors

- Patients with multiple tumors are often treated as though each tumor were a primary lesion: i.e., surgery with wide surgical margins for each tumor is recommended.
- In cases where this would be difficult, consider adjunctive therapy with one of the chemotherapy protocols described above.

Table 7.4.   Vinblastine/prednisolone protocol for canine MCT

Week	1	2	3	4	5	6	7	8	9	10	11	12
Vinblastine 2 mg/m^2	X	X	X	X		X		X		X		X
Prednisolone 1 mg/kg daily	X	X										
Prednisolone 1 mg/kg e.o.d			X	X	X	X	X	X	X	X	X	X

Table 7.5.   Single-agent CCNU protocol for canine MCT

Week	1	2	3	4	5	6	7	8	9	10	11	12
CCNU 70 mg/m^2	X			X			X			X		

Other Treatments

- Prednisolone alone (systemically or intralesionally)
  - As palliative therapy to control inflammation.
  - There is in vitro evidence that glucocorticoids have an effect on MCT proliferation, but their clinical efficacy on survival rate is variable.
- Cimetidine or ranitidine and other GI protectants are recommended as supportive therapy to protect the GI tract against ulceration.
- Deionized water instilled into the surgery bed (at the time of surgery or where the pathologist reports "incomplete margins") has been described.
  - In theory the hypotonic solution causes mast cell lysis.
  - Clinical efficacy is unproven and controversial.
  - Reported success may be related more to the fact that a significant group of tumors reported with incomplete margins do not grow back.

See also the algorithm to aid decision making in treatment in Figure 7.3.

Part 2: Feline Mast Cell Disease

Introduction

- Two major anatomical forms of mast cell tumors exist in cats:
  - Cutaneous
  - Visceral
- Intestinal only
- Diffuse splenic with mastocytosis
- Generalized visceral

Cutaneous Feline MCTs

- Cutaneous MCTs are relatively common:
  - 20% of feline cutaneous tumors in the U.S.
  - 8% of feline cutaneous tumors in a U.K. study of 1986

Visceral (Splenic and Intestinal) MCTs

- Primary MCTs of the feline gastrointestinal tract is reported as third most common tumor at this site (after lymphoma and adenocarcinoma).
- Splenic MCT (diffuse involvement) is a major cause of splenomegaly in the cat.
- Visceral primary MCT can have disseminated cutaneous metastases.

Pathology and Behavior

There are three cutaneous presentations (Tables 7.6, 7.7).
- The more common is the **mastocytic** form:
  - Seen in older cats, subdivided into

Table 7.6.   Histological criteria used in determining grade of feline mast cell tumors*

Grade	Histological Criteria
Compact	Monomorphic round cells with abundant eosinophilic cytoplasm, and intracytoplasmic granules easily identified on toluidine blue staining. No mitotic figures noted. Few eosinophils associated with the lesions. Tumor infiltrating mid and deep dermis but well circumscribed.
Diffuse	As above, but some giant cells and marked anisocytosis/anisokaryosis. Mitotic figures are 2–3 per high-power field. Tumor infiltrating mid and deep dermis.
Histiocytic	Sheets of histiocyte-like mast cells with abundant eosinophilic vacuolated cytoplasm with fine or not obvious intracytoplasmic granules. Numerous eosinophils and lymphocyte aggregates. Tumor in the junction of dermis and subcutis.

* Wilcock et al., 1986.

Table 7.7.   Estimated frequency of each type of feline cutaneous mast cell tumor

Grade	Frequency
Compact	70–85%
Diffuse	5–10%
Histiocytic	10–20%

- ○ The more common **compact mastocytic** does not metastasize and has locally limited invasion
  - ○ The rarer **diffuse mastocytic** forms are more locally aggressive and can metastasize. (Visceral metastasis is rare.)
- The rarer **histiocytic** form of MCTs
  - Is typically seen in cats under 4 years old.
  - Siamese cats are overrepresented.
  - Presents as multiple lesions.
  - The neoplastic cells resemble histiocytes histologically.
  - Spontaneous regression over a period of 4–24 months is common.

Clinical Presentation

- Cutaneous MCTs of cats are reportedly more common on the head and neck.
- They can be single or multiple, nodular or plaquelike (not dissimilar to eosinophilic granuloma complex) but typically appear as round, hairless lesions.
  - Like dogs, the vasoactive granules within the mast cell can cause the lesion to appear erythrematous, cause paraneoplastic gastrointestinal signs and cause the lesion to be pruritic, leading to self trauma, ulceration and bleeding. Cats can also present with systemic signs alone.

Diagnostic Investigations

- Biopsy (excisional) is preferred to FNA.
  - Unlike dogs, feline MCTs frequently have poorly staining intracytoplasmic granules.
  - Mast cells are often seen associated with eosinophils in both eosinophilic granuloma complex or MCT, and therefore a biopsy rather than FNA may be more useful to distinguish the two.

Staging

- As about 5–10% of cats with cutaneous MCT are secondary to primary visceral disease, all cats with diffuse or multiple MCTs should be staged by abdominal palpation, ultrasonography, and routine hematology.
  - Peripheral eosinophilia and up to 40% of cats with visceral disease have mast cell–positive buffy coats.

Treatment Options

Surgery

- Compact tumors have limited local infiltration and a low metastatic rate; therefore, excision with a narrow margin is usually successful.
- Diffuse tumors have a higher incidence of recurrence and need a wider margin of excision, although nowhere in the literature is that margin defined.
  - The completeness of margin is not thought to be a useful prognostic indicator as to recurrence.
  - Cats with mastocytosis and diffuse splenic involvement can achieve durable remission following splenectomy.

Radiotherapy

- Anecdotally external beam RT has been used for "incompletely" resected tumors.
- Strontium 90 plesiotherapy has been used very successfully to control multiple cutaneous mast cell tumors.

Chemotherapy

- In theory, cats with metastatic disease or with intestinal disease could benefit from chemotherapy.
- Chemotherapy for feline MCT is as yet unproven. Discuss with an oncologist.
  - Vinblastine—but efficacy unproven.
    - 2 mg/m^2 dose (used in dogs) causes neutropenia in cats.
    - Unpublished reports suggest that 1.5 mg/m^2 may be better tolerated.
  - CCNU has been used to treat an oral MCT (single case).
  - CCNU has been used for GI tract MCT (unpublished) at 50 mg/m^2 q. 28d.

Other Treatments

- Prednisolone has been tried for unresectable tumors but with little effect.
  - If there is any splenic involvement and splenectomy is planned, steroids should not be used postoperatively because the postulated immuno-modulating effect of splenectomy would be lost.

Prognostic Factors

- Histological grading does not appear to be of prognostic value.

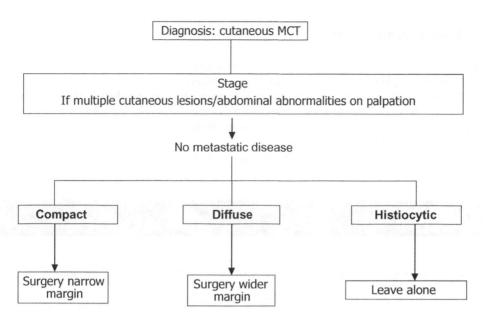

Figure 7.5. Decision making in feline cutaneous MCT.

Cutaneous

- Clinical stage
  - Stage I or II—MST not reached
  - Stage III or IV—MST = 582d and 283d, respectively
- Single vs. multiple
  - Cats with multiple tumors had a shorter survival time (median 375 days) than those with single masses (MST not reached).

An algorithm to aid decision making is shown in Figure 7.5.

Splenic Mast Cell Tumors

- MCT primary to the spleen in cats is most common in older non-purebred cats.
- Signs include nonspecific illness or chronic vomiting due to histamine release causing gastroduodenal ulceration.
- Liver, lymph nodes, and bone marrow are also commonly affected.
- Staging includes a CBC, biochemical profile, urinalysis, FeLV, FIV, thoracic radiographs, abdominal ultrasonography, and bone arrow aspirate.
- Fine needle aspiration cytology or biopsy of spleen is indicated. The diagnosis is sometimes made from ascitic fluid or blood smear.
- As initial treatment, splenectomy normalizes other disease within 5 weeks. The median survival is 12 months.
- As adjunctive therapy, the use of corticosteroids is controversial. Chemotherapy (CCNU, vinblastine) has not been reported.
- Supportive therapy consists of preoperative H_1 and H_2 antihistamines to reduce risk of gastrointestinal damage and shock, especially during surgery.
- The same drugs may be palliative for clinical signs but results are variable.

Intestinal Mast Cell Tumors

- Intestinal MCT are most common in the small intestine, causing vomiting, inappetance, and weight loss.
- Staging is the same as splenic MCTs. Metastasis is very common.
- Prognosis is poor. Initial treatment consists of a wide surgical excision including 5–10 cm of normal bowel.
- Adjunctive therapy has not been described, but consider chemotherapy with prednisolone or CCNU. Other drugs such as vincristine or L-asparaginase may have anecdotal success.
- Supportive care is as for other intestinal tumors.
- Prednisolone may be palliative after wound healing is complete.

Further Reading

Part 1

Bostock D. 1973. The prognosis following surgical removal of mastocytomas in dogs. Journal of Small Animal Practice 14:27–40.

Dobson J.M., Samuel S., Milstein H., Rogers K., Wood J.L. 2002. Canine neoplasia in the UK: Estimates of incidence rates from a population of insured dogs. Journal of Small Animal Practice 43(6):240–246.

Frimberger A., Moore A., LaRue S. et al. 1997. Radiotherapy of incompletely resected moderately differentiated mast cell tumours in the dog: 37 cases (1989–1993). Journal of the American Animal Hospital Association 33:320–323.

Fulcher R.P., Ludwig L.L., Bergman P.J., Newman S.J., Simpson A.M., Patnaik A.K. 2006. Evaluation of a two-centimeter lateral surgical margin for excision of grade I and grade II cutaneous mast cell tumors in dogs. Journal of the American Veterinary Medical Association 15;228:210–215.

Hayes A., Adams V., Smith K., Maglennon G., Murphy S. Vinblastine and prednisolone chemotherapy for surgically excised grade III canine cutaneous mast cell tumours. Veterinary and Comparative Oncology. In press.

Jaffe M., Hosgood G., Kerwin S. et al. 2000. Deionised water as an adjunct to surgery for the treatment of canine cutaneous mast cell tumors. Journal of Small Animal Practice 41:1–7.

LaDue T., Price G., Dodge R. et al. 1998. Radiation therapy for incompletely resected canine mast cell tumours. Veterinary Radiology and Ultrasound 39:57–62.

McManus P. 1999. Frequency and severity of mastocytemia in dogs with and without mast cell tumors: 120 cases (1995–1997). Journal of the American Veterinary Medical Association 215:355–357.

Miller D. 1995. The occurrence of mast cell tumours in young sharpeis. Journal of Veterinary Diagnostic Investigation 7:360–363.

Murphy S., Sparkes A.H., Smith K.C., Blunden A.S., Brearley M.J. 2004. Relationships between the histological grade of cutaneous mast cell tumours in dogs, their survival and the efficacy of surgical resection. Veterinary Record 12; 154:743–746.

Northrup N.C., Howerth E.W., Harmon B.G., Brown C.A., Carmicheal K.P., Garcia A.P., Latimer K.S., Munday J.S., Rakich P.M., Richey L.J., Stedman N.L., Gieger T.L. 2005. Variation among pathologists in the histologic grading of canine cutaneous mast cell tumors with uniform use of a single grading reference. Journal of Veterinary Diagnostic Investigation 7(6):561–564.

Patnaik, A.K., Ehler W., MacEwan G. 1984. Canine cutaneous mast cell tumor: Morphologic grading and survival time in 83 dogs. Veterinary Pathology 21:469–474.

Rassnick K.M., Moore A.S., Williams L.E., London C.A., Kintzer P.P., Engler S.J., Cotter S.M. 1999. Treatment of canine mast cell tumors with CCNU (lomustine). Journal of Veterinary Internal Medicine 13(6):601–606.

Seguin, B., Leibman, N.F., Bregazzi, V.S. et al. 2001. Clinical outcome of dogs with grade-II mast cell tumors treated with surgery alone: 55 cases (1996–1999). Journal of the American Veterinary Medical Association 218:1120–1123.

Simpson A.M., Ludwig L.L., Newman S.J., Bergman P.J., Hottinger H.A., Patnaik A.K. 2004. Evaluation of surgical margins required for complete excision of cutaneous mast cell tumors in dogs. Journal of the American Veterinary Medical Association 15;224(2):236–240.

Thamm D.H., Mauldin E.A., Vail D.M. 1999. Prednisolone and vinblastine chemotherapy for canine mast cell tumor—41 cases (1992–1997). Journal of Veterinary Internal Medicine 13(5):491–497.

Thamm D.H., Turek M.M., Vail D.M. 2006. Outcome and prognostic factors following adjuvant prednisolone/vinblastine chemotherapy for high-risk canine mast cell tumour: 61 cases. Journal of Veterinary Medical Science 68(6):581–587.

Turrell J.M., Kitchell B., Miller L.M., et al. 1988. Prognostic factors for radiation treatment of mast cell tumor in 85 dogs. Journal of the American Veterinary Medical Association 193:936–940.

Weisse C., Shofer F.S., Sorenmo K. 2002. Recurrence rates and sites for grade II canine cutaneous mast cell tumors following complete surgical excision. Journal of the American Animal Hospital Association 38:71–73.

Withrow and MacEwan's Small Animal Clinical Oncology, 4th edition. 2007. W.B. Saunders, Encinitas, CA, pp. 402–416.

Part 2

Buerger R.G., Scott D.W. 1987. Cutaneous mast cell neoplasia in cats: 14 cases (1975–1985). Journal of the American Veterinary Medical Association1;190(11):1440–1444.

Johnson T.O., Schulman F.Y., Lipscomb T.P., Yantis L.D. 2002. Histopathology and biologic behavior of pleomorphic cutaneous mast cell tumors in fifteen cats. Veterinary Pathology 39(4):452–457.

Litser A., Sorenmo K.U. 2006. Characterisation of the signalment, clinical and survival characteristics of 41 cats with mast cell neoplasia. Journal of Feline Medicine and Surgery 8(3):177–183.

Molander-McCrary H., Henry C.J., Potter K., Tyler J.W., Buss M.S. 1998. Cutaneous mast cell tumors in cats: 32 cases (1991–1994). Journal of the American Animal Hospital Association 34(4):281–284.

Turrel J.M., Farrelly J., Page R.L., McEntee M.C. 2006. Evaluation of strontium 90 irradiation in treatment of cutaneous mast cell tumors in cats: 35 cases (1992–2002). Journal of the American Veterinary Medical Association 15;228(6):898–901.

Wilcock B.P., Yager J.A., Zink M.C. 1986. The morphology and behavior of feline cutaneous mastocytomas. Veterinary Pathology 23(3):320–324.

Withrow and MacEwan's Small Animal Clinical Oncology, 4th edition. 2007. W.B. Saunders, Encinitas, California, pp. 416–420.

Wright Z.M., Chretin J.D. 2006. Diagnosis and treatment of a feline oral mast cell tumor. Journal of Feline Medicine and Surgery 8(4):285–289.

8
CANINE AND FELINE HISTIOCYTIC DISORDERS

David J. Argyle and Laura Blackwood

Introduction

Canine histiocytic proliferative disorders represent a diagnostic and therapeutic challenge. This chapter will describe the main clinicopathological features of this disease and therapeutic options.

Key Points
- Histiocytic proliferative disorders represent a range of disorders with different pathologies and clinical behaviors.
- For simplicity we can consider these disorders as manifesting as one of four well-defined syndromes (Table 8.1).
- Although originally considered a histiocytic disorder, malignant fibrous histiocytoma (MFH) is now considered a soft-tissue sarcoma (Chapters 6 and 18).
- To understand these diseases, we must first consider the origins of the histiocyte (Figure 8.1).

Histiocyte Biology

- Histiocytes are derived from bone marrow stem cells and can be either macrophages (antigen processing) or dendritic cells (antigen presenting).
- Dendritic cells can be further subdivided:
  - Langerhans cells (epithelial dendritic cells), found in the skin
  - Interstitial dendritic cells, found in many organ systems
  - Interdigitating dendritic cells, antigen presenting cells found in the T cell zone of peripheral lymphoid organs
- Dendritic cells are derived from CD34+ hematopoietic stem cells.
- Macrophages are derived from CD34– blood monocytes.
- Both dendritic cells and macrophages are derived from a common hematopoietic stem cell (granulocyte monocyte progenitor).
- The formation of these cells in the bone marrow requires interaction between the stem cell and the bone marrow stroma, orchestrated by specific cytokines:
  - M-CSF and GM-CSF promote the development of macrophages.
  - GM-CSF, TGF-β, TNF-α and IL-4 promote dendritic cell development.

Canine Cutaneous Histiocytoma (Figures 8.2, 8.3)

- This is considered benign.
- These lesions represent up to 14% of all skin tumors.

Table 8.1. Histiocytic diseases

Disease	Description	Proposed Origins
Canine cutaneous histiocytoma	Considered benign Fast-growing raised, hairless lesions Affects young dogs Affects extremities, ears, neck Resolves spontaneously	Epidermal Langerhans cells
Reactive histiocytosis		Interstitial dendritic cell
• Cutaneous	Lesions of the face, ears, nose, neck, trunk, extremities, perineum, and scrotum Lesions wax and wane	
• Systemic	Ocular and nasal mucosa Peripheral lymph nodes Pulmonary, spleen/liver, bone marrow involvement Lesions wax and wane	
Histiocytic sarcoma		Myeloid dendritic cell
• Localized	Rapidly growing soft tissue mass Can involve bone Usually occurs in the limbs (often near a joint) Flat-coated retrievers are commonly affected (also Rottweilers)	
• Disseminated	Previously described as malignant histiocytosis Disseminated disease, affecting multiple organs and rapidly fatal	
Hemophagocytic histiocytic sarcoma	Similar clinical picture to disseminated/local histiocytic sarcoma but with marked hemophagocytosis leading to anemia	Macrophage

- Cutaneous hystiocytoma occurs mainly in young dogs (<3 years).
- This has been reported in older dogs. However, whether this is a more malignant variant has yet to be elucidated.
- Breed predilection has been reported in Boxers, dachshunds, cocker spaniels, and bull terriers.
- Cytology reveals pleomorphic round cells, often with an inflammatory (lymphoid) infiltrate (suggesting regression).
- Histology often demonstrates a high mitotic index (despite benign course), with a heavy infiltrate of lymphocytes (CD8+ cytotoxic T cells) in regressing lesions.
- Surface markers for this disease are shown in Table 8.2.
- These are self-regressing lesions, and prognosis is excellent (even in multiple lesions with lymph node involvement).

Reactive Histiocytosis

The cause of this syndrome is unknown, but considered to be a dysregulation of the proliferation and activation of dendritic cells, and their interaction with T cells (Figure 8.4).

Two forms are recognized in the dog:
- **Cutaneous Histiocytosis**
  - Confined to the skin and subcutis (lymph node involvement is rare)
  - Multiple cutaneous nodules
  - Depigmentation of lesions is common.
  - Face, ears, nose, neck, trunk, perineum, and scrotum
  - Waxing and waning clinical course

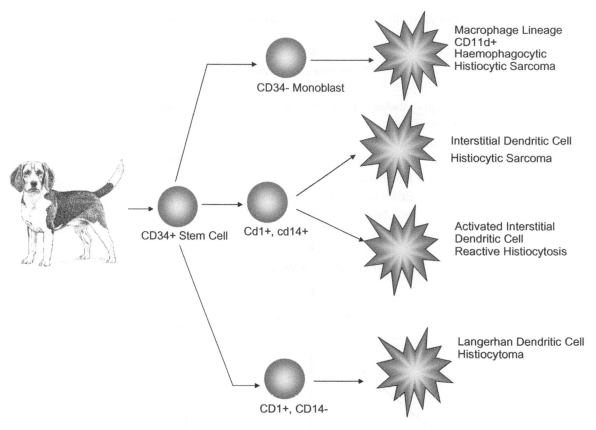

Figure 8.1. The cellular origins of canine histiocytic disease.

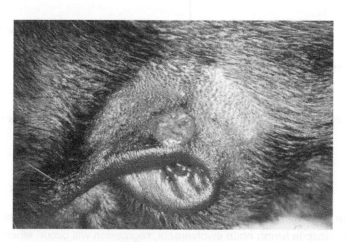

Figure 8.2. Canine cutaneous histiocytoma affecting the canine lip.

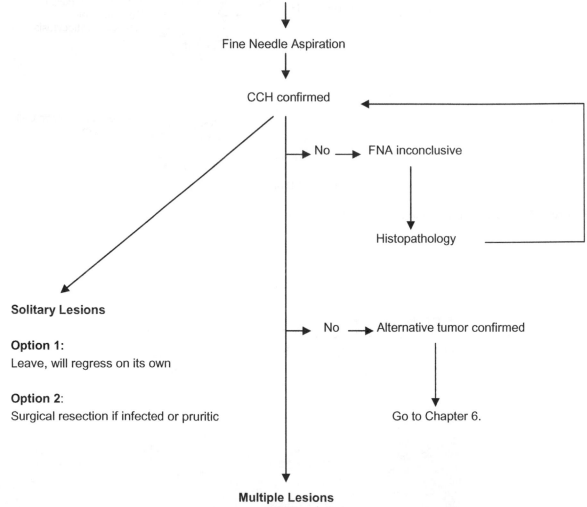

Solitary, rapidly growing, raised, buttonlike, hairless lesion

↓

Differential Diagnosis

- Benign epithelial tumor of the skin (e.g., benign adenoma, or inclusion cyst)
- Malignant tumor
  - Round cell (mast cell, lymphoma, histiocytoma)
  - Melanoma
  - Epithelial tumor (sebaceous gland)
  - Soft tissue sarcoma

↓

Fine Needle Aspiration

↓

CCH confirmed

No → FNA inconclusive

↓

Histopathology

Solitary Lesions

Option 1:
Leave, will regress on its own

Option 2:
Surgical resection if infected or pruritic

No → Alternative tumor confirmed

↓

Go to Chapter 6.

Multiple Lesions
- Some dogs with multiple lesions also have lymph node involvement.
- Leave alone; despite lymph node involvement, regression will occur, albeit slower.

Figure 8.3. Canine cutaneous histiocytoma decision tree.

Table 8.2. Surface markers in canine histiocytic disease

Histiocytic Disease	CD1a	CD1b	CD1c	CD4	CD11c	CD11d	CD18	CD45	CD45RA	MHC II	Thy1	E-Cadherin
Histiocytoma	+	+	+	−	+					+	−	+
Reactive histiocytosis		+	+	+	+					+	+	
Histiocytic sarcoma		+	+	−	+	−	+	+		+	−	−
Hemophagocytic histiocytic sarcoma				−		+	+	+	−	+		

+ = positive.
− = negative.

- Absence of systemic clinical signs
- Often associated with a prolonged clinical course
- Systemic Histiocytosis
  - Skin is affected (especially mucocutaneous junctions).
  - Ocular and nasal mucosa are affected.
  - Peripheral lymph node involvement occurs.
  - Lungs, spleen, bone marrow, and liver can be affected.
  - Clinical signs can vary depending on affected areas.
  - Systemic signs including lethargy and anorexia can develop.
  - Polygenic inheritance has been demonstrated in the Bernese Mountain dog and a breed predilection has been documented for Rottweilers and retriever breeds.
  - Clinical progression tends to occur more rapidly

Histiocytic Sarcoma

- This is a disease complex that often carries a grave prognosis in dogs.
- Etiology is unknown but there is a clear genetic link, with some breeds being particularly predisposed (flat-coated retriever, Bernese Mountain dog, Golden Retriever, and Rottweiler).

We can consider two forms of the disease (Figure 8.5): localized histiocytic sarcoma and disseminated histiocytic sarcoma.

Localized Histiocytic Sarcoma (Figure 8.6)

- A tumor occurs at a focal site, usually affecting the limbs.
- Dogs present with a rapidly growing soft tissue mass.
- Dogs with lesions on the limbs often present with lameness.
- Lameness is often associated with one joint. It has been suggested that the association with a joint is because the tumor arises from the dendritic cells of the synovial lining.
- Primary, localized lesions have also been reported in stomach, lungs, liver, spleen, pancreas, and central nervous system.
- Clinical signs depend on the affected sites (e.g., seizures in CNS histiocytic sarcoma).
- Localized lesions are considered to be highly metastatic.

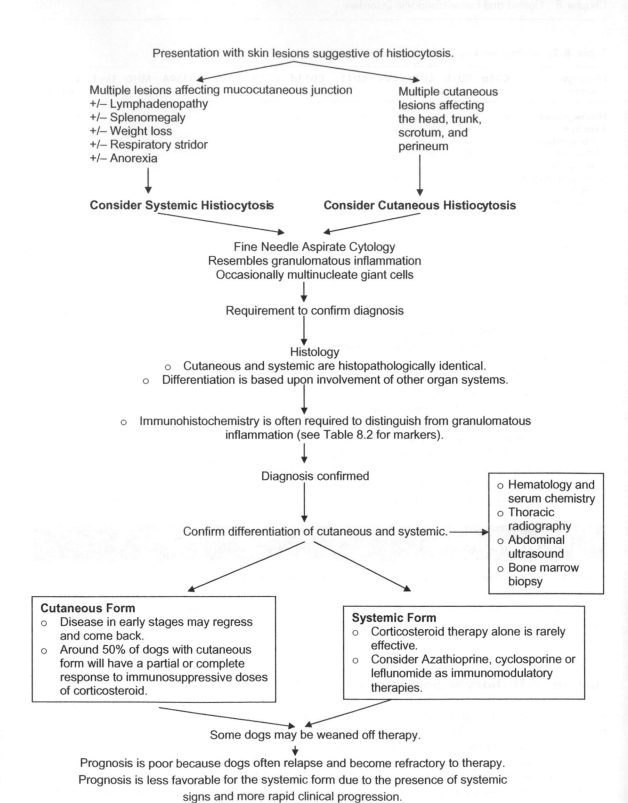

Figure 8.4. Histiocytosis decision tree.

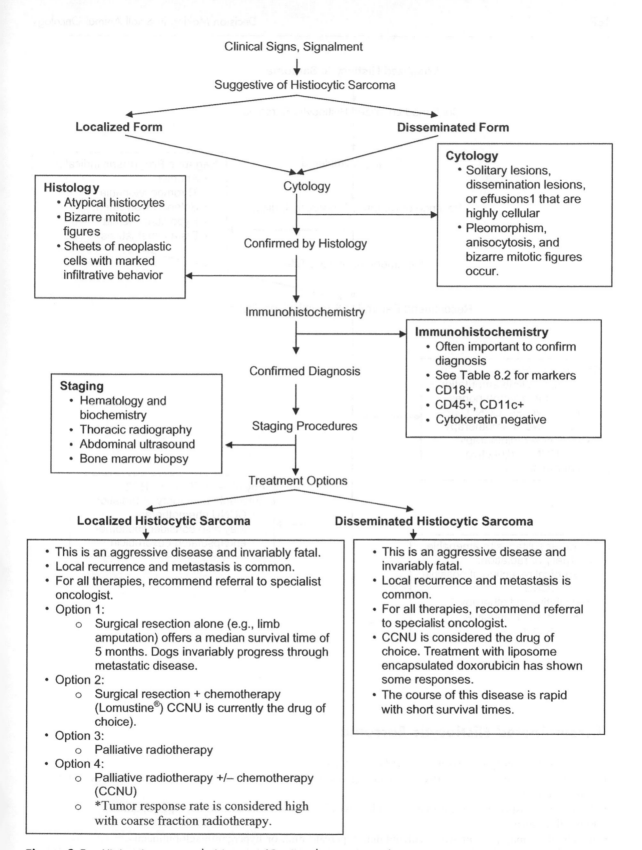

Clinical Signs, Signalment

↓

Suggestive of Histiocytic Sarcoma

Localized Form ← → **Disseminated Form**

Cytology

Histology
- Atypical histiocytes
- Bizarre mitotic figures
- Sheets of neoplastic cells with marked infiltrative behavior

Confirmed by Histology

Cytology
- Solitary lesions, dissemination lesions, or effusions1 that are highly cellular
- Pleomorphism, anisocytosis, and bizarre mitotic figures occur.

Immunohistochemistry

Confirmed Diagnosis

Immunohistochemistry
- Often important to confirm diagnosis
- See Table 8.2 for markers
- CD18+
- CD45+, CD11c+
- Cytokeratin negative

Staging
- Hematology and biochemistry
- Thoracic radiography
- Abdominal ultrasound
- Bone marrow biopsy

Staging Procedures

Treatment Options

Localized Histiocytic Sarcoma — **Disseminated Histiocytic Sarcoma**

- This is an aggressive disease and invariably fatal.
- Local recurrence and metastasis is common.
- For all therapies, recommend referral to specialist oncologist.
- Option 1:
    - Surgical resection alone (e.g., limb amputation) offers a median survival time of 5 months. Dogs invariably progress through metastatic disease.
- Option 2:
    - Surgical resection + chemotherapy (Lomustine®) CCNU is currently the drug of choice).
- Option 3:
    - Palliative radiotherapy
- Option 4:
    - Palliative radiotherapy +/– chemotherapy (CCNU)
    - *Tumor response rate is considered high with coarse fraction radiotherapy.

- This is an aggressive disease and invariably fatal.
- Local recurrence and metastasis is common.
- For all therapies, recommend referral to specialist oncologist.
- CCNU is considered the drug of choice. Treatment with liposome encapsulated doxorubicin has shown some responses.
- The course of this disease is rapid with short survival times.

Figure 8.5. Histiocytic sarcoma decision tree. (Continued on next page.)

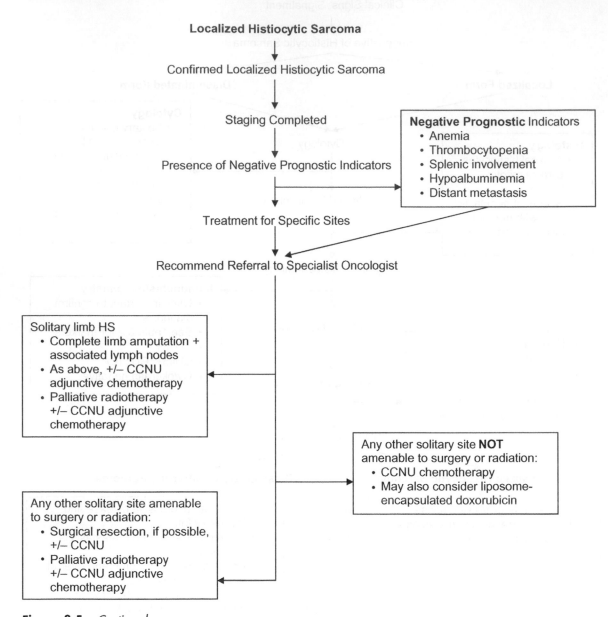

Figure 8.5. *Continued.*

Disseminated Histiocytic Sarcoma

- This was previously termed *malignant histiocytosis*.
- Multiple organ systems are affected, including spleen, liver, lungs, lymph nodes, central nervous system, and bone marrow.
- There are nonspecific clinical signs, including weight loss, anemia, thrombocytopenia, and hypoalbuminemia.
- Rarely, dogs may present with neutrophilia, hypercalcemia, or hypergammaglobulinemia.
- Hyperferritinemia has been reported in people and one dog with histiocytic sarcoma. However, its value as a diagnostic marker has yet to be demonstrated.

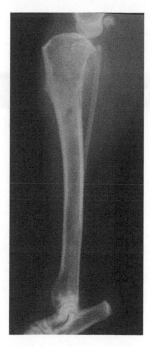

Figure 8.6.   Lysis of the tibia in the dog associated with histiocytic sarcoma.

Hemophagocytic Histiocytic Sarcoma

- This is a distinct subtype of histiocytic sarcoma characterized by
  - Hemophagocytosis
  - Coomb's negative regenerative anemia
- Clinical features, breed predilection, and clinical course are near identical to that of localized and disseminated forms.
- Surface markers of these tumors are indicative of a tumor of splenic and bone marrow macrophages (CD11d positive) and not dendritic cells (CD1c and CD11c negative).
- Typically:
  - Anemia
  - Thrombocytopenia
  - Hypoalbuminemia
  - Hypocholesterolemia
  - Rapid clinical course with survival times of 7 weeks from diagnosis to death
- Currently, very little is known about this disease, and most cases are treated as for disseminated histiocytic sarcoma (e.g., CCNU-based protocols).

Feline Histiocytic Sarcoma

- Rare in cats
- Typically multifocal and disseminated
- Multiorgan involvement

- Anemia and thrombocytopenia are typical findings
- There are no reported successful therapies
- Recommend referral to specialist oncologist

Selected Further Reading

Withrow, S.J., Vail, D.M. 2007. Small Animal Clinical Oncology, 4th edition. W.B. Saunders, Encinitas, California.

9
CANINE LYMPHOMA AND LEUKEMIA

Michelle M. Turek, Corey Saba, Melissa C. Paoloni, and David J. Argyle

Canine Lymphoma

Introduction

Lymphoma is one of the most common forms of malignancy encountered in small animal practice. It is characterized by the malignant proliferation of lymphoid cells, which can arise in any organ containing lymphoid tissue. Lymphoma (*syn.* malignant lymphoma, lymphosarcoma) is one of the more common canine neoplasms.

> **Key Points**
> - The annual, age-adjusted incidence of lymphoma has been estimated to be 13 to 24 per 100,000 dogs at risk. Lymphoma occurs most commonly in middle-aged animals (median age 6 to 9 years), although very young and old dogs are affected. There is no sex predilection. Airedales, Basset hounds, Boxers, Bulldogs, St. Bernards, and Scottish terriers are at increased risk.
>   - The etiology of lymphoma is unknown. An association between herbicide exposure and canine lymphoma has been reported. Repeated efforts to identify a retroviral etiology have so far been unsuccessful.

Clinical Presentation

The presentation and clinical manifestations of lymphoma are due to either
- **The presence of a solid mass**
  - **Multicentric:** Localized or generalized lymphadenopathy ± hepatosplenomagaly. Can cause respiratory embarrassment or edema formation if lymph nodes are reducing venous flow (e.g., precaval syndrome).
  - **Thymic:** Anterior mediastinal mass ± pleural effusion leading to respiratory signs (e.g., dyspnea)
  - **Alimentary:** Vomiting, diarrhea, weight loss, ± palpable abdominal mass
  - **Cutaneous forms:** Cutaneous tumors, which rapidly progress to cause systemic disease
  - **Hepatosplenic:** Vomiting, diarrhea, weight loss, hepatosplenomegaly
  - **Nasal:** Nasal discharge, epistaxis, epiphora, facial deformity
  - **Ocular:** Uveitis ± hyphema
- **The systemic effects of the tumor**
  - Anemia
  - Thrombocytopenia
  - Hypercalcemia (Chapter 2)
  - Organ failure due to lymphoid infiltration

Diagnosis and Staging

- The most frequent anatomical form of canine lymphoma is multicentric; patients present with painless, generalized lymphadenopathy (Figure 9.1, Table 9.1).
- In decreasing order of frequency, other forms include cranial mediastinal, gastrointestinal, cutaneous, and other extranodal forms (eye, CNS, bone, nasal cavity).

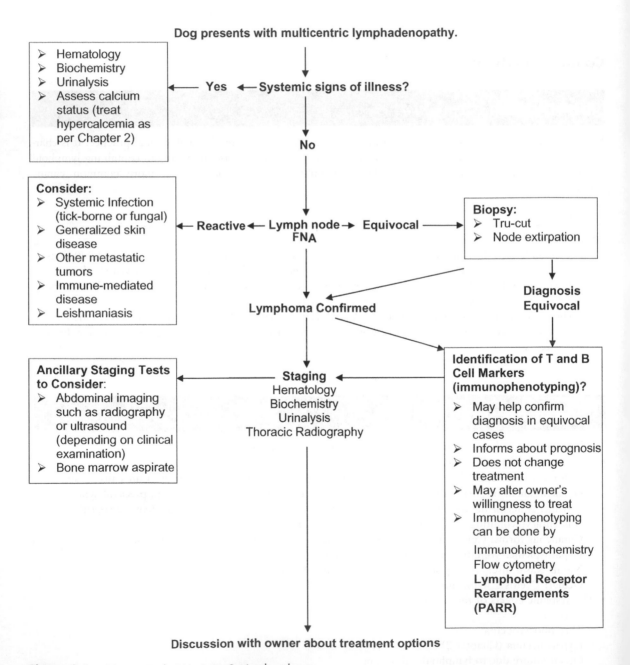

Figure 9.1. Diagnostic decision tree: Canine lymphoma.

Table 9.1. Differential diagnosis

Clinical Features	Differential Diagnosis
Signs indicative of multicentric lymphoma (e.g., generalized lymphadenopathy)	Multicentric lymphoma
	Tumor metastasis to nodes
	Disseminated infections (tick-borne disease, fungal infection)
	Immune-mediated disease
	Generalized cutaneous disease (e.g., generalized pyoderma)
	Other hematopoietic tumors (leukemia, histiocytosis)
	Leishmaniasis
Signs indicative of thymic lymphoma (e.g., dyspnea)	Thymic lymphoma
	Thymoma
	Other tumors (chemodectoma, ectopic thyroid carcinoma)
	Granulomatous disease
	Pyothorax
	Chylothorax
	Hemothorax
	Congestive cardiac failure
	Pneumonia/lung disease
	Branchial cyst
Signs Indicative of alimentary tract lymphoma (e.g., weight loss, vomiting, diarrhea, and inappetence)	Other GI tumors
	Lymphangectasia
	Foreign body
	Inflammatory/infiltrative bowel disease
	Pancreatitis
	Renal or hepatic disease
Signs Indicative of cutaneous lymphoma	Pyoderma
	Immune-mediated skin disease
	Other skin tumors

- Diagnosis, suspected from history, physical examination and/or imaging studies may be confirmed by biopsy. Fine needle aspiration of an enlarged lymph node or other mass will often provide a definitive diagnosis. Sometimes, a tissue biopsy for histopathology is required for confirmation.
- A number of histopathological classification schemes have been developed, although most veterinary pathologists will only classify canine lymphoma as "low-grade" (also called *small-cell* or *lymphocytic*) or "intermediate- to high-grade" (also called *intermediate- to large-cell*, or *lymphoblastic*).

The Minimum Diagnostic Database

- History and physical examination
- Complete blood count and serum chemistry
- Urinalysis
- Thoracic radiography
  - Three-view thoracic radiographs
- Cytology/histopathology of the appropriate lesions
  - Lymph nodes
    - ○ Fine needle aspirate (FNA) for cytology
    - ○ Tru-cut needle biopsy for histopathology
    - ○ Whole node extirpation for histopathology
  - Thymus
    - ○ Ultrasound/CT-guided FNA or Tru-cut needle biopsy
    - ○ Surgical biopsies obtained by thoracoscopy/thoracotomy

- Alimentary tract
  - Endoscopic biopsy
  - Laparotomy and full thickness biopsy
- Cutaneous
  - Touch preparation (also called *impression smear*) cytology
  - FNA
  - Punch biopsy

Additional Procedures

- **Abdominal ultrasound**: if a clinical examination reveals a potential abnormality
- **Bone marrow biopsy**:
  - If hematology reveals unexplained cytopenias
  - If hematology reveals abnormal circulating cells
- **Immunophenotyping**: Immunophenotyping of canine lymphoma tissue is straightforward. Laboratories can classify tumors as T cell (CD3 positive) or B cell (CD79 positive); the latter is more common and the former is associated with a poorer prognosis. In the clinic, the fact that a tumor may be T or B cell does not alter the type of conventional therapy that is offered. However, it may alter an owner's willingness to treat and can be offered as part of the diagnostic workup. It is possible, however, as we progress to classification systems based upon molecular and immunological markers, that we may adopt different treatment protocol tailored to subclassifications. Immunophenotype can be determined using immunohistochemistry, flow cytometry, or polymerase chain reaction for antigen receptor rearrangement (PARR, see below).
- **Lymphoid Receptor Rearrangements**: The monoclonality of a population of neoplastic lymphoid cells lends itself to providing supporting evidence for a diagnosis of lymphoma. Both B and T cells have cognate receptors that enable them to take part in the immune response. PCR amplification of either the T cell receptor (TCR) or Immunoglobulin chains on B cells will demonstrate either a mixed population (i.e., in the case of a reactive lymphadenopathy) or a clonal population of cells (as is the case with lymphoma). Therefore, this technique, called *PARR* (*PCR* for antigen receptor rearrangement), allows for 1) confirmation of neoplasia by demonstrating clonality and 2) immunophenotyping by identifying T cell or B cell receptors.

Clinical Staging

- Once a definitive diagnosis is achieved, clinical staging can be done to allow more accurate prognostication.
- The widely used World Health Organization staging scheme is appropriate for dogs with multicentric lymphoma and takes into account the extent of peripheral lymph node involvement, involvement of liver or spleen, involvement of bone marrow, and involvement of nonlymphoid organs (eye, lung, CNS, etc.) in the disease process (Tables 9.2, 9.3).

Table 9.2. Clinical stage for multicentric lymphoma

Stage	Criteria
Stage I	A single node affected
Stage II	Two or more nodes affected in a regional area (i.e., cranial or caudal to the diaphragm)
Stage III	Generalized lymph node involvement
Stage IV	Stage III plus liver and spleen involvement
Stage V	Bone marrow and/or nonlymphoid organ involvement such as eye, CNS, or lung (with or without stage I–IV disease)
Suffix "a"	At all stages denotes no systemic clinical signs
Suffix "b"	At all stages denotes presence of systemic clinical signs

Table 9.3. Prognostic factors for canine lymphoma

Factor	Description
Immunophenotype	B cell median survival time (MST) 12 months T cell MST 5–6 months
WHO substage	"a" MST 12 months "b" MST 2–6 months
Stage	Previously considered to be important but likely related to extent of diagnostic testing performed Stage I/II is associated with a more favorable prognosis than higher stages; stage I disease may be treated locally with surgery or radiation therapy instead of chemotherapy. Stage III/IV MST 12–14 months Stage V MST 5–6 months
Grade	Intermediate- or high-grade (lymphoblastic) lymphoma is rapidly progressive and responds favorably to chemotherapy. It has a more aggressive clinical course than low-grade (lymphocytic) lymphoma, which is an indolent, chemoresistant disease. The median survival time is longer for dogs with low-grade lymphoma compared to those with high-grade lymphoma.
Site of Disease	Dogs with CNS, gastrointestinal, hepatosplenic, or cutaneous lymphoma have a worse prognosis than those with multicentric disease.
Prolonged single-agent steroid treatment	This is a poor prognostic indicator because it leads to multidrug resistance. Clients should be warned that use of prednisolone before chemotherapy can make these regimes less effective.
MDR (multidrug resistance)	This is more common in relapse disease. Collies and other at-risk breeds should have their MDR status assessed before treatments with drugs transported by the p glycoprotein pump. Substitute alkylating agents until status is known. Only those homozygous for the mutation require dose/drug modulations.

- There are five main stages, designated by uppercase Roman numerals. Most dogs are presented with advanced disease (stage III–V).
- Dogs that are presented apparently feeling well are designated substage "a." Those presented with clinical signs of illness (lethargy, anorexia, vomiting, diarrhea) are designated substage "b."
- Paraneoplastic hypercalcemia is designated substage "b."

Treatment Options (Figures 9.2, 9.3)

- Irrespective of treatment modality, a cure is rarely attained and this must be explained to the owner.
- The aim of therapy is to give the patient a good quality of life by putting the lymphoma into remission for as long as possible. Without treatment, most dogs succumb to disease 4–6 weeks following diagnosis. Because lymphoma is a systemic disease it requires systemic therapy to achieve the best possible outcomes.
- In general, the best response to treatment in dogs is seen with multicentric lymphoma. Therapy for thymic often gives a good initial response and alleviation of clinical signs, but remission duration is shorter than for the multicentric form. Alimentary forms are often difficult to treat, as are the hepatosplenic and cutaneous forms. Rarely, a local, extranodal lymphoma is diagnosed that can be treated with surgery (or radiation) alone.

Therapeutic Regimes

1. **No treatment**
2. **Single-agent therapy (Tables 9.4, 9.5 and 9.6)**
   - **Prednisolone:** Dogs can be treated with *prednisolone* alone (2 mg/kg PO daily for 7 days tapering to 1 mg/kg daily), but this will provide only a short remission (typically 2 to 4 months). Moreover, dogs pretreated

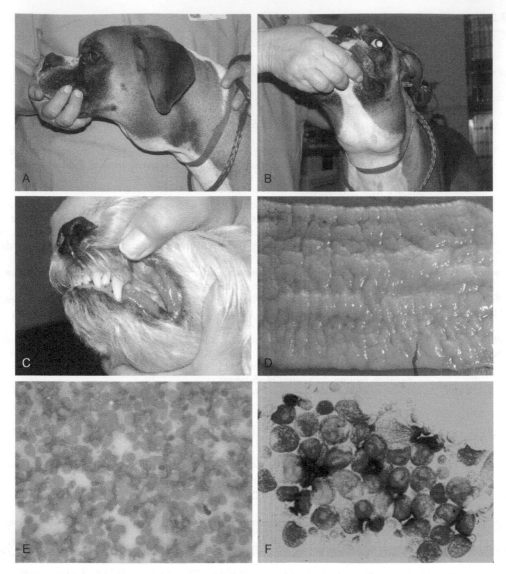

Figure 9.2. Multicentric lymphoma (A and B) affecting the mandibular lymph nodes. Epitheliotopic lymphoma (C) affecting the mucocutaneous junctions; diffuse infiltration of the large bowel in alimentary tract lymphoma (D) and cytology from affected lymph nodes (E, F).

with steroids are less likely to enter into complete remission if the owner subsequently decides to opt for more aggressive chemotherapy.

- **Doxorubicin:** This is the best agent to use if the client desires the simplicity and convenience of single-agent use and is willing to accept a shorter predicted survival. The complete remission (CR) rate is likely to be between 70 and 85% with median survival between 8 and 10 months. The drug is given every 21 days as a slow IV infusion (over at least 15 minutes). Typically, 5 doses are given over 15 weeks. The dose used is 30 mg/m^2 in dogs >15 kg, 25 mg/m^2 in dogs <15 kg, and 1 mg/kg in toy-breed dogs. Dogs with preexisting heart disease causing decreased cardiac contractility should not be treated with Doxorubicin because of its potential cardiotoxicity (see Chapter 5). Equally, cats with poor renal function should not receive doxorubicin.
- **CCNU (Lomustine®):** This may be considered for use as a first-line single-agent therapy if the client desires the simplicity and convenience of single-agent use and is willing to accept a shorter predicted survival.

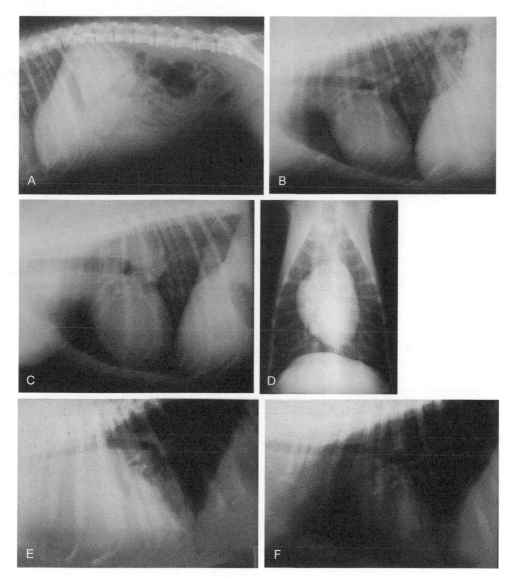

Figure 9.3. Lateral radiographs of lymphoma infiltration of liver and spleen causing hepatosplenomegaly (A), lateral radiograph of Interstitial lymphoma infiltrate of the lungs with perihilar lymph node enlargement (B), lateral (C) and dorsoventral (D) radiographic views of pulomonary infiltrate of lymphoma with mediastinal lymph node enlargement; thymic lymphoma before treatment (E) and 1-week posttreatment (F).

Table 9.4. Single-agent therapies

Single Agent	Regime
Prednisolone	2 mg/kg PO daily for 7 days, then 1.5 mg/kg daily for 7 days, then 1 mg/kg daily
Doxorubicin (±Prednisolone)	30 mg/m² (25 mg/m² for dogs below 15 kg and 1 mg/kg for toy breeds) IV every 3 weeks for 5 cycles (total of 5 treatments over 15 weeks)
Lomustine (CCNU) (±Prednisolone)	65–70 mg/m² PO once every 3 weeks until progressive disease or hepatotoxicity develops

Table 9.5. Low-dose COP

Vincristine (0.5–0.7mg/m^2) weekly for 8 weeks then as shown in the table. Cyclophosphamide (50 mg/m^2) every other day (during treatment weeks). Prednisolone (2mg/kg daily for 7 days and then 1mg/kg every other day).

Week	Vincristine	Cyclophosphamide	Prednisolone
1	•	•	•
2	•	•	•
3	•	•	•
4	•	•	•
5	•	•	•
6	•	•	•
7	•	•	•
8	•	•	•
9			
10	•	•	•

At 8 weeks, COP administration is reduced to every second week for 4 months. At 6 months (if the disease is still in CR), treatments are reduced to every 3 weeks until 1 year. If still in CR at 1 year, treatments are reduced to every 4 weeks for a further 6 months. In many cases, it is prudent to replace cyclophosphamide with chlorambucil at 6 months to prevent hemorrhagic cystitis.

Table 9.6. High-dose COP

Vincristine (0.5–0.7 mg/m^2) weekly for 4 weeks then as shown in the table. Cyclophosphamide (250 mg/m^2) once, every third week. Prednisolone (2mg/kg daily for 7 days and then 1mg/kg every other day).

Week	Vincristine	Cyclophosphamide	Prednisolone
1	•	•	•
2	•		•
3	•		•
4	•	•	•
5			•
6			•
7	•	•	•
8			•
9			•
10	•	•	•

At 4 weeks, a three weekly cycle of Vincristine and Cyclophosphamide is continued until 1 year. After this, the cycle is extended to every 4 weeks for a further 6 months unless the disease becomes progressive.

CCNU is more commonly used for relapse multicentric lymphoma and for epitheliotropic cutaneous lymphoma (mycosis fungoides). The dose is 60–70 mg/m^2 every 3 weeks orally.

3. **Multidrug chemotherapy**
   - Many chemotherapeutic protocols are available for use in the treatment of lymphoma. In general, the protocol used will be based upon available drugs and facilities. Protocols are based on the following drugs: cyclophosphamide (Cytoxan®), vincristine (Oncovin®), prednisolone, and doxorubicin (hydroxydaunorubicin or Adriamycin®).
   - **COP protocol for canine lymphoma:** This is an effective treatment for lymphoma. Complete remission (no evidence of detectable gross disease) occurs in approximately 60–70% of dogs with multicentric lymphoma, and median survival times are around 6–7 months. The two regimes below have equal efficacy in treatment and are inexpensive and relatively well tolerated. The drug is available in injectable form for IV use and in tablet form. On a practical point, cyclophosphamide tablets are produced in limited doses and should not be divided. This may limit the dose that can be delivered orally.

Table 9.7.   19-week University of Wisconsin-Madison CHOP protocol for dogs

Week	V	P1	P2	P3	P4	C	D
1	X	X					
2			X			X	
3	X			X			
4					X		X
5							
6	X						
7						X	
8	X						
9							X
10							
11	X						
12						X	
13	X						
14							X
15							
16	X						
17						X	
18	X						
19							X

V (vincristine) = 0.5–0.7 mg/m^2 IV.
P (prednisolone), 1 = 2 mg/kg PO sid; P2 = 1.5 mg/kg sid. P3 = 1 mg/kg sid; P4 = 0.5 mg/kg sid.
C = cyclophosphamide (Cytoxan) at 250 mg/m^2 IV, or PO over 2–4 days.
D = doxorubicin at 30 mg/m^2 (25 mg/m^2 for dogs below 15 kg and 1 mg/kg for toy breeds) IV.
Treatments no. 8–16 may be delivered on a q 2-week schedule if this is more tolerable for the dog or convenient for the client. The duration of the protocol is 25 weeks in this case.

- **CHOP-based protocols:** Although COP is a reasonable combination to use in general practice, it has been clearly established that the best combination protocols also include doxorubicin. University and specialist practices dealing with oncology patients should be using protocols containing doxorubicin as "Standard of Care." Protocols using doxorubicin (CHOP protocols) generally result in an 80–90% remission rate and median survival times of 12 months. Although several protocols are in operation worldwide, the author has included the University of Wisconsin-Madison (UW-M) protocol for illustration (see Table 9.7, later in this chapter).

The Role of Maintenance Therapy

- The role of sustained maintenance therapy in management of canine lymphoma has recently come under scrutiny. It has been reported that a 25-week CHOP protocol (i.e., the. UW-M short protocol) followed by routine reexamination and reinitiation of chemotherapy at time of relapse provides results similar to a CHOP protocol with sustained maintenance treatments.
- Similar clinical results are achieved when the UW-M protocol is delivered in 19 weeks rather than 25 weeks. The 19-week protocol uses the same number of treatments but they are delivered in a shorter period of time. (See protocol in Table 9.7.)

Protocols for Therapy

- It is important to educate clients on the expectations and side effects of therapy for lymphoma.
- Chemotherapy is not a cure for canine lymphoma, and 90% of dogs will eventually relapse even with gold standard therapy such as multiagent (CHOP-based) chemotherapy. It is important that clients understand

Table 9.8. Treatment options based upon anatomical site

Anatomical Site	Treatment Options	Prognosis Median Survival Time (MST)
Multicentric	No treatment	4–6 weeks MST
	Single-agent prednisolone	50–66% response rate (RR), 1–2 months MST
	Single-agent doxorubicin	70–80% RR, 8–10 months MST
	Systemic multiagent chemotherapy	80–90% complete remission rate, 8–13 months MST*, 25% 2 years+
	CHOP (vincristine, cyclophosphamide, doxorubicin, prednisolone)	60–70% RR, 5–7 months MST
	COP (cyclophosphamide, vincristine, prednisolone)	
Mediastinal	Systemic multiagent chemotherapy	May require RT and chemotherapy especially in cases of precaval syndrome
	Radiation	Rare single site
		MST 5–8 months
Alimentary**	Systemic multiagent chemotherapy	Poor: 4 months MST
Hepatosplenic	Systemic multiagent chemotherapy	Poor when isolated to these sites due to low RR
Cutaneous	Prednisolone	Palliative when used alone
	CCNU	Most active single agent, tumor responses last for a few to several months; treatment of choice for mycosis fungoides***
	Retinoids	40–50% RR, responses 5–13 months, difficult to obtain
Extranodal (in particular, CNS)	Chemotherapy (include Cytosar or CCNU-agents that cross the blood-brain barrier)	Multimodality therapy often indicated, survival depends on response to treat and is poorly reported, prognosis considered poor
	Radiation therapy	May be useful for focal lesions
	Surgery	May be required for decompression

*Varies based on prognostic indicators.
**Alimentary tract lymphoma: Solitary lesions can be treated with surgical resection of the affected bowel, (including mesenteric lymph node). However, due to the multifocal nature of lymphoma, surgical resection is rarely performed other than in cases of chemotherapy-resistant obstructive tumors. Response to chemotherapy is generally poor or short-lived. If an alimentary tract lymphoma is to be treated with chemotherapy, owners need to be warned that gastrointestinal perforation is a potential complication.
***Mycosis fungoides is epitheliotropic, lymphocytic, T-cell cutaneous lymphoma. This form of cutaneous lymphoma is usually not associated with systemic involvement.

that if nonmaintenance protocols are used, reported median survival times reflect multiple courses of chemotherapy (i.e., reinitiation of chemotherapy at the time of relapse if relapse occurs after chemotherapy has been discontinued).

- Quality of life for dogs on chemotherapy is largely good; hence, the treatment is generally well tolerated. Treatment protocols and prognosis based on anatomical site are listed in Table 9.8, later in this chapter.

COP-Based Protocols

1. **Low-dose COP regime:** Vincristine (0.5–0.7 mg/m^2) weekly for 8 weeks and then as shown in Table 9.5. Cyclophosphamide (50 mg/m^2) PO every other day (during treatment weeks).
Prednisolone (2 mg/kg PO daily for 7 days and then tapered to 1 mg/kg every other day).
2. **High-dose COP regime**
Vincristine (0.5–0.7 mg/m^2) IV weekly for 4 weeks and then as shown in Table 9.6.
Cyclophosphamide (250 mg/m^2) PO divided over 2–5 days, every third week.
Prednisolone (2 mg/kg daily for 7 days and taper to 1 mg/kg every other day)

Single-Agent Therapy Versus Combination Chemotherapy.

When would you choose a single agent over combination chemotherapy?
- Single-agent corticosteroids when only short-term palliation is desired
- When finances, owners' circumstances, or practice facilities dictate that combination therapy has to be avoided

COP Versus CHOP

When should you choose COP over CHOP?
- CHOP is considered the protocol of choice because it is associated with a higher remission rate and longer survival time. This is because doxorubicin is the most active chemotherapy agent against lymphoma.
- COP may be considered when practice experience/facilities dictate that doxorubicin should be avoided (due to its vesicant potential), or for dogs with decreased cardiac contractility and/or severe arrythmias.

High-Dose Versus Low-Dose COP Regime

- There is very little difference in disease-free interval with either high-dose or low-dose COP regimes.
- Often choice is based upon
  - Owner circumstances
  - Size of the animal: often it is easier to more accurately dose smaller dogs with the high-dose COP regime.

Monitoring Therapy

- It is necessary to perform serial assessments of all patients being treated for lymphoma.
- The nature of these assessments will vary on the original site and extent of disease, chosen treatment protocol, and current clinical status.
- Reevaluations must focus on documenting a response to treatment as well as ensuring that the patient may safely be administered a scheduled therapy.

Monitoring Regime for Chemotherapy Patients

Treatment Day
- Physical examination   Ensure remission.
- Vital signs: temperature, HR, RR   Ensure afebrile, stable vitals.
- CBC   Treat if PMN >1500 ($\times 10^6$),
                                    and plt >75,000 ($\times 10^6$)

7–10 Days After Chemotherapy
- Physical examination   Ensure remission.
- Vital signs: temperature, HR, RR   Ensure afebrile, stable vital signs.
- CBC
  - If temperature >103° F and PMN <2000
    - Admit to hospital for IV fluids and IV antibiotics
  - If temperature <103° and PMN <2000
    - Prescribe antibiotics
    - Owner to take temperature twice daily and return if T >103° or if dog shows clinical signs of illness

Table 9.9. Categories for response

Complete response (CR)	Complete disappearance of all detectable lesions
Partial response (PR)	A 50% or > decrease in the size of the measured lesion
Minor response (MR)	A 25–49% decrease in the size of the measured lesion
Stable disease (SD)	A 0–24% change in size of the measured lesion
Progressive disease (PD)	An increase of >25% in the size of the measured lesion or formation of new lesions

Assessing Response

Assessing response is necessary for therapeutic decision-making. Response should be gauged on resolving clinical signs, improved hemataologic or biochemical values and resolution of physical examination/imaging abnormalities (Table 9.9).

For the typical dog with multicentric lymphoma response, measurements are based on lymph node size as assessed by physical examination.

If lymphadenopathy resolves with treatment and nodes are palpably normal, this is termed a complete response (CR).

Failure to Respond to Therapy

- Dogs whose lymphoma fails to respond to chemotherapy have a grave prognosis.
- Failure to respond is defined as persistent lymphadenopathy or other clinical manifestation of disease after all drugs in the protocol have been administered once.
- For multiagent chemotherapy, protocols begin to repeat after one cycle. For the UW-M CHOP protocol, cycles repeat starting at week 6. Hence, if lymphadenopathy has not resolved by this juncture, rescue therapy should be sought.
- For other protocols, such as single-agent doxorubicin, remission must be obtained after two cycles of the drug in order to justify continuing therapy with that drug. It is critical to recognize when patients fail to respond to therapy so that other chemotherapy agents (so-called *rescue therapy*) can be sought.

Reinduction Versus Rescue

- Since lymphoma is treated with chemotherapy, the goal is to induce remission.
- Remission is the resolution of the clinical signs of disease, and in initial treatment this is known as *induction*.
- If relapse occurs after chemotherapy is discontinued, the goal is to attempt to reinduce remission by restarting the front-line therapy.
- Reinduction chemotherapy can be successful; 80–90% of patients who received a CHOP-based protocol can be reinduced with these same drugs.
- In general, the duration of subsequent remissions is often less than the first. If the cancer fails to respond to therapy while on protocol, rescue therapy or new drugs must be sought to combat the disease. There are a variety of rescue protocols for lymphoma patients and some are listed in Table 9.10.

Rescue Protocols

- Overall: 30–50% response rate, median response duration of 1–3 months
  - CCNU (Lomustine) (Table 9.11)
  - L-asparaginase (Elspar)

Table 9.10.   Rescue protocols

Treatment Failure	Action
Patient is on single-agent prednisolone with disease progression within 4–6 weeks.	This protocol is palliative. Failure at this juncture is expected and owners should be counseled.
Patient is on single-agent chemotherapy (e.g., doxorubicin) and fails to achieve remission by the third dose.	Instigate rescue therapy. A good alternative is a combination protocol of CCNU and L-asparaginase.
Patient is on multidrug chemotherapy and fails to achieve remission at the end of the first cycle of treatment (e.g., at week 6 of the UW-M protocol).	Instigate rescue therapy.
Patient achieves remission on protocol, but comes out of remission prior to the end of the protocol.	Instigate rescue therapy.
Patient achieves CR and completes protocol and then lymphoma relapses while the patient is off treatment.	Instigate reinduction therapy using the same protocol that was used to induce the first remission.

Table 9.11.   Lomustine/L-aspariginase protocol for lymphoma rescue

Drug	Day 0	Day 21	Day 42*
CCNU (Lomustine) 65–70 mg/m2 PO	X	X	X
L-asparaginase (Elspar) 400 IU/kg SQ	X	X	
Prednisolone	X (2 mg/kg PO daily)	X (1 mg/kg PO daily)	X (1 mg/kg PO eod)

*Repeat q 3 weeks as long as remission is maintained and drug is tolerated. Monitor liver enzyme activity regularly for CCNU-hepatotoxicity.

- Mitoxantrone
- DMAC (dexamethasone, melphalan, actinomycin, cytosar)
- DTIC (dacarbazine)
- MOPP (mustargen, vincristine, procarabazine, prednisolone)
- Cytosar

Other Strategies Beyond Chemotherapy

- Lymphoma is exquisitely sensitive to the effects of radiation.
- For stage-negative, solitary lesions (e.g., a single, cutaneous lesion that does not lend itself to wide surgical resection, or nasal lymphoma), radiotherapy is an effective modality because lymphoid tissue is highly radiation-sensitive.
- Despite the sensitivity of lymphoma to the effects of radiation, the use of total body irradiation to treat multicentric disease has been limited by the lack of hematological support and autologous bone marrow transplantation that would be required to treat complications.
- The use of half-body irradiation is being investigated in combination with multidrug chemotherapy as a possible alternative strategy to reap the benefits of radiation but limit the side effects. In this regime, half of the body is irradiated at a time point and then the other half is irradiated 4 weeks later.

Canine Leukemia

This section describes the main clinical and pathological features of leukemia in dogs, including diseases affecting both the lymphoid and myeloid cell lineages.

Key Points
- Leukemia refers to a malignant neoplastic disease affecting the cells of the bone marrow (but sometimes originating in the spleen).
- Neoplastic cells may or may not circulate in the peripheral bloodstream.
- The classification of leukemias is difficult in dogs because they are often associated with mixed lineages.
- The clinical signs of leukemia in dogs are referable to
  - Marrow replacement with neoplastic cells (leading to cytopenias) and
  - Infiltration of organs systems (mainly liver, spleen, and sometimes lymph nodes).
- Clinically, the important distinction is whether the disease is **acute** or **chronic**.
- Acute leukemia refers to a disease in which the majority of neoplastic cells are immature or blastic. This disease carries a grave prognosis.
- Chronic leukemia refers to a disease in which the majority of neoplastic cells are mature and well differentiated. This disease carries a better prognosis.

The Pathophysiology of Leukemia

- Normal bone marrow contains stem cells that divide and differentiate through either the **myeloid lineage** (red cells, platelets, neutrophils, eosinophils, basophils, and monocytes), or **lymphoid lineage** (T cells, B cells, NK cells, plasma cells).
- Stem cells differentiate into committed colony forming-units, from which neutrophils, eosinophils, monocytes, basophils, RBCs, and platelets arise. In normal adults hematopoiesis is restricted to bone marrow within the proximal ends of long bones, the pelvis, the vertebrae, and the sternum, but when necessary can take place in the spleen and liver (so-called "extramedullary hematopoiesis").
- The complex orchestration of hematopoiesis requires three physiologic components:
  - The *stem cell* pool
  - *hematopoietic cytokines*, which are the hormones that regulate hematopoiesis through both endocrine and paracrine mechanisms
  - The *hematopoietic inductive microenvironment*, which is made up of the bone marrow stroma and vasculature.
- In leukemia, marrow infiltration due to uncontrolled proliferation results in crowding out of normal marrow elements, competition for nutrients, the failure of the marrow to elaborate normal stimulatory factors and the buildup of inhibitory factors released by the neoplastic cells (myelophthisis).
- As a result of this, normal blood cell production is reduced. The first manifestation of this is neutropenia, followed by thrombocytopenia.
- It is considered that leukemia is a true stem cell disease, i.e., that malignant transformation takes place in the stem cell. The nature of that change will dictate the lineage affected and the degree by which differentiation is blocked.
- The pathophysiology of leukemia allows for varying effects on a patient's hematology and serum biochemistry profile (Figure 9.4).

Main Clinical Features (Depending on Subtype)
(Tables 9.12 and 9.13)

The various abnormalities described in the preceding section give rise to varying degrees of clinical signs depending on whether the leukemia is acute or chronic. In general, acute leukemic patients often present quite sick with marked clinical signs. In contrast, dogs with chronic leukemias often feel quite well, and in many cases the leukemia is an incidental finding.

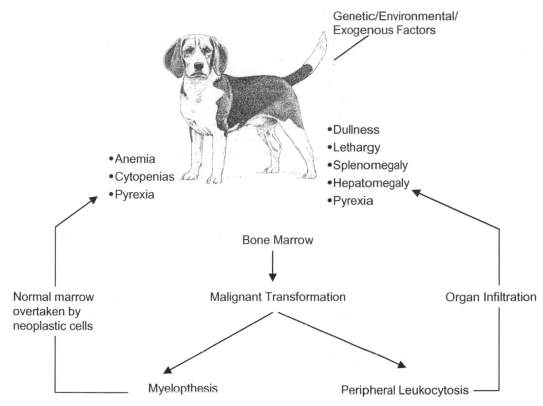

Figure 9.4.   The clinical consequences of leukemia.

Clinical Features: Acute Leukemias

- Acute onset of clinical signs
- Dullness and lethargy
- Anorexia
- Anemia
- ± Pallor of mucous membranes
- Splenomegaly, ± hepatomegaly, ± lymphadenopathy
- Febrile episodes

Clinical Features: Chronic Leukemias

- Longer duration of illness
- More indolent in nature
- Mild anemia
- ± Splenomegaly, ± hepatomegaly, ± lymphadenopathy
- Often, there are no clinical signs of illness and the leukemia is detected incidentally during routine blood screening.

Table 9.12. General hematological features of leukemia

Anemia	Nonregenerative (normochromic, normocytic, low reticulocyte count) due to myelopthesis and effects of chronic disease
	or
	Regenerative anemia:
	• Immune-mediated secondary to tumor (Coomb's +ve)
	• Hemorrhage secondary to thrombocytopenia and/or DIC
Neutropenia	$<3 \times 10^9$/L there is an increased risk of infection
	$<1 \times 10^9$/L risk of life-threatening septicemia
Leukocytosis	Large numbers of atypical,neoplastic cells in peripheral blood
	Grossly visible increased buffy coat on hematocrit tube
	Possible sludging of blood and hyperviscosity
Thrombocytopenia	Risk of spontaneous hemorrhage:
	$<50 \times 10^9$/L in dog
	$<30 \times 10^9$/L in cat
	Usually due to marrow ablation (myelopthesis) or secondary immune-mediated mechanisms
Bleeding diathesis	DIC as a terminal event
	As a complication of elevated gammaglobulins (see below)
	Liver failure
	Thrombocytopenia
Hyperviscosity syndrome	Hyperviscosity of the blood can occur when there are vastly elevated numbers of cells in the circulation or due to hypergammaglobulinemia, which results from aberrant production of immunoglobulins by neoplastic B cells. IgA- and IgM-producing tumors cause more severe hyperviscosity than IgG because the former are multimeric molecules. Clinical consequences of hyperviscosity syndrome include
	• Bleeding diatheses (due to interference of para-proteins with platelet function and clotting factors)
	• Ocular changes (especially retinal detachment and hemorrhage, retinal vessel dilation, and tortuosity)
	• Neurological signs due to poor perfusion of the brain (e.g., seizures, depression)
	• PU/PD due to poor perfusion and renal tubular and glomerular damage
	• Thromboembolism
	• Plasmapharesis is the emergency treatment for hyperviscosity. Red cells should be returned to the patient (unless the cause is polycythemia).

Table 9.13. General biochemical abnormalities associated with leukemia

Hypercalcemia	Lymphoproliferative diseases are the most common cause of paraneoplastic hypercalcemia.
Azotemia	Secondary to hypercalcemia or hyperviscosity, which can result in renal tubular and glomerular damage or poor renal perfusion.
Monoclonal gammopathy	Associated with multiple myeloma and some B lymphoid leukemias and lymphomas.
Hypoproteinemia	Gastrointestinal protein loss due to tumor infiltration of the gut.
Elevated liver enzyme activity	May be a consequence of hepatic infiltration.
Hyperkalemia	When there are large numbers of atypical lymphoid cells in the circulation, potassium may become artifactually increased due to release from friable cells after sampling.
Hypoglycemia	Uncommonly associated with lymphoproliferative disease. When there are large numbers of abnormal white blood cells, these cells may continue to metabolize glucose after sampling producing an artifactually low glucose.

Leukemia Classification

For simplicity we can divide the leukemias as either lymphoid or myeloid. Clinically we are considering the following:

Lymphoid Tumors:

- **Acute Lymphoblastic Leukemia**
  - Poorly differentiated lymphoblasts in blood and bone marrow.
  - Usually CD34 positive (cell surface marker).
  - Hepatosplenomegaly and lymphadenopathy are typical clinical features.
  - Grave prognosis. Treatment is often unrewarding even in the short term.
- **Chronic Lymphocytic Leukemia**
  - Abnormally elevated numbers of mature lymphocytes in blood and bone marrow
  - Lymphocyte counts in the blood usually in excess of 30,000/uL
  - Usually CD34 negative
  - Predominantly T cell
  - Hepatosplenomegaly and lymphadenopathy
  - Prognosis is reasonably good. Treatment is rewarding. Long-term survival can occur, especially in cases that are diagnosed incidentally.
  - Some oncologists do not advocate treatment for chronic lymphocytic leukemia unless 1) the circulating lymphocyte count is >60,000/uL, 2) clinical signs of illness are present, or 3) lymphadenopathy or organomegaly are present.
- **Multiple Myeloma**
  - Malignant transformation and clonal expansion of a plasma cell (B lymphocytes become antibody-secreting plasma cells).
  - This is often not detectably leukemic (i.e., cancer cells are usually not detected in circulation on routine CBC).

Myeloproliferative Disease (Figure 9.5)

- Myeloproliferative disease encompasses all the nonlymphoid dysplastic and neoplastic conditions arising from the hemopoietic stem cells or their progeny.
- The individual conditions are described according to the cell lineage involved, i.e., erythroid, granulocytic monocytic, or megakaryocytic. However, although only one cell line may be predominantly affected, usually other cell lineages are involved.
- In addition to a morphological classification, myeloproliferative disease can be classified according to the degree of differentiation of the neoplastic cells as either acute or chronic (as described above). The commonly recognized myeloproliferative diseases include
  - Granulocytic leukemia
  - Monocytic leukemia
  - Myelomonocytic leukemia
  - Eosinophilic leukemia
  - Basophilic leukemia
  - Polycythemia rubra vera
  - Erythroleukemia
  - Thrombocytothemia
  - Megakaryocytic leukemia
  - Myelofibrosis
  - Myelodysplasia
  - Hypereosinophilic syndromes

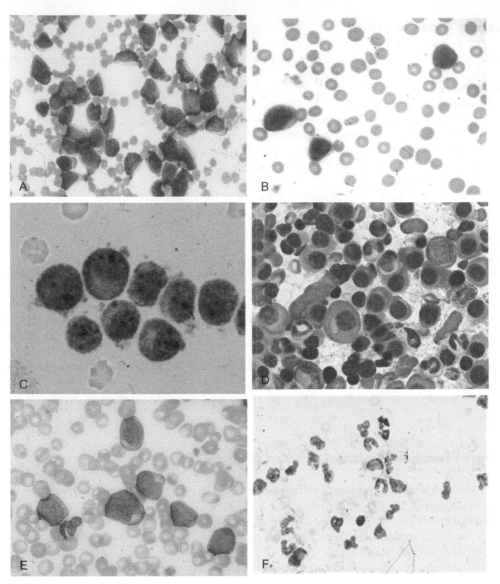

Figure 9.5. Cytological features of canine ALL (A) and CML (B), canine plasma cell leukemia (C) and myeloma affected bone marrow (D); and canine AML (E) and CGL (F).

The Diagnosis and Treatment of Leukemia (Figure 9.6)

Lymphoid Leukemias

- Acute Lymphoblastic Leukemia
  - In this condition, clones of poorly differentiated neoplastic lymphoblasts proliferate with great rapidity within the bone marrow.
  - Diagnosis is based upon hematology and bone marrow aspiration (based on the presence of many [>50%] blast cells in the marrow. These may be so poorly differentiated that they cannot be distinguished from myeloid blast cells without special stains).

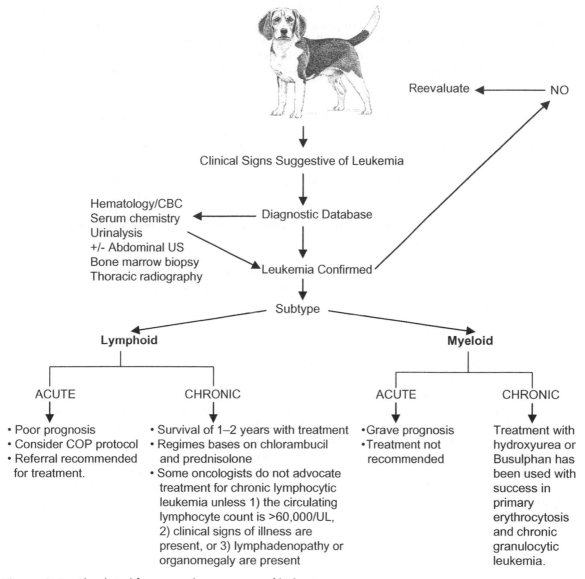

Figure 9.6. The clinical features and management of leukemia.

- Treatment of these cases is fraught with difficulties because many cytotoxic drugs may exacerbate cytopenias in the short term due to their myelosuppressive effects. The prognosis is poor even with aggressive chemotherapy regimes. Only about 30–40% of dogs respond to treatment; median survival time is approximately 4 months for responders and considerably less for the majority that do not respond. Sepsis, hemorrhage, or organ failure are the most common causes of death. Treatment, if attempted, must be tailored to the individual. Vincristine, L-asparaginase, cytosine arabinoside, prednisolone, cyclophosphamide, and doxorubicin are most commonly used. Supportive therapy must also be given (often systemic antibiotics, blood transfusions, etc.). This is a rapidly fatal disease. The clinical signs are usually associated with the concomitant cytopenias and the infiltration of organ systems with neoplastic cells.
- **Chronic Lymphocytic Leukemia**
  - In this condition there is an uncontrolled proliferation of morphologically normal small lymphocytes in the bone marrow and blood. These cells are functionally abnormal. Again, they may secondarily infiltrate the liver, spleen, and lymph nodes.

- Diagnosis is usually suggested by a lymphocytosis of 5 to 100×10^9/L or more. There may be mild to moderate anemia with mild thrombocytopenia or neutropenia. Bone marrow aspiration is necessary for diagnosis as well as to rule out a group of cells lurking there that is not as well differentiated. (A quarter of cases have a monoclonal gammopathy.) Immunohistochemical staining or flow cytometry for CD34 can also be performed to help distinguish ALL versus CLL in samples that are confounding to the clinical pathologist.
- Treatment
  - ○ Chlorambucil   0.2 mg/kg PO daily for 1 to 2 weeks, and then 0.1 mg/kg PO continuously. Long-term maintenance at 2 mg/m² every other day can also be used.
  - ○ Prednisolone   30 mg/m² daily for 7 days, and then 20 mg/m² PO SID, then 10 mg/m² PO every other day.
  - ○ The maintenance dose can be reduced gradually based on hematological monitoring, aiming to keep the lymphocyte count within normal limits and to eliminate the cytopenias. Dogs that do not respond to chlorambucil and prednisolone should be treated with a COP regime. The prognosis for CLL is reasonably good, with median survival times of about 12 months. Longer remissions ranging from 1–3 years are not uncommon).
- **Multiple Myeloma**
  - This form of lymphoproliferative disease encountered does not represent a common diagnosis. The disease arises as a result of malignant transformation of plasma cells in the bone marrow.
  - Clinical features are described in Table 9.14.
- **Diagnosis**
  - Diagnosis of myeloma requires two of the following criteria:
    - ○ Plasmacytosis of the bone marrow
    - ○ Serum monoclonal gammopathy (occasionally biclonal)
    - ○ Osteolytic lesions
    - ○ Bence-Jones proteinuria
  - Multiple myeloma is characterized by plasmacytosis of the bone marrow. Examination of marrow reveals clusters of plasma cells. These plasma cells can be well differentiated or poorly differentiated. A halo of pink proteinaceous material may be seen around some of these cells (flame cells).
  - Multiple myeloma is associated with a high globulin level and a low albumin to globulin ratio. Serum electrophoresis classically shows a monoclonal gammopathy, i.e., a monoclonal spike in the gamma region (Figure 9.7). THIS IS NOT PATHOGNOMONIC OF MYELOMA. Note that lymphoid leukemias, lymphomas, and infectious diseases such as Ehrlichia canis can also cause monoclonal gammopathies. Idiopathic gammopathies also occur.

Table 9.14. Clinical features of multiple myeloma

Hypergammaglobulinemia	This is a relatively consistent feature of multiple myeloma and arises because the neoplastic cells retain their secretory ability and cause a monoclonal (occasionally biclonal) gammopathy. IgG gammopathies often have no effect on blood viscosity, but the IgM/IgA gammopathies can increase the viscosity of the blood because they are multimeric molecules. Clinical consequences of hyperviscosity include bleeding diathesis, retinal detachment, and neurological problems.
Osteolytic bone lesions	Osteolysis can result in pain and may ultimately lead to pathological fracture. Collapse of affected vertebrae can result in paralysis or paresis due to spinal cord compression. These lytic lesions are often poorly defined or sharply "punched out" and may affect either the appendicular or axial skeleton at sites of active hematopoesis. (Bone resorption is thought to be due to release of osteoclast activating factor from tumor cells).
Bone marrow infiltration with plasma cells	This can result in cytopenias affecting neutrophils, platelets, and red blood cells. Plasma cells are not seen in the circulation.
Hypercalcemia	This is a common paraneoplastic syndrome associated with multiple myeloma and can result in anorexia, vomiting, PU/PD, constipation, and neurological signs.

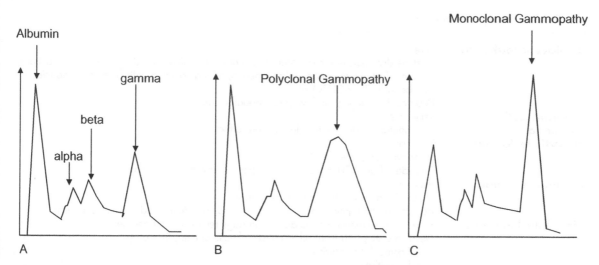

Figure 9.7. Serum protein electrophoresis of normal serum (A), serum with a polyclonal gammopathy (B), and serum from a patient with a monoclonal gammopathy (C). In (C), the albumin is reduced through renal loss. Circulating antibody complexes may cause a membranous glomerulonephropathy leading to a protein-losing nephropathy.

- Urinalysis: The presence of Bence-Jones proteins (light chain fragments) in the urine is not pathgnomonic for myeloma. These proteins are immunoglobulin light chain fragments that are small enough to pass through the glomerular barrier. B-J proteins are not always found in myeloma, and they can be found in urine in other conditions. Note that dipstix do not detect Bence-Jones proteins. Urine electrophoresis will produce the same spike as seen on serum electrophoresis, or it can be detected using the sulphosalicylic acid test.
- Paraneoplastic hypercalcemia resulting in azotemia may occur.
- **Treatment**

Key Points
- The aim of therapy is to lower the plasma immunoglobulin concentration to within normal limits. This is achieved in approximately 50% of patients. The other 50% achieve a partial remission with improved clinical signs.
- Treat the hyperviscosity if present (phlebotomy/fluid replacement).
- Chemotherapy:
  - Melphalan 0.1 mg/kg PO SID for 10–14 days, and then 0.05 mg/kg PO SID continuously. An alternate pulse dosing schedule of 7 mg/m² PO for 5 days every 3 weeks can also be used if significant myelosuppression occurs using the initial dosing regime.
  - Prednisolone 0.5 mg/kg PO SID for 10 days, then 0.5 mg/kg PO every other day. If in remission this is sometimes discontinued after 60 days.
- If there is a poor response to melphalan and prednisolone, cyclophosphamide may be added to the regime, or the VAD (vincristine, doxorubicin, dexamethasone) regime may be substituted.
- The aim of treatment is to reduce the globulin level enough to see clinical improvement, or ideally to return it within the normal range. Reduction of Ig levels or B-J proteinuria can take 3–6 weeks. This is due to the long half-life of some Ig. Subjective improvement in clinical signs can occur sooner. Radiographic improvement of bony lesions can take months or never occur.
- The prognosis for myeloma patients can be quite good; 85% of patients respond to melphalan/prednisolone and the median survival time is 18 months, although these patients can require a significant amount of supportive care in the initial stages of their disease.
- Biphosphonates may be considered to alleviate discomfort associated with osteolytic lesions and/or to reduce paraneoplastic hypercalcemia. Pamidronate is the most commonly used bisphosphonate in veterinary oncology. It is administered IV as a 4-hour infusion at a dose of 1 mg/kg every 3–4 weeks.

Table 9.15. The myeloid leukemias

Granulocytic leukemia	Rare
	Must be distinguished from other causes of neutrophilia, including leukemoid reactions from infections or paraneoplastic neutrophilia associated with other malignancies
	Can be ACUTE or CHRONIC
	Hepatosplenomegaly and lymphadenopathy can occur.
Myelomonocytic leukemia	Very rare
	Both neutrophil and monocyte lines are affected.
Monocytic leukemia	Very rare
	Monocytes only are affected.
	Considered an ACUTE leukemia irrespective of cell morphology
Basophilic leukemia	Very rare
	Should be distinguished from mastocytosis
	Hepatosplenomegaly, lymphadenopathy, thrombocytosis, and anemia can occur.
Eosinophilic leukemia	Rare – true existence of this disease in dogs remains questionable.
	Need to distinguish from other causes of eosinophilia, including
	• Eosinophilic enteritis
	• Parasitism
	• Allergy
	• Hypereosinophilic syndrome
Primary erythrocytosis (polycythemia vera)	Rare
	PCV >65–85%
	Characterized by increased RBC mass, increased PCV, increased hemoglobin concentration, and low/normal EPO levels
	Hyperplastic bone marrow but often normal M : E
	Rule out secondary causes of polycythemia (e.g., chronic hypoxia)
Erythroleukemia	Rare
	Primitive erythroid precursors in the blood
	Considered **acute** and carries a grave prognosis
Primary thrombocythemia	Very rare
	Platelet counts >1,000,000/uL
	Giant platelets in the periphery often with bizarre morphology
	Increased numbers of megakaryocytes/megakaryoblasts in bone marrow
	Rule out secondary causes of thrombocytosis.
Megakaryocytic leukemia	Very rare
	Abnormal megakaryocytes in the bone marrow
	Leads to either thrombocytopenia or thrombocytosis
Myelofibrosis	Occurs secondary to myeloproliferative disorders, radiation damage, and congenital hemolytic anemias in dogs
	Often results in pancytopenia

Acute Myeloproliferative Disease (Acute Myeloid Leukemia) (Table 9.15)

The treatment of acute myeloid leukemia is fraught with difficulty. It would require the complete obliteration of the bone marrow population using high dose chemotherapy or radiation. The marrow would then have to be repopulated via marrow transplant. This is not, at the present time, feasible in veterinary medicine. Chemotherapy is often unrewarding because, although the cells may be sensitive to the drugs used, they also obliterate the marrow. The resulting cytopenias are difficult to control and the animals often die fairly quickly. A new approach is to try and use differentiating agents, but this is only at the experimental stage at the moment. Once acute myeloid leukemia has been diagnosed, survival time is rarely longer than a few weeks.

Chronic Myeloproliferative Disease

In terms of treatment, the most important chronic myeloproliferative diseases are chronic granulocytic leukemia and polycythemia vera (primary erythrocytosis).

Chronic granulocytic leukemia (CGL) versus leukamoid reaction: A diagnostic challenge

Leukemoid reactions are characterized by a significant leukocytosis ranging from 50,000 to 100,000 cell/uL. There is usually an orderly left shift sometimes demonstrating toxic change. Cell counts in excess of 100,000 cells/uL with a mild left shift are referred to as **extreme neutrophilic leukocytosis** and must be distinguished from chronic granulocytic leukemia. The presence of toxic changes or Dohl bodies is suggestive of a leukemoid response rather than true leukemia (Figure 9.8). These reactions can be seen in inflammatory conditions such

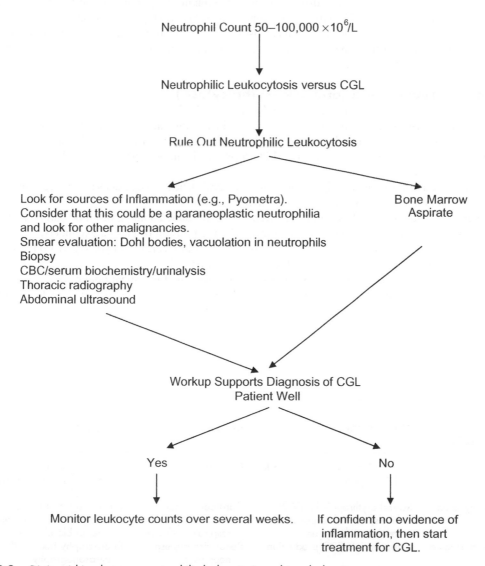

Figure 9.8. Distinguishing between neutrophilic leukocytosis and true leukemia.

as closed pyometra. However, these extreme counts may also be observed as paraneoplastic syndromes, reactive responses to immune-mediated hemolysis or as part of canine granulocytopathy syndrome.

- Often the peripheral blood smear will appear identical in both conditions. However, in CGL there may be some disorderly maturation identified by an experienced hematologist. In CGL cases there is no clinical evidence of inflammation.
- Bone marrow morphology may be suggestive of CGL, but this can be difficult to interpret.
- In CGL there is usually no toxic change in the peripheral neutrophils (Dohl bodies and vacuolation).
- Despite these criteria it is still very difficult to distinguish between these two conditions. If the clinician can rule out any obvious life-threatening inflammatory causes (e.g., pyometra) and the animal is clinically well, serial blood samples may be required to monitor changes in white cell dynamics before a diagnosis of leukemia can be made.

Chronic granulocytic leukemia

- The aim of treatment is to reduce the granulocyte count to normal levels and attempt to correct any other hematological abnormality. The drug of choice is busulphan (Mleran). This is an alkylating agent that is specific to the granulocytic series. The drug is given at 2–6 mg/m^2 daily to effect and the dose is gradually reduced to a maintenance dose. Hematology is monitored regularly. Dogs can usually be maintained for months (and occasionally years) on this regime. Cases, however, invariably go into blast crisis where differentiation is lost and the animals become acutely leukemic. The story in cats is a little different; these respond very poorly to treatment.

Polycythemia rubera vera (primary erythrocytosis)

- Diagnosis is based upon ruling out secondary polycythemia (Table 9.16).
- In a clinical approach to the investigation of the polycythemic animal, it is important to rule out any secondary causes of polycythemia, before a diagnosis of primary polycythemia can be made. EPO assays are useful because in secondary polycythemia, EPO levels are high, but they are normal or low in the case of primary polycythemia.
- The clinical signs associated with polycythemia (neurological deficits, visual defects, lethargy, and dullness) are often due to an increased PCV and resulting hyperviscosity.
- In the emergency situation the PCV can be reduced by phlebotomy. 20 ml/kg of blood can be removed every 3 days, the circulating volume being maintained by the infusion of plasma expanders.
- Primary erythrocytosis can be controlled with the use of the oral medication hydroxyurea (Hydrea). This is given at 30 mg/kg daily for 10 days, after which the dose is halved.
- A radioactive isotope of phosphorus (phosphorus-32) has been used investigationally.
- The aim of therapy is maintenance of a normal PCV. Toxic side effects of hydroxyurea include anorexia, vomiting, and myelosuppression. Despite this the drug is usually well tolerated.

Table 9.16. Diagnosis of erythrocytosis

Type of Erythrocytosis	Mechanism	Cause	Diagnosis
Relative	Relative increase in PCV due to fluid depletion	Dehydration	Clinical signs of dehydration, elevated serum total protein, prerenal azotemia, etc.
Secondary: hypoxia	Raised erythropoietin (EPO) levels, normal response to low arterial oxygen	Cardiopulmonary disease, e.g., VSD, respiratory disease	Clinical signs of hypoxia, thoracic adiography, echocardiography, arterial blood gases
Secondary: normoxia	Inappropriate EPO production	Renal disease, esp. neoplasia	Radiography (plain/IVU), ultrasonography

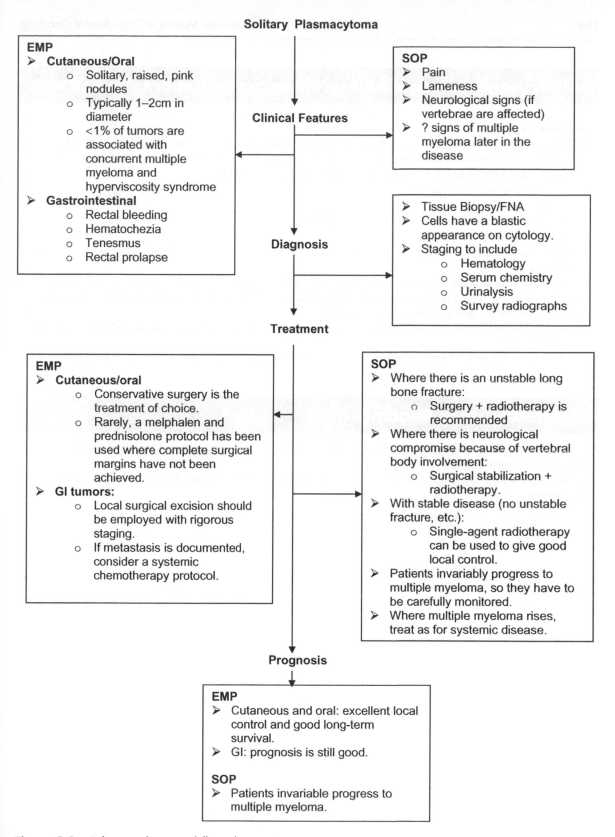

Solitary Plasmacytoma

EMP
➢ **Cutaneous/Oral**
  o Solitary, raised, pink nodules
  o Typically 1–2cm in diameter
  o <1% of tumors are associated with concurrent multiple myeloma and hyperviscosity syndrome
➢ **Gastrointestinal**
  o Rectal bleeding
  o Hematochezia
  o Tenesmus
  o Rectal prolapse

Clinical Features

SOP
➢ Pain
➢ Lameness
➢ Neurological signs (if vertebrae are affected)
➢ ? signs of multiple myeloma later in the disease

Diagnosis

➢ Tissue Biopsy/FNA
➢ Cells have a blastic appearance on cytology.
➢ Staging to include
  o Hematology
  o Serum chemistry
  o Urinalysis
  o Survey radiographs

Treatment

EMP
➢ **Cutaneous/oral**
  o Conservative surgery is the treatment of choice.
  o Rarely, a melphalen and prednisolone protocol has been used where complete surgical margins have not been achieved.
➢ **GI tumors:**
  o Local surgical excision should be employed with rigorous staging.
  o If metastasis is documented, consider a systemic chemotherapy protocol.

SOP
➢ Where there is an unstable long bone fracture:
  o Surgery + radiotherapy is recommended
➢ Where there is neurological compromise because of vertebral body involvement:
  o Surgical stabilization + radiotherapy.
➢ With stable disease (no unstable fracture, etc.):
  o Single-agent radiotherapy can be used to give good local control.
➢ Patients invariably progress to multiple myeloma, so they have to be carefully monitored.
➢ Where multiple myeloma rises, treat as for systemic disease.

Prognosis

EMP
➢ Cutaneous and oral: excellent local control and good long-term survival.
➢ GI: prognosis is still good.

SOP
➢ Patients invariable progress to multiple myeloma.

Figure 9.9. Solitary and extramedullary plasmacytic tumors.

Solitary and Extramedullary Plasmacytic Tumors (Figure 9.9)

Key Points
- Whereas multiple myeloma is considered a "liquid" tumor arising in the bone marrow, a plasmacytic tumor is a solid, solitary collection of plasma cells originating in the soft tissues (extramedullary plasmacytoma, **EMP**) or in bone (solitary osseous plasmacytoma, **SOP**).
- The most common locations are
  - Cutaneous (86%)
  - Mucous membranes of the oral cavity and lip (9%)
  - The rectum and colon (4%)
- Cutaneous and oral forms of EMP tend to have a benign behavior, with local excision often being curative.
- Plasmacytomas at other sites (e.g., the GI tract) tend to have a more aggressive behavior in the dog, with metastasis to the lymph nodes commonly reported. However, bone marrow involvement and monoclonal gammopathies are **not** a feature of these tumors.
- On contrast, SOP tumors eventually progress to multiple myeloma, but over a protracted time course of months to years.

Selected Further Reading

Souhami, Tannock, Hohenberger, and Horiot, editors. 2002. Oxford Textbook of Oncology, 2nd edition. Oxford University Press.

Withrow, S.J., Vail, D.M. 2007. Small Animal Clinical Oncology, 4th edition. W.B. Saunders, Encinitas, California.

10
FELINE LYMPHOMA AND LEUKEMIA

David J. Argyle, Corey Saba, and Melissa C. Paoloni

Feline Lymphoma

The goal of this section is to describe the main clinical and pathological features of feline lymphoma. It should provide the mechanism for the diagnosis and staging of cats with lymphoma as well as a clinical plan for their management. Since it is an overview and not an exhaustive text, further references or referral to a specialist is indicated in complicated cases.

Key Points
- Lymphoma is a systemic neoplasm of the lymphoid system that can involve multiple anatomic sites.
- Etiology is often unknown but retroviral infection (FeLV, FIV) can increase risk.
- The anatomic site of origin is important in prognosis hence definitive staging is indicated. Organ involvement can include: gastrointestinal, renal, CNS, nasal, mediastinal, extranodal, or multicentric.
- Systemic chemotherapy is indicated for treatment in diffuse disease or multiorgan involvement.
- Small-cell (also called *lymphocytic* or *low-grade*) gastrointestinal lymphoma is an indolent neoplasm that carries a good prognosis with treatment compared to gastrointestinal large-cell (also called *lymphoblastic* or *high-grade*) lymphoma. Biopsy is often necessary to differentiate between these two variations but this distinction is important because treatment regimes differ.
- Mitigating side effects of therapy versus disease recurrence is more complicated in cats than in dogs.
- Rescue protocol results are not as well established in literature for cats.
- Recommend that patients be offered referral to a specialist.

The Role of FeLV in Lymphoma

- Hemopoietic tumors are the most commonly diagnosed neoplasms of the cat, accounting for around 30–40% of all tumors, and this is directly related to FeLV.
- FeLV isolates are classified into three distinct subgroups (A, B, and C) on the basis of viral interference with superinfection.
- These subgroups most likely define envelope subtypes that use different cellular receptor molecules for viral entry. FeLV A is ecotropic (can only infect feline cells) and represents the dominant form of FeLV. FeLV B is polytropic (can also infect human cells) and is overrepresented in cases of virally induced lymphoma in cats. FeLV B isolates are thought to arise de novo, from recombination events between FeLV A and feline endogenous sequences present in the feline genome. FeLV C is also thought to arise de novo by mutation of the *env* gene in FeLV A and are not transmitted in nature. They are uniquely associated with the development of pure red cell aplasia (PRCA) in cats.
- Persistently viremic cats are the main source of infection. The virus is secreted continuously in the saliva and is spread by intimate social contact.
- The virus can also be spread congenitally from an infected queen to her kittens. In the first few weeks after viral exposure, interactions between the virus and the host's immune system determine the outcome of infection.

- The potential outcomes of infection include persistent viral infection, latent infection and the establishment of complete immunity and viral clearance. It is the persistently viremic cats that go on to develop FeLV-associated diseases (Figure 10.1).
- Malignant diseases associated with FeLV include lymphomas and leukemias.
- Lymphoma is the most common tumor of cats and can present most commonly in thymic, multicentric and alimentary forms (Figure 10.2, Table 10.1).

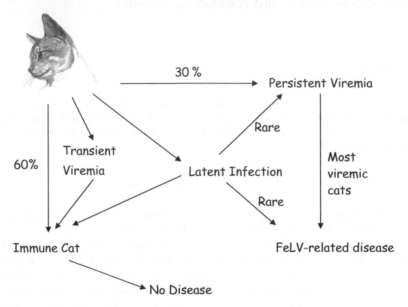

Figure 10.1. Feline persistent viremia.

Lymphoma Anatomic Sites

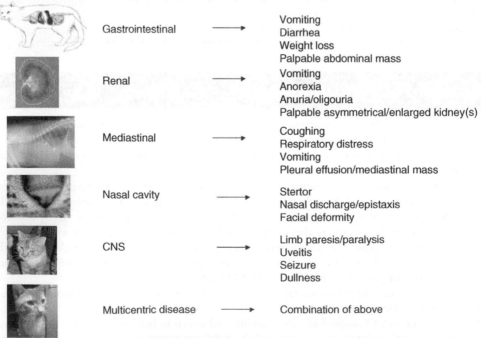

Figure 10.2. Clinical signs associated with the various anatomical forms of lymphoma.

Table 10.1. Staging recommendations for lymphoma subtypes

Anatomic Site	Bloodwork	Imaging	Further Diagnostics

Gastrointestinal
Also includes
• hepatic
• splenic
	CBC
	• cytopenias
	• lymphocytosis
	Chemistry profile
	• hepatic enzymopathy
	• icterus
	• hypoalbuminemia
	Urinalysis
	• r/o concurrent UTI
	• FIV/FeLV test
		Abdominal radiographs
		• mass effect
		Abdominal ultrasound
		• GI mass/wall thickening
		  with loss of normal tissue
		  layering
		• lymphadeopathy
		• splenomagaly
		• hepatomegaly or
		  echogenicity changes
		• peritoneal effusion
		Chest radiographs (staging)
			FNA of gastrointestinal
			  mass/LN/liver/spleen
			• via ultrasound guidance
			• cytologic evaluation
			Surgical biopsy (full
			  thickness preferred)
			• surgery indicated only in
			  perforations or difficult-to-
			  diagnose patients, or for
			  chemoresistant obstructive
			  tumors

Renal Can be • unilateral • bilateral	CBC • cytopenias Chemistry profile • azotemia Urinalysis • specific gravity • r/o concurrent UTI FIV/FeLV test	Abdominal ultrasound • renal asymmetry • renomegaly • renal mass(es) Chest radiographs (staging)	FNA abnormal kidney(s) • cytologic evaluation
Mediastinal	CBC • cytopenias • lymphocytosis Chemistry profile Urinalysis • r/o concurrent UTI FIV/FeLV test • often positive in young cats	Chest radiographs • mediastinal mass • pleural effusion Abdominal ultrasound (staging)	Thoracocentesis • fluid analysis FNA of mass • via ultrasound guidance • cytologic evaluation

Nasal
Can be
• unilateral
• bilateral
	CBC
	• cytopenias
	• lymphocytosis
	Chemistry profile
	Urinalysis
	• r/o concurrent UTI
	• FIV/FeLV test
		Chest radiographs (staging)
		Abdominal ultrasound
		  (staging)
		CT scan of head
		• mass effect in nasal cavity
		  and/or sinuses
		• ocular displacement
			Nasal flush
			• cytologic evaluation
			• Rhinoscopy
			• transnostril biopsy

CNS	CBC
	• cytopenias
	• lymphocytosis
	Chemistry profile
	Urinalysis
	• r/o concurrent UTI
	• FIV/FeLV test
		Chest radiographs (staging)
		Abdominal ultrasound
		  (staging)
		Spinal radiographs if lesion is
		  localized to spine based on
		  neurologic exam
		MRI/CT scan of brain or
		  spinal cord
		• mass effect
		• multiple, diffuse lesions
			CNS tap
			• fluid analysis
			Surgery
			• biopsy
			• decompress

Multicentric	CBC
	• any abnormalities
	Chemistry profile
	• any abnormalities
	Urinalysis
	• r/o concurrent UTI
	FIV/FeLV test
		Chest radiographs (staging)
		Abdominal ultrasound
		  (staging)
		±Bone marrow aspiration or
		  biopsy if lymphocytosis or
		  cytopenias
		Lymph node FNA or biopsy
		  by extirpation
			Any of the above as
			  indicated by disease site

- Essentially the mechanism of tumorogenesis includes both immunosuppression of the host and insertional effects of proviral DNA on cellular oncogenes such as *myc*.
- It is important to note that FeLV is not isolated from all cats with lymphoma. Only 80% of cats with thymic lymphoma are viremic; only 60% and 30% are viremic in the multicentric and alimentary forms, respectively. There is some evidence to suggest, however, that these viruses may be involved as an initiating event before being cleared by the animal's immune system.
- FeLV is also associated with nonmalignant diseases such as bone marrow failure, immunosuppression, and reproductive failure. The pathogenesis of these conditions is poorly understood.

Feline Immunodeficiency Virus (FIV) and Tumorogenesis

- In contrast to the oncogenic retroviruses, FIV is a lentivirus.
- These are retroviruses that classically cause diseases with a slow incubation period and include FIV, HIV, maedi visna, and equine infectious anemia.
- FIV has been associated with neoplastic disease in cats, especially lymphomas. These can largely be explained by the immunosuppression caused by the virus; however, a direct effect associated with viral insertional mutagenesis has been postulated.

Table 10.1 describes the staging recommendations and possible abnormalities associated with each anatomic subtype of lymphoma. In some cases additional staging will be necessitated based on individual patient complications.

Prognostic Factors for Feline Lymphoma

- Most important is response to treatment.
- FeLV Status. FeLV positive status has been shown by some groups to have a negative prognostic effect. However, FeLV per se does not alter the effects of chemotherapy drugs on a tumor, but it may be associated with hastened drug resistance.
- Anatomic stage.
- Compared to dogs, Immunophenotype is **NOT** considered prognostic.

Treatment of Feline Lymphoma

- The various anatomical forms of feline lymphoma (mediastinal, alimentary, renal, multicentric and extranodal) have been well described.
- For multicentric, renal, high-grade gastrointestinal, and thymic forms of the disease, the treatment options are similar to that described for canine patients (Chapter 9). COP regimes (as in Chapter 9) provide extended remission and median survival times. It has been suggested that, as in dogs, protocols that include doxorubicin afford better clinical outcomes. This is not strongly supported by clinical experience and, considering that doxorubicin can be nephrotoxic in cats, many oncologists use a COP-based protocol for cats with lymphoma. Doxorubicin should not be used in cats with compromised renal function.
- Low-grade GI lymphoma is best treated with oral prednisolone and chlorambucil.

COP-Based Protocols: High-Dose COP Regime

Vincristine ($0.5–0.7$ mg/m²) IV weekly for 4 weeks and then as shown in Table 10.2.
  Cyclophosphamide ($200–250$ mg/m²) PO over 2 days once every third week.
  Table 10.3 lists protocols for therapy based on anatomical location.

Table 10.2. Combination therapy

Week	Vincristine	Cyclophosphamide	Prednisolone
1	•	•	•
2	•		•
3	•		•
4	•	•	•
5			•
6			•
7	•	•	•
8			•
9			•
10	•	•	•

Continue this cycle until progressive disease develops. After 1 year of complete remission, discontinuation of chemotherapy may be considered, but the effect on clinical outcome is not known.

Table 10.3. Protocols for therapy based on anatomical location

Anatomic Site	Treatment Options	Prognosis Median Survival Time (MST)
Gastrointestinal* (large-cell or lymphoblastic or high-grade)	Multiagent chemotherapy (vincristine, cyclophosphamide, prednisolone, ±doxorubicin)	6–8 months
Gastrointestinal* (small-cell or lymphocytic or low-grade)	Chlorambucil and prednisolone	90% response rate and 1–2 years MST
Renal	Multiagent chemotherapy, including Cytosar	3–6 months
Mediastinal	Systemic multiagent chemotherapy	Although some reports suggest very short MSTs (2–3 months), long-term remissions are possible.
Nasal	Multiagent chemotherapy and/or radiation therapy	MST 12–14 months
CNS	Multiagent chemotherapy to include agents that cross the blood-brain barrier (Cytosar, CCNU)	Poor
	Radiotherapy for focal spinal lesions	Focal spinal lesions may respond favorably to radiotherapy.
Multicentric	Multiagent chemotherapy	3–6 months
Overall for all sites	Multiagent chemotherapy	50% response rate MST 6–8 months 30% of cats will achieve a sustainable complete remission for >1 year.

***Feline Gastrointestinal Lymphoma** is characterized by gastric and/or intestinal infiltration with or without mesenteric lymph node involvement. This is one of the more common forms of feline lymphoma. Gastrointestinal lymphoma may present as a solitary mass lesion or as a diffuse infiltration of extensive areas of bowel. Clinical signs are nonspecific, including anorexia, weight loss, vomiting, and diarrhea. Animals previously diagnosed with lymphoplasmacytic gastroenteritis have been reported to go on to develop gastrointestinal lymphoma. Most cats with alimentary lymphoma are FeLV ELISA negative. Surgical excision of apparent solitary lesions is not recommended because disease often extends well beyond the detectable lesion and, in many cases, is diffuse. Surgical excision must be considered for perforated lesions or for chemoresistant obstructive lesions. Multiagent chemotherapy is the treatment of choice for high-grade feline GI lymphoma. For cats with low-grade or small-cell lymphoma, a protocol consisting of oral prednisolone and chlorambucil offers a good treatment modality (see Table 10.7). In some cases it is difficult to distinguish inflammatory bowel disease from low-grade small-cell lymphoma purely on pathological assessment of the affected gut. However, a number of groups have described a PCR (polymerase chain reaction) based test that determines the clonality of biopsied tissues by analyzing, for example, the T cell receptor gamma variable gene. Tumor lesions are clonal in origin and therefore have a different PCR pattern to polyclonal inflammatory lesions.

Therapeutic Regimes

1. No treatment
2. Single-agent therapy (Table 10.4)
    - **Prednisolone:** Cats can be treated with *prednisolone* alone at a dose of 2 mg/kg PO daily for 2 weeks, and then 1 mg/kg daily thereafter. This may provide varying degrees of palliation.
    - **CCNU (Lomustine®):** CCNU may be considered for single-agent therapy if the client desires the simplicity and convenience of single-agent use and is willing to accept a possible shorter predicted survival. Response rate to CCNU is variable; some cats and their lymphomas respond better to CCNU than to COP-based protocols. The dose is 55–65 mg/m2 PO once every 3–6 weeks depending on the duration of myelosuppression.
    - **Doxorubicin:** Doxorubicin may be considered for single-agent therapy, but it rarely is because of the risk of nephrotoxicity in cats.
3. Combination chemotherapy (Table 10.2)
    - Many chemotherapeutic protocols are available for use in the treatment of lymphoma. In general, the protocol used will be based upon available drugs and facilities. All protocols are based upon the standard COP regime (cyclophosphamide, oncovin [vincristine], and prednisolone).
    - **COP protocol for feline lymphoma:** Largely speaking, the high-dose COP regime is used in cats to allow for more accurate dosing.
    - **CHOP-based protocols:** Although CHOP-based protocols are considered standard of care in dogs with lymphoma, the addition of doxorubicin to a COP-based protocol is not considered to be as effective in cats. If a complete remission is not achieved with COP alone, doxorubicin should be strongly considered. Doxorubicin may be administered at a dose of 1 mg/kg IV once every 2 weeks. It should not be used in cats with compromised renal function. The author has included the University of Wisconsin-Madison (UW-M) long-term maintenance CHOP-based protocol for illustration (Table 10.5) and the UW-M 25-week CHOP protocol, but efficacy has not been evaluated in cats (Table 10.6).
    - **Chlorambucil and Prednisolone for Low-Grade Feline Lymphoma:** Small-cell (lymphocytic) alimentary lymphoma is best treated with a combination protocol of chlorambucil and daily prednisolone (Table 10.7). The protocol is included below.

The Role of Maintenance Therapy

- Unlike in dogs, discontinuation of chemotherapy after an extended period of remission has not been evaluated for its effect on clinical outcome in cats. Most feline lymphoma chemotherapy protocols include a maintenance phase (Table 10.5). As mentioned above, some oncologists use the canine UW-M 25-week CHOP protocol, but efficacy has not been evaluated in cats (Table 10.6). Furthermore, the

Table 10.4. Single-agent therapy

Single Agent	Regime
Prednisolone	Provides palliative care only for high-grade lymphoma
	May provide durable resolution of clinical signs in cats with low-grade, epitheliotropic GI lymphoma
	2 mg/kg PO daily for 14 days, then 1 mg/kg daily thereafter
Doxorubicin (±Prednisolone)	1 mg/kg IV every 2–3 weeks
	Monitor renal values. Do not use in cats with compromised renal function.
CCNU (Lomustine) (±prednisolone)	

Table 10.5. University of Wisconsin-Madison long-term maintenance protocol for cats

Week	V	As	C	D	M	P
1	X	X				x
2			X			x
3	X					x
4				X		x
5						X
6	X					X
7			X			X
8	X					X
9				X		X
10						X
11	X					X
12	x					X
13			X			X
14						X
15	X					X
16						X
17					x	X
18						X
19	X					X
20						X
21			X			X
22						X
23	X					X
24						X
25				X		X

This protocol is continued biweekly as described for weeks 11–25 for 12 months, and then triweekly for 6 months, and then monthly for 6 months.
V = vincristine at 0.5–0.7 mg/m^2 IV once on the appropriate treatment week
As = L-Asparaginase at 400 U/kg SC once on the appropriate treatment week
C = cyclophosphamide at 250 mg/m^2 IV once on the appropriate treatment week
D = doxorubicin at 1 mg/kg IV once on the appropriate treatment week
M = methotrexate 0.8 mg/kg IV once on the appropriate treatment week
P = prednisolone 2 mg/kg daily for the first 2 weeks, and then 1 mg/kg daily

proportion of feline patients that experience a prolonged remission in which discontinuation of chemotherapy is an option is considerably lower than in dogs. Therefore, the decision to discontinue therapy is often made on a case-by-case basis.

Monitoring Therapy

- It is necessary to perform serial assessments of all patients being treated for lymphoma.
- The nature of these assessments will vary on the original site and extent of disease, chosen treatment protocol, and current clinical status.

Table 10.6. 25-week University of Wisconsin-Madison CHOP protocol for cats

Week	V	As	C	D	P
1	X	X			x
2			X		x
3	X				x
4				X	x
5					X
6	X				X
7			X		X
8	X				X
9				X	X
10					X
11	X				X
12					X
13			X		X
14					X
15	X				X
16					X
17				X	X
18					X
19	X				X
20					X
21			X		X
22					X
23	X				X
24					X
25				X	X

V = vincristine at 0.5–0.7 mg/m² IV once on the appropriate treatment week
As = L-Asparaginase at 400 IU/kg SC. once on the appropriate treatment week
C = cyclophosphamide at 250 mg/m² IV once on the appropriate treatment week
D = doxorubicin at 1 mg/kg IV once on the appropriate treatment week
P = prednisolone at 2 mg/kg PO daily for 14 days, and then 1 mg/kg PO daily thereafter

Table 10.7. Chlorambucil and prednisolone for low-grade feline lymphoma

Chlorambucil	20 mg/m2 PO once every 2 weeks Available in 2 mg tablets that should not be split
Prednisolone	2 mg/kg PO daily for 14 days, and then 1 mg/kg PO daily thereafter

• Regular reevaluations must focus on documenting a response to treatment as well as ensure that the patient may safely be administered a scheduled therapy.

Chemotherapy patients:

Treatment Day

• Physical examination and history   Ensure remission
• Vital signs: temperature, HR, RR   Ensure afebrile, stable vitals
• CBC   Treat if PMN >1500; plt >75,000

Table 10.8.   Categories for response

Complete response (CR):	Complete disappearance of all detectable lesions
Partial response (PR):	A 50% or > decrease in the size of the measured lesion
Minor response (MR):	A 25–49% decrease in the size of the measured lesion
Stable disease (SD):	A 0–24% change in size of the measured lesion
Progressive disease (PD):	An increase of >25% in the size of the measured lesion or formation of new lesions

- 7–10 Days After Chemotherapy
- Physical examination and history   Ensure remission
- Vital signs: temperature, HR, RR   Ensure afebrile, stable
- CBC
  - If temperature >103°F and PMN <2000
    - Admit to hospital for IV fluids and IV antibiotics.
  - (If temperature <103°F and PMN <2000
    - Prescribe antibiotics.
    - Owner takes temperature twice daily and returns if T >103°F

Assessing Response

Assessing response is necessary in order to continue therapy. Response should be guaged on resolving clinical signs, improved hematologic or biochemical values and resolution of physical examination/imaging abnormalities (Table 10.8).

- In cats, failure of the lymphoma to respond to appropriate chemotherapy is a poor prognostic indicator.
- For most cats with lymphoma a response should be documented within 3–6 weeks of therapy. If no or inadequate response is evident at that juncture, rescue therapy should be sought or euthanasia considered.
- Failure to remain in remission is also a poor prognostic factor. This is defined as progressive disease after remission (CR or PR) has already been achieved with appropriate therapy. In this situation, rescue therapy should be sought or euthanasia considered.
- Chemoresistance is the cause of both failure to respond to therapy as well as progression of disease after an initial remission.

Feline Leukemia

This section describes the main clinical and pathological features of leukemia in cats, including diseases affecting both the lymphoid and myeloid cell lineages (Figure 10.3, Table 10.9).

Key Points
- Leukemia refers to a malignant neoplastic disease affecting the blood cells of the bone marrow (but sometimes originating in the spleen).
- Neoplastic cells may or may not circulate in the peripheral bloodstream.
- The classification of leukemias is difficult in cats because they are often associated with mixed lineages.
- The clinical signs of leukemia in cats are referable to marrow replacement with neoplastic cells (leading to cytopenias) and infiltration of organs in the periphery (mainly liver and spleen) (Figure 10.4).
- Clinically, the important distinction is whether the disease is **ACUTE** or **CHRONIC.**
- Acute leukemia refers to a disease in which the majority of neoplastic cells are immature or blastic. This disease carries a grave prognosis.
- Chronic leukemia refers to a disease in which the majority of neoplastic cells are mature and well differentiated. This disease carries a better prognosis (Figure 10.5, Table 10.10).
- Lymphoid leukemias are most common.

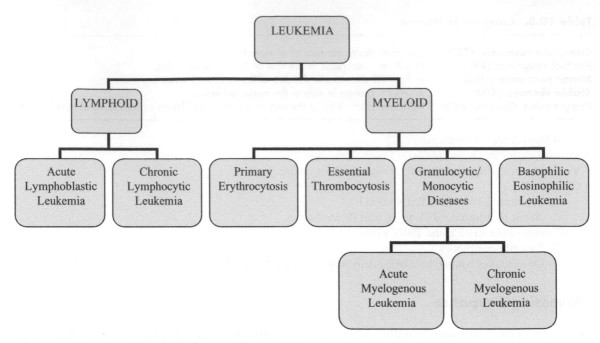

Figure 10.3. Classification of leukemias in the cat.

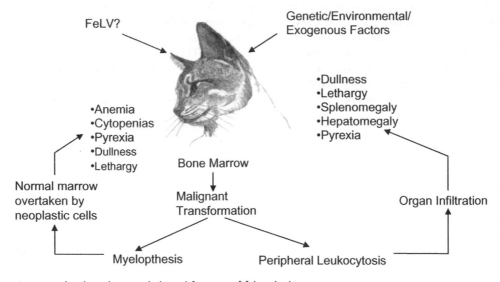

Figure 10.4. Pathophysiology and clinical features of feline leukemias.

Main Clinical Features (Depending on Subtype)

1. **Acute leukemias**
   - Dullness and lethargy
   - Anorexia
   - Anemia
   - Splenomegaly
   - Febrile episodes

Table 10.9. Leukemia in the cat

Leukemia	Features
Acute lymphoid leukemia	Most common leukemia
	Poorly differentiated lymphoblasts in blood and bone marrow
	Usually T cell
	75% are FeLV positive
	Grave prognosis
Chronic lymphoid leukemia	Rare
	Mature lymphocytes in blood and bone marrow
	Must be differentiated from reactive (benign) mature lymphocytosis in blood and bone marrow, which can be secondary to the following conditions:
	• Red cell aplasia, immune-mediated anemia
	• Inflammatory diseases, stress
	Lymphocyte counts in the blood usually in excess of 50,000/uL
	Predominantly FeLV negative
Myeloid leukemias	
Granulocytic leukemia	Rare
	Must be distinguished from leukemoid reactions from infections
	Can be **ACUTE** or **CHRONIC**
Myelomonocytic leukemia	Both neutrophil and monocyte lines affected
Monocytic leukemia	Monocytes only
	Considered an **ACUTE** leukemia irrespective of cell morphology
Basophilic leukemia	Very rare
	Probably a variant of chronic granulocytic leukemia
Eosinophilic leukemia	Rare
	Eosinophil counts usually >15,000/uL
	Need to distinguish from other causes of high eosinophil counts, including
	• Eosinophilic Enteritis
	• Parasitism
	• Allergy
	• Hypereosinophilic syndrome
Primary erythrocytosis	Rare
	PCV > 65 l/L
	Low/normal EPO levels
	Rule out secondary causes of polycythemia (e.g., chronic hypoxia)
Erythroleukemia	Rare
	Primitive erythroid precursors in the blood
	Considered **ACUTE** and carries a grave prognosis
Primary thrombocytopenia	Very rare
	Platelet counts >1,000,000/uL
	Giant platelets in the periphery often with bizarre morphology
Megakaryocytic leukemia	Very rare
	Abnormal megakaryocytes in the bone marrow
	Leads to either thrombocytopenia or thrombocytosis
Myelofibrosis	Abnormal growth and differentiation of erythroid, myeloid, and megakaryocytic cell types
	Proliferation of bone marrow stroma
	May be associated with FeLV
	Often considered a preleukemic event
Erythremic myelosis	Excessive proliferation of erythroid elements in the bone marrow
	Often excessive production of nucleated red blood cells
	May progress to erythroleukemia

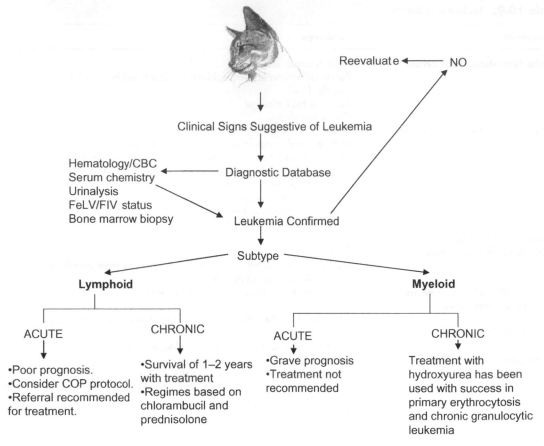

Reevaluate ◄──── NO

Clinical Signs Suggestive of Leukemia

Hematology/CBC ◄──── Diagnostic Database
Serum chemistry
Urinalysis
FeLV/FIV status
Bone marrow biopsy ──► Leukemia Confirmed

Subtype

Lymphoid   **Myeloid**

ACUTE   CHRONIC   ACUTE   CHRONIC

•Poor prognosis.   •Survival of 1–2 years   •Grave prognosis   Treatment with
•Consider COP protocol. with treatment   •Treatment not   hydroxyurea has been
•Referral recommended   •Regimes based on   recommended   used with success in
for treatment.   chlorambucil and   primary erythrocytosis
                        prednisolone   and chronic granulocytic
                                                                        leukemia

Figure 10.5. Diagnosis and treatment of leukemias.

Table 10.10. Treatment regimes

Acute Lymphoid Leukemia	Responses are poor. 27% response rate has been reported with feline COP regime. Recommend referral to a specialist oncologist if treatment is being considered.
Chronic Lymphoid Leukemia	Chlorambucil: • 0.2 mg/kg or 2 mg/cat PO every other day Prednisolone: • 1 mg/kg daily 1–2 years survival have been reported
Acute Myeloid Leukemia	Treatment is not recommended because it is usually ineffective. Prognosis is grave.
Chronic Myeloid Leukemia: • Chronic myeloid leukemia • Primary erythrocytosis	Hydroxyurea is the treatment of choice. It is difficult to dose cats because they are 500 mg capsules. Refer to a specialist center that has access to reformulated hydroxurea (125 mg capsules) Recommend 125 mg daily and then every other day for maintenance. Phlebotomy can be used in cases of primary erythrocytosis, in the early stages of treatment

2. **Chronic leukemias**
   - Longer duration of illness
   - Mild anemia
   - ±Splenomegaly

Feline Multiple Myeloma

- This is a rare disease.
- It most commonly affects older cats.
- Clinical signs and hematological/biochemical abnormalities are similar to those of dogs: however, skeletal lesions are less common.
- Prognosis is usually not as favorable in the cat as compared to the dog.
- Cats often transiently respond to melphalan/prednisolone protocols.
- Most responses are partial and not durable.
- Median survival times are short (2–4 months), but durable remissions have been reported.

11
SPLENIC TUMORS

Malcolm J. Brearley and Suzanne Murphy

This chapter describes the main clinical and pathological features of splenic tumors in dogs and cats.

Key Points
- The canine spleen can be the site for both malignant and benign tumors and nonneoplastic disease (Table 11.1).
- Splenic tumors tend to occur in middle-aged to older patients.
- Clinical signs of splenic neoplasia can be vague or nonexistent, or dramatic in the case of splenic rupture and bleeding.
- Approximately two-thirds of canine splenic lesions are neoplastic and of those, two-thirds are hemangiosarcoma.
- 50% of feline splenic lesions are neoplastic.
- Splenic lesions may be generalized or localized.
- Splenomegaly may be described in a similar manner (Table 11.2).
- Splenic abnormalities may be identified on clinical examination, but ultrasound will give better categorization.
- Cytology is not always accurate. A recent study showed about 60% agreement of cytology with subsequent histopathology.
- If a splenectomy or exploratory laparotomy is performed, multiple sites of the spleen should be sampled.
- Hemangiosarcoma frequently has areas of hemorrhage and fibrosis associated with it, which may lead to a misdiagnosis (Figure 11.1). Alternatively larger samples can be sliced like a loaf to ensure even penetration of formalin saline.

Table 11.1. Differential diagnoses for splenic masses in the dog and cat

Benign/Nonneoplastic	Malignant
Hematoma	Hemangiosarcoma
Abscess	Fibrosarcoma
Nodular hyperplasia	Leiomyosarcoma
Extramedullary hemopoeisis	Histiocytic sarcoma
Myelolipoma	Metastatic disease
Hemangioma	
Splenic thromboses or infarcts	

Table 11.2. Differential diagnoses for uniform splenomegaly in the dog and cat

Nonneoplastic	Neoplastic
Normal for breed (GSDs are reported to have relatively larger spleens than would be anticipated for their size)	Leukemia
Congestion	Lymphoma
Inflammation	Multiple myeloma
Immune-mediated disease	Primary mast cell tumor (common in cats)
Infectious agents	Mast cell tumor metastasis
Some anesthetic agents	Disseminated (malignant) histiocytosis
Splenic torsion in dogs	Polycythemia vera

It should be noted that sometimes disease processes that are described as uniformly infiltrative can give mass lesions and vice versa.

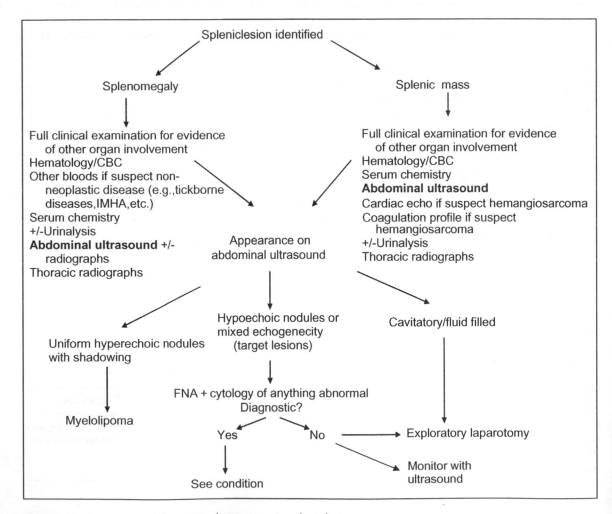

Figure 11.1. A general diagnostic decision tree in splenic lesions.

Canine Splenic Tumors – Hemangiosarcoma

Key Point
- Malignant tumor arising from vascular endothelium.
- Spleen is the most common primary site of hemangiosarcoma.
- The classical presentation is a solitary cavitated lesion that bleeds, causing hemoperitoneum and hypovolemic collapse.
- This tumor readily metastasizes to liver and other areas of the abdominal cavity and to lungs.
- Cutaneous metastases can be seen, but this tumor also has a primary cutaneous form.
- Splenic lesions are found concurrently with right atrial lesions in about 25% of cases.
- Hemangiosarcoma is seen more commonly in large-breed dogs and is particularly associated with the German Shepherd dog.
- The median age of affected animals is 10 years old.
- Dogs with hemangiosarcoma frequently have coagulation abnormalities such as DIC (50% of cases) or thrombocytopenia (75% of cases) and often are anemic.
- CBC and coagulation profile; serum biochemistry; ultrasonography of abdomen, especially liver as well as spleen; and assessment of heart for right atrial lesions is necessary to stage these cases.
- Hematology may show polychromasia, hypochromasia, reticulocytosis, schistocytes, and nucleated RBCs on blood smears.
- Even with treatment the prognosis is grave. Low-grade and stage 1 have a slightly improved prognosis (Tables 11.3, 11.4).

Treatment

Table 11.3.   Survival times for dogs treated for splenic hemangiosarcoma

Treatment	Median Survival Times
Splenectomy alone (stage1 or 2)	86 days
Splenectomy plus VAC*	164 days
Splenectomy plus AC*	179 days
Splenectomy plus doxorubicin	60 days if evidence of gross disease after splenectomy
	172 days if no evidence of further disease

*Stage unknown.
VAC: vincristine, doxorubicin, cyclophosphamide, (plus chlorambucil and methotrexate).
AC: Doxorubicin, cyclophosphamide.

Table 11.4. WHO staging system for canine hemangiosarcoma*

T—Primary tumor	
T0	No evidence of tumor
T1	Tumor confined to spleen
T2	Tumor confined to spleen but ruptured
N—Regional lymph nodes	
N0	No regional lymph node involvement
N1	Regional lymph node involvement
N2	Distant lymph node involvement
M—Distant metastasis	
M0	No evidence of distant metastasis
M1	Distant metastasis

* Wood et al. 1998. Prognosis for dogs with stage I or II splenic hemangiosarcoma treated by splenectomy alone: 32 cases (1991–1993). Journal of the American Animal Hospital Association 34(5):417–421.

Stage	
I	T0 or T1, N0, M0
II	T1 or T2, N0 or N1, M0
III	T2 or T3, N1 or N2, M1

Primary Splenic Nonangiomatous, Nonlymphoid Tumors

- Benign
  - Myelolipomas are benign tumors composed of a mixture of mature adipose tissue and normal hematopoietic cells.
  - Lipomas have also been recorded in spleens.
  - Both conditions are associated with long survival times after splenectomy.
- Malignant
  - Fibrosarcoma, undifferentiated sarcoma, leiomyosarcoma, osteosarcoma, myxosarcoma, and liposarcoma have a guarded prognosis with a median survival of 4 months Figure 11.2.
  - Splenic neoplasms of this type with a mitotic index <9 showed significantly longer survival intervals than those with an index >9.
- Histiocytic disease (see Chapter 8)
  - The spleen can be the site of primary or disseminated histiocytic sarcoma.
  - Primary splenic histiocytic sarcoma has been associated with a Coombs test–negative anemia due to erythrophagia by the neoplastic histiocytes.
  - Disseminated histiocytic sarcoma (also referred to as malignant histiocytosis) is a rare condition in most dog breeds but very common in Bernese Mountain dogs (estimated 600-fold increase in risk relative to other dog breeds). Flat-coated retrievers (and less so Golden Retrievers) are also at increased risk.
  - All of these conditions have a guarded or poor prognosis.

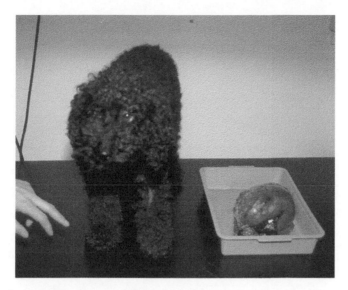

Figure 11.2.   Canine leiomyosarcoma. (Image courtesy of Suzanne Murphy)

Tumors Usually Associated with Metastatic Disease in the Spleen

- Lymphoma (see Chapters 9 and 10)
  - Lymphoma can arise in the spleen but, more often, as part of multicentric lymphoma.
  - Lymphoma often gives a "Swiss cheese" appearance on ultrasonography, but diffuse patterns can also be seen.
- Other myeloproliferative diseases (can involve the spleen)
  - Multiple myeloma
  - Leukemia
  - Polycythemia vera
- Mast cell tumors
  - In dogs, high-grade MCTs can metastasize to the spleen.
  - In cats, the spleen may be a primary site for MCT with secondary mastocytosis (Chapter 7).

12
GASTROINTESTINAL TUMORS

David J. Argyle and Corey Saba

This section describes the main clinical and pathological features of gastrointestinal tumors in dogs and cats, including tumors of the liver and exocrine pancreas.

Key Points
- Gastrointestinal tumors most commonly occur in middle-aged to older patients.
- Clinical signs of gastrointestinal tumors are typically organ-dependent and may be nonspecific.
- The site of the primary tumor will influence the clinical presentation (Figures 12.1, 12.2).
- The clinical features are often associated with the physical effects of the mass.
- The gastrointestinal tract can be the site for both malignant and benign tumors.

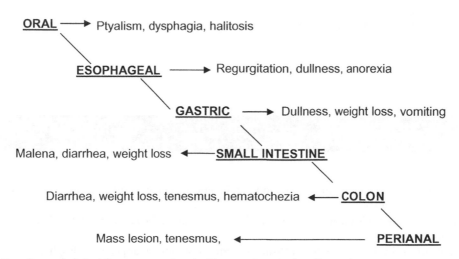

Figure 12.1. General clinical features associated with gastrointestinal malignancies.

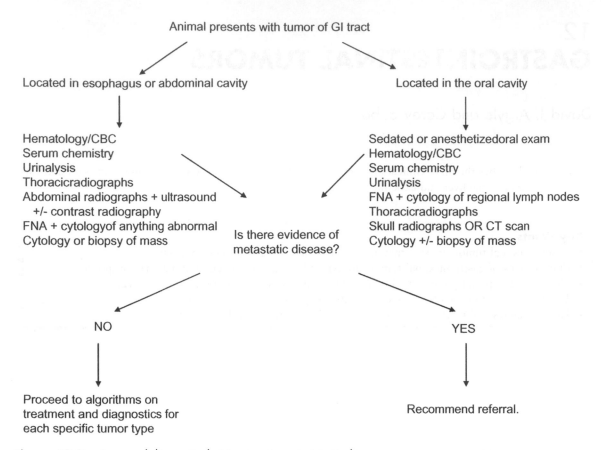

Animal presents with tumor of GI tract

Located in esophagus or abdominal cavity

Located in the oral cavity

Hematology/CBC
Serum chemistry
Urinalysis
Thoracicradiographs
Abdominal radiographs + ultrasound
 +/- contrast radiography
FNA + cytologyof anything abnormal
Cytology or biopsy of mass

Sedated or anesthetizedoral exam
Hematology/CBC
Serum chemistry
Urinalysis
FNA + cytology of regional lymph nodes
Thoracicradiographs
Skull radiographs OR CT scan
Cytology +/- biopsy of mass

Is there evidence of
metastatic disease?

NO

YES

Proceed to algorithms on
treatment and diagnostics for
each specific tumor type

Recommend referral.

Figure 12.2. A general diagnostic decision tree in gastrointestinal tumors.

Oral Tumors

Key Points
- The most common oral tumors in dogs include **malignant melanoma, squamous cell carcinoma, fibro-sarcoma,** and the **epulides.**
- Squamous cell carcinoma is the most common feline oral tumor. Fibrosarcoma and melanoma occur, but are less common.
- Clinical signs of oral tumors include ptyalism (sometimes bloody), inappetence, dysphagia, weight loss, halitosis, exophthalmus, epistaxis, and/or loose teeth (Tables 12.1, 12.2; Figures 12.3, 12.4).
- Biologic behavior and prognosis of oral tumors are best predicted by histologic type, tumor location, tumor size, and stage of disease (Figures 12.5–12.7, Table 12.3–12.6).

Table 12.1. Clinical features of oral tumors in the dog

Histologic Type	Features
Malignant melanoma (OMM)	Most common canine oral tumor. Golden Retrievers, Scottish terriers, poodles, and dachshunds are overrepresented. Immunohistochemistry may be necessary to diagnose some melanomas, especially amelanotic tumors. In general, locally invasive and highly metastatic. True metastatic rate is dependent on size, location, and grade of the tumor. Common sites of metastasis: regional lymph nodes and lungs.
Squamous cell carcinoma (SCC)	Second most common canine oral tumor. Locally invasive. Metastatic rate is variable and dependent on location. Tonsillar SCC has a much higher metastatic rate than more rostral tumors. At diagnosis, ~10–20% of patients with tonsillar SCC have overt evidence of metastatic disease; ~90% have micrometastatic disease. Sites of metastasis: Tonsil, regional lymph nodes, and lungs.
Fibrosarcoma (FSA)	Occurs less commonly than OMM and SCC. There is a specific variant: "Histologically low grade, biologically high grade" FSA appears benign histologically, but it is very locally aggressive and grows rapidly. Metastatic rate of FSA is <20%. Lungs are the most common site of metastasis, but spread to regional lymph nodes can occur.
Epulides	Arise from the periodontal ligament. Tend to be slow-growing and firm. May appear similar to gingival hyperplasia. Subtypes include • **Acanthomatous** (previously termed *basal cell carcinoma* or *adamantinoma*): This is a locally aggressive tumor that frequently invades the underlying bone. The most common site is the rostral mandible. • **Fibromatous:** Slow-growing firm masses. Often found around the maxillary premolar teeth. • **Ossifying:** Slow-growing firm masses. Often found around the maxillary premolar teeth. • **Giant Cell:** Rare form. Are locally aggressive, often invading underlying bone. Bony invasion is typically dependent on the type of epulis. Never metastasize.

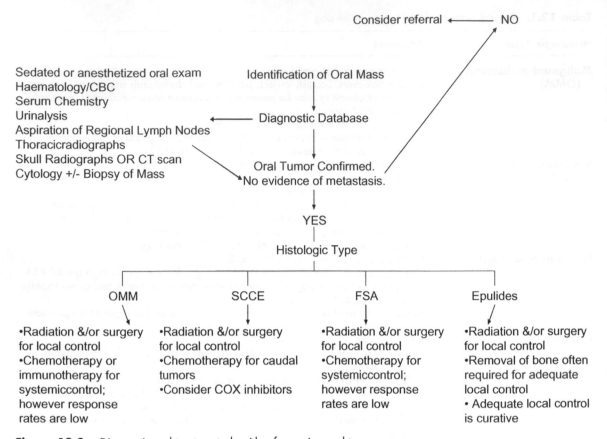

Sedated or anesthetized oral exam
Haematology/CBC
Serum Chemistry
Urinalysis
Aspiration of Regional Lymph Nodes
Thoracicradiographs
Skull Radiographs OR CT scan
Cytology +/- Biopsy of Mass

Consider referral ← NO

Identification of Oral Mass

Diagnostic Database

Oral Tumor Confirmed.
No evidence of metastasis.

YES

Histologic Type

OMM

SCCE

FSA

Epulides

•Radiation &/or surgery
for local control
•Chemotherapy or
immunotherapy for
systemiccontrol;
however response
rates are low

•Radiation &/or surgery
for local control
•Chemotherapy for caudal
tumors
•Consider COX inhibitors

•Radiation &/or surgery
for local control
•Chemotherapy for
systemiccontrol;
however response
rates are low

•Radiation &/or surgery
for local control
•Removal of bone often
required for adequate
local control
• Adequate local control
is curative

Figure 12.3. Diagnostic and treatment algorithm for canine oral tumors.

Table 12.2. Clinical staging (TNM) of oral tumors in dogs and cats

Primary Tumor

T	Tumor in situ
T1	Tumor < 2 cm in diameter at the greatest dimension
T2	Tumor 2–4 cm in diameter at the greatest dimension
T3	Tumor > 4 cm in diameter at the greatest dimension
Suffix a	Without evidence of bony invasion
Suffix b	With evidence of bony invasion

Regional Lymph Node

N0	No regional lymph node metastasis
N1	Movable ipsilateral lymph nodes
N2	Movable contralateral lymph nodes
N3	Fixed lymph nodes
Suffix a	No evidence of lymph node metastasis
Suffix b	Evidence of lymph node metastasis

Distant Metastasis

M0	No distant metastasis
M1	Distant metsastasis

Table 12.3. Treatment regimes and prognosis for canine oral tumors

OMM
Recommend surgical excision for tumors easily excised with wide (at least 2 cm) margins. Removal of bone is often required for good local control.

For nonresectable tumors, consider coarse-fractionated radiation therapy (e.g., 9 Gy × 4 fractions). Reported response rates: 83–95%. Complete response rates: 53–70%. MST: 21–31 weeks.

For medical management, consider carboplatin chemotherapy. Reported response rate: 28%. (Mostly partial responses reported.) MST: 165 days.

Alternatively, for medical management, consider immunotherapy. Several tumor vaccines are currently under clinical investigation.

Overall prognosis is poor; however, size and stage of disease are important predictors.

One-year survival rate: 25–35%.

MST for dogs who stage negatively and have tumors <2 cm: 511 days.

MST for dogs with metastasis and/or tumors >2 cm: 164 days.

Metastasis is commonly the cause of death, especially when the primary tumor is well controlled.

SCC
Recommend surgical excision for tumors easily excised with wide (at least 2 cm) margins. Removal of bone is often required for good local control. Rostral tumors are easier to completely excise.

For incompletely excised or nonresectable tumors, consider radiation therapy (definitive **OR** palliative).

For medical management, consider piroxicam (0.3 mg/kg PO every 24 hours). Reported response rate: 18%.

Cisplatin in combination with piroxicam has also been reported. Reported response rate: 55%. **HOWEVER,** both drugs are nephrotoxic and incidence of kidney damage/failure is high. **USE THIS PROTOCOL WITH CAUTION.** Discontinuation of piroxicam around the time of cisplatin administration is recommended. **CONSIDER REFERRAL.**

Carboplatin is an alternative to cisplatin chemotherapy and is less nephrotoxic. Careful monitoring of BUN/creatinine is still recommended.

In general, prognosis is good for completely excised rostral tumors. However, for tonsillar SCC, the metastatic rate is high and prognosis is poor.

FSA
Recommend surgical excision for tumors easily excised with wide (at least 2 cm) margins. Removal of bone is often required for good local control.

For incompletely excised tumors, consider definitive radiation therapy (MST: 540 days).

Inadequate local control results in death more commonly than distant metastasis.

Role of chemotherapy is unknown.

Prognosis guarded.

Epulides
Recommend surgical excision for tumors easily excised. Removal of bone is often required for good local control, especially for acanthomatous epulides.

Alternatively, consider definitive radiation therapy. Reported control rates are up to 90%.

Adequate local control is curative. Prognosis is excellent.

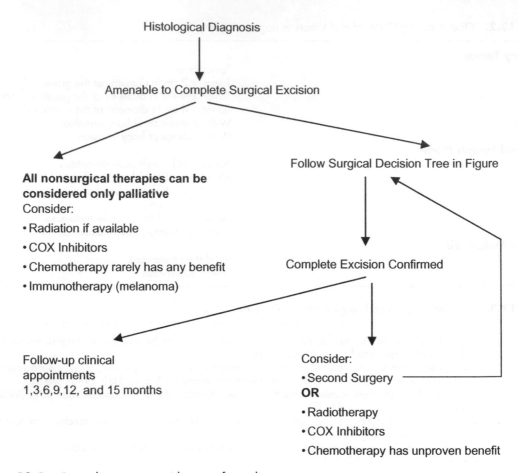

Histological Diagnosis

Amenable to Complete Surgical Excision

**All nonsurgical therapies can be
considered only palliative**
Consider:

• Radiation if available

• COX Inhibitors

• Chemotherapy rarely has any benefit

• Immunotherapy (melanoma)

Follow Surgical Decision Tree in Figure

Complete Excision Confirmed

Follow-up clinical
appointments
1,3,6,9,12, and 15 months

Consider:

• Second Surgery
OR

• Radiotherapy

• COX Inhibitors

• Chemotherapy has unproven benefit

Figure 12.4.   General treatment considerations for oral tumors.

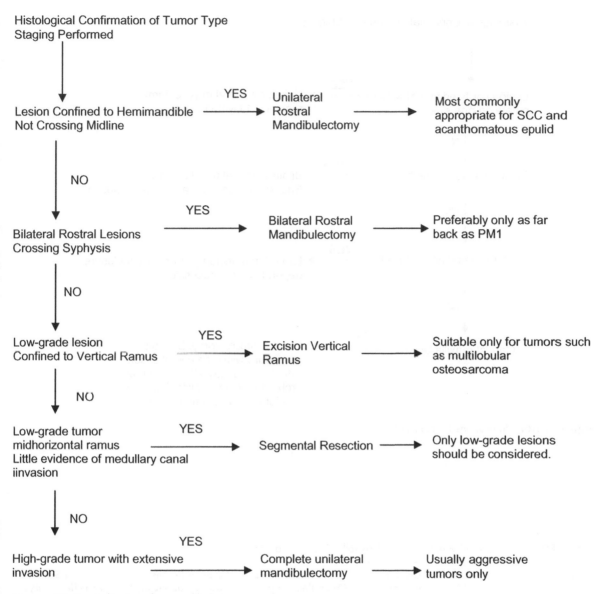

Histological Confirmation of Tumor Type
Staging Performed

Lesion Confined to Hemimandible
Not Crossing Midline

YES → Unilateral Rostral Mandibulectomy → Most commonly appropriate for SCC and acanthomatous epulid

NO

Bilateral Rostral Lesions Crossing Syphysis

YES → Bilateral Rostral Mandibulectomy → Preferably only as far back as PM1

NO

Low-grade lesion Confined to Vertical Ramus

YES → Excision Vertical Ramus → Suitable only for tumors such as multilobular osteosarcoma

NO

Low-grade tumor midhorizontal ramus Little evidence of medullary canal iinvasion

YES → Segmental Resection → Only low-grade lesions should be considered.

NO

High-grade tumor with extensive invasion

YES → Complete unilateral mandibulectomy → Usually aggressive tumors only

Figure 12.5. Indications for mandibulectomy.

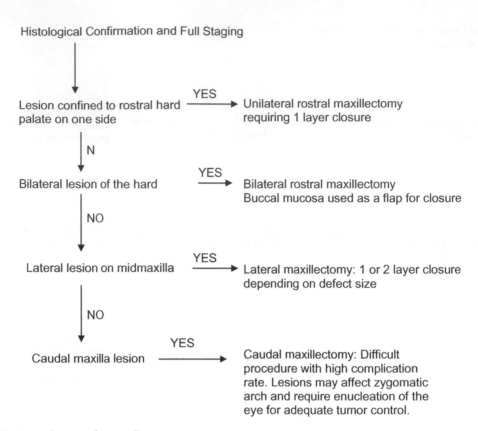

Figure 12.6. Indications for maxillectomy.

Table 12.4. Postoperative outcomes in dogs following surgical resection

Tumor Type	Local Recurrence (Mandibulectomy)	Local Recurrence (Maxillectomy)	Median Survival (Mandibulectomy)	Median Survival (Maxillectomy)
Malignant melanoma	0–40%	21–48%	7–17 months	5–10 months
Squamous cell carcinoma	0–23%	29–50%	9–26 months	19 months
Fibrosarcoma	31–60%	35–57%	11–12 months	10–12 months
Osteosarcoma	15–44%	27–100%	6–18 months	4–10 months
Acanthomatous epulide	0–3%	0–11%	>28–64 months	>26–30 months

Table 12.5. Clinical features of oral tumors in the cat

Histologic Type	Features
Squamous cell carcinoma (SCC)	Most common feline oral tumor.
	Risk factors include use of flea products (collars and dips), diet (canned food, especially tuna), and possibly second-hand tobacco smoke.
	Extremely locally invasive.
	Successful treatment often difficult due to advanced nature of local disease at time of diagnosis.
	Although uncommon, sites of metastasis include regional lymph nodes and lungs.
Fibrosarcoma (FSA)	Second most common feline oral tumor.
	Tumors are locally aggressive, but metastatic rate is typically low.
	Lungs are the most common site of metastasis, but spread to regional lymph nodes can occur.
Malignant melanoma (OMM)	Rare in cats.

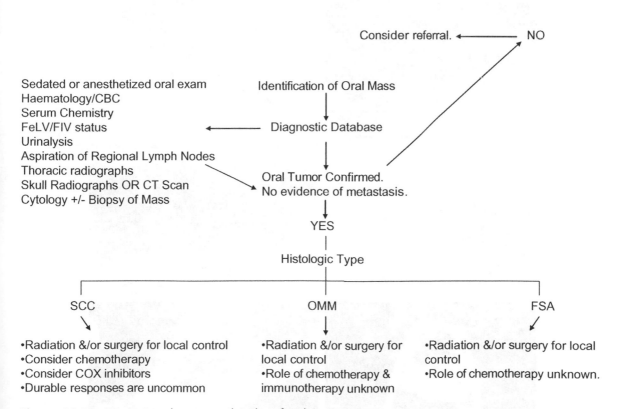

Figure 12.7. Diagnosis and treatment algorithm of oral tumors in cats.

225

Table 12.6. Treatment recommendations for oral tumors in cats (Figure 12.8)

SCC	Recommend surgical excision for tumors easily excised with wide margins. Removal of bone is often required for good local control.
	For nonresectable tumors, consider radiation therapy, but durable responses are uncommon.
	For medical management, consider piroxicam and/or chemotherapy.
	Various chemotherapeutic drugs have been used for SCC in cats (most anecdotally). These include carboplatin, gemcitabine, doxorubicin, and mitoxantrone. **DO NOT USE CISPLATIN IN CATS.**
	Prognosis is poor; <10% of cats will survive >1 year.
	Death is commonly due to poor local control rather than metastasis.
FSA	Recommend surgical excision for tumors easily excised with wide margins. Removal of bone is often required for good local control.
	For incompletely excised tumors, consider definitive radiation therapy.
	Death is commonly due to poor local control rather than metastasis.
	Prognosis is guarded.
OMM	Few reports in the veterinary literature.
	Recommend surgical excision for tumors easily excised with wide margins. Removal of bone is often required for good local control.
	For nonresectable tumors, consider coarse-fractionated radiation therapy. Response rate appears lower than in dogs, and responses typically are not durable. Reported MST with radiation therapy: 146 days.
	Role of chemotherapy is unknown.
	Prognosis is guarded.

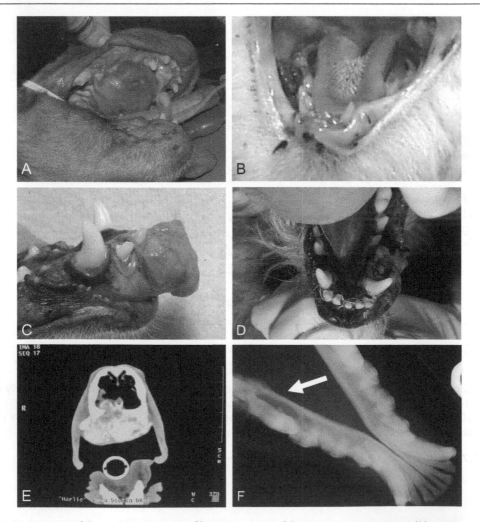

Figure 12.8. Tumors of the oral cavity: canine fibrosarcoma (A), feline squamous carcinoma (B), canine acanthomatous epulid (C), canine malignant melanoma (D), CT image of palantine fibrosarcoma eroding into the nasal cavity (E), and squamous carcinoma of the mandible causing bony erosion (F). Images courtesy of Nicole Northup and Karen Cornell.

Salivary Tumors in Dogs and Cats

- Salivary tumors are rare in dogs and cats.
- Major differential diagnosis:
  - Lipoma
  - Abscess
  - Sialadenitis
  - Salivary mucocele
- Diagnosis:
  - History and clinical signs
  - Imaging (ultrasound/CT)
  - Biopsy (FNA/incisional)
- In the cats, Siamese and male cats may be overrepresented.
- Adenocarcinoma is the most common histological type. Benign salivary tumors are very rare.
- While any gland may be affected, salivary tumors most commonly occur in the mandibular glands.
- Salivary tumors are locally invasive. Wide surgical excision is the treatment of choice, and radiation therapy is a viable option for incompletely resected tumors.
- The metastatic rate is moderate (8–17% for dogs and 16–39% for cats). Common metastatic sites include regional lymph nodes and lungs.
- The role of chemotherapy is unknown.
- In one report, the median survival time for dogs with salivary tumors treated with surgery, with or without postoperative radiation therapy, was 550 days. For cats, the reported MST was 516 days.

Esophageal Tumors in Dogs and Cats

- Extremely rare in dogs and cats.
- Signs associated with esophageal tumors include weight loss, regurgitation, and anorexia.
- Histologic types include squamous cell carcinoma, leiomyosarcoma, leiomyoma, fibrosarcoma, lymphoma, and mast cell tumor.
- *Spirocera lupi* infestation has been linked to esophageal sarcoma development.
- Typically, surgery is the treatment of choice. However, resection is often difficult in this location.
- For malignant esophageal tumors, prognosis is guarded due to the inability to control the primary tumor and the high metastatic rate of esophageal cancer.
- Roles of radiation therapy and chemotherapy are unknown.

Gastric Tumors in Dogs and Cats

- The most common gastric tumor in the dog is adenocarcinoma, and the most common gastric tumor in the cat is lymphoma. Other gastric tumor types include leiomyosarcoma, gastrointestinal stromal tumor (GIST), and mast cell tumor. (Mast cell tumor and lymphoma and are covered in Chapters 7, 9, and 10.)
- Clinical signs include vomiting, weight loss, and inappetence (Table 12.7).
- Microcytic hypochromic anemia is common due to chronic GI blood loss.
- Typically, surgery is the treatment of choice. However, resection is often difficult in this location (Table 12.8).
- The role of chemotherapy other than with lymphoma is unknown.

Table 12.7. Features of gastric tumors

Histologic Type	Features
Adenocarcinoma	Most common histologic type in dogs.
	Commonly occurs along the lesser curvature and at the gastric antrum.
	Reported metastatic rate: 74–80%. Sites of metastasis include regional lymph nodes, liver, omentum, spleen, and lungs.
Leiomyoma/ leiomyosarcoma	Leiomyomas more common in very old dogs (~15 years).
	Paraneoplastic hypoglycemia reported.
	Reported metastatic rate is high. Sites of metastasis include liver and duodenum.
Gastrointestinal stromal tumor (GIST)	19% of GIST occur in the stomach.
	~50% of GIST stain positively for CD117 (c-Kit).

Table 12.8. Treatment regimes and prognosis for canine and feline gastric tumors

Adenocarcinoma	Surgical excision is the treatment of choice. However, successful treatment is often difficult due to tumor location and advanced nature of disease at time of diagnosis.
	Role of chemotherapy is unknown.
	Prognosis is good for benign tumors, but poor for malignant tumors.
Leiomyoma/leiomyosarcoma	Surgical excision is the treatment of choice.
	Complete excision is curative for leiomyoma.
	Successful treatment of leiomyosarcoma is more difficult due to tumor location and advanced nature of disease at time of diagnosis.
	Prognosis is good for benign tumors but guarded to poor for malignant tumors.
Gastrointestinal stromal tumors (GIST)	Surgical excision is the treatment of choice.
	Prognosis is guarded to poor.

Intestinal and Rectal Tumors

- Lymphoma is the most common intestinal tumor in dogs and cats; discussion of this cancer is covered in Chapters 9 and 10. Other intestinal tumors include adenocarcinoma, leiomyoma, leiomyosarcoma, gastrointestinal stromal tumor (GIST), and mast cell tumor (more common in cats and discussed in Chapter 7).
- Leiomyoma/leiomyosarcoma occurs more commonly in male dogs.
- In reports of intestinal adenocarcinoma in cats, Siamese cats are overrepresented.
- Clinical signs include weight loss, inappetence, vomiting, diarrhea, melena, and/or hematochezia (Tables 12.9, 12.10; Figure 12.9).
- Microcytic hypochromic anemia is also common due to chronic GI blood loss.
- Smooth muscle tumors have been associated with paraneoplastic hypoglycemia.
- Typically, surgery is the treatment of choice (Table 12.11). However, resection is often difficult in this location.
- The role of chemotherapy is unknown.

Table 12.9. Intestinal tumors in the dog

Histologic Type	Features
Adenocarcinoma	Most commonly occurs in the large intestine. In the small intestine, the most common location is the jejunum. Metastatic rate is moderate (>44%). Most common site of metastasis is regional lymph nodes. Other sites include mesentery, omentum, and lungs.
Leiomyoma/leiomyosarcoma	Second most common intestinal tumor in dogs. Most common intestinal locations are jejunum and cecum. Polyuria, polydipsia, anemia, and hypoglycemia are common clinical findings. Metastatic rate for leiomyosarcoma is low to moderate (16–50%). Metastasis most commonly occurs to abdominal viscera. Sites include mesentery, spleen, liver, and lymph nodes.
Gastrointestinal stromal tumors (GIST)	52% express CD117 (c-KIT). Large intestine is the most common location. Metastatic rate for GIST is moderate (29%). Metastasis most commonly occurs to abdominal viscera. Sites include liver, lymph nodes, and other abdominal organs.

Table 12.10. Intestinal tumors in the cat

Histologic Type	Features
Adenocarcinoma	Most commonly occurs in the small intestine. Sites of metastasis include regional lymph nodes and lungs. Poor prognosis.
Leiomyoma/leiomyosarcoma/GIST	Rare/not reported in cats.

Lymphoma is covered in Chapter 10, and mast cell tumor is covered in Chapter 7.

Table 12.11. Treatment regimes and prognosis for canine and feline intestinal tumors (Figure 12.10)

Adenocarcinoma	Surgical excision with wide margins (5 cm on either side of the tumor) is the treatment of choice. Chemotherapy for systemic disease is reasonable; however, exact role of chemotherapy is unknown. Reported MST for canine SI adenocarcinoma without metastasis: 15 months. MST with metastasis: 3 months.
Leiomyoma/ leiomyosarcoma	Surgical excision with wide margins (5 cm on either side of the tumor) is the treatment of choice. Complete excision is curative for leiomyoma. Chemotherapy for systemic disease is reasonable; however, exact role of chemotherapy is unknown. Reported MST for canine leiomyosarcoma without metastasis: 15–21 months. MST with metastasis: 2–21. (Mixed reports about the prognostic significance of metastasis at diagnosis.)
Gastrointestinal stromal tumors (GIST)	Surgical excision with wide margins (5 cm on either side of the tumor) is the treatment of choice. Chemotherapy for systemic disease is reasonable; however, exact role of chemotherapy is unknown. Prognosis is guarded.

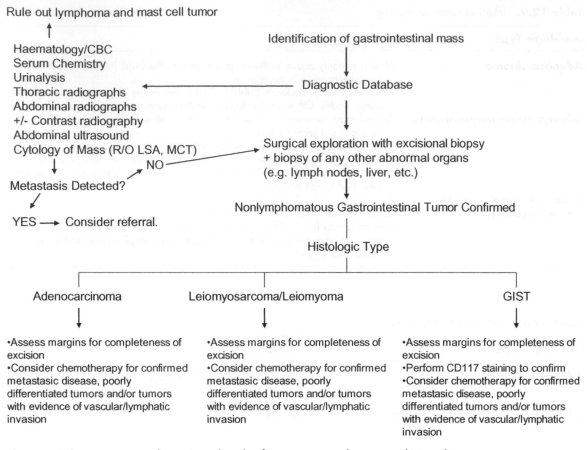

Rule out lymphoma and mast cell tumor

↑

Haematology/CBC
Serum Chemistry
Urinalysis
Thoracic radiographs
Abdominal radiographs
+/- Contrast radiography
Abdominal ultrasound
Cytology of Mass (R/O LSA, MCT)

Identification of gastrointestinal mass

↓

Diagnostic Database

↓

Metastasis Detected?

NO

Surgical exploration with excisional biopsy
+ biopsy of any other abnormal organs
(e.g. lymph nodes, liver, etc.)

↓

Nonlymphomatous Gastrointestinal Tumor Confirmed

YES → Consider referral.

Histologic Type

Adenocarcinoma

•Assess margins for completeness of excision
•Consider chemotherapy for confirmed metastasic disease, poorly differentiated tumors and/or tumors with evidence of vascular/lymphatic invasion

Leiomyosarcoma/Leiomyoma

•Assess margins for completeness of excision
•Consider chemotherapy for confirmed metastasic disease, poorly differentiated tumors and/or tumors with evidence of vascular/lymphatic invasion

GIST

•Assess margins for completeness of excision
•Perform CD117 staining to confirm
•Consider chemotherapy for confirmed metastasic disease, poorly differentiated tumors and/or tumors with evidence of vascular/lymphatic invasion

Figure 12.9. Diagnosis and treatment algorithm for gastrointestinal tumors in dogs and cats.

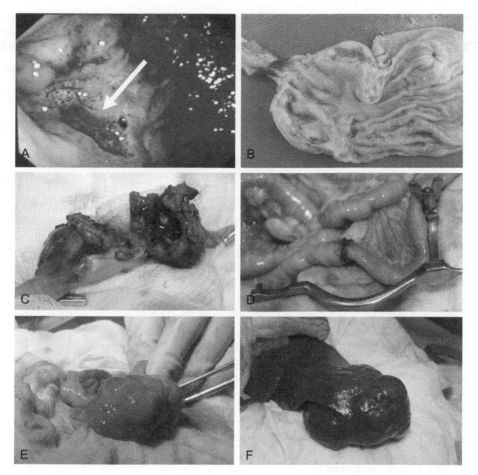

Figure 12.10. Endoscopy of canine gastric adenocarcinoma (A), feline gastric lymphoma (B), small bowel perforation associated with small intestinal lymphoma (C) and after repair (D), small intestinal adenocarcinoma (E), and a solitary hepatobiliary carcinoma in the dog (F). Image courtesy of Nicole Northup and Karen Cornell.

Perianal Tumors

- Hepatoid tumors (perianal adenomas/perianal adenocarcinomas) arise from sebaceous glands located in the dermis around the anus (Table 12.12, Figure 12.11).
- Apocrine gland adenocarcinomas arise from the anal sacs located at the 4 o'clock and 8 o'clock positions on either side of the anus (Figure 12.12).
- Perianal adenoma is the most common histologic type in intact male dogs. Perianal adenocarcinomas occur less commonly in both sexes.
- Apocrine gland adenocarcinomas are the most common histologic type in female dogs. Contrary to prior reports, recent reports suggest that this tumor type occurs with equal frequency in neutered males and females. It is least common in intact males.
- Apocrine gland adenocarcinomas are frequently associated with paraneoplastic hypercalcemia.
- Castration is the treatment of choice for perianal adenomas in intact male dogs. Otherwise, conservative excision is often adequate.
- Wide surgical excision is the treatment of choice for perianal adenocarcinomas. Although the exact roles of radiation and chemotherapy are unknown, these treatment options should be considered for incompletely excised and/or metastatic tumors.
- Wide surgical excision is the treatment of choice for perianal adenocarcinomas. Due to the high rates of local recurrence and metastasis, radiation and chemotherapy should also be considered in conjunction with surgery (Table 12.13).
- Perianal tumors are rare in cats.
- In reports of intestinal adenocarcinoma in cats, Siamese cats are overrepresented.
- Clinical signs include weight loss, inappetence, vomiting, diarrhea, melena, and/or hematochezia (Tables 12.9, 12.10; Figure 12.9).
- Microcytic hypochromic anemia is also common due to chronic GI blood loss.
- Smooth muscle tumors have been associated with paraneoplastic hypoglycemia.
- Typically, surgery is the treatment of choice (Table 12.11). However, resection is often difficult in this location.
- The role of chemotherapy is unknown.

Table 12.12. Perianal tumors

Histologic Type	Features
Perianal adenoma	Most common perianal tumor in older, intact male dogs.
	Development is thought to be androgen-dependent.
	These tumors tend to grow slowly and do not metastasize.
	Prognosis is good.
	Rare in cats.
Perianal adenocarcinoma	Occurs in older intact and neutered male and female dogs.
	Metastatic rate at diagnosis is low (15%), but tumors may metastasize more frequently later in the course of the disease.
	Sites of metastasis include regional lymph nodes, lungs, liver, and bone.
	Rare in cats.
Apocrine gland adenocarcinoma of the anal sac	Most common perianal tumor in older female dogs.
	Occurs in older dogs. Equal sex distribution.
	Paraneoplastic hypercalcemia commonly occurs with this tumor type. Reported incidence is 25–53%.
	Presenting complaints include tenesmus and/or constipation secondary to mass effect from the tumor. Polyuria-polydipsia may also occur secondary to hypercalcemia.
	Is locally invasive with a moderate to high metastatic rate (36–96%).
	Sites of metastasis include sublumbar lymph nodes, lungs, liver, and bone.
	Rare in cats.

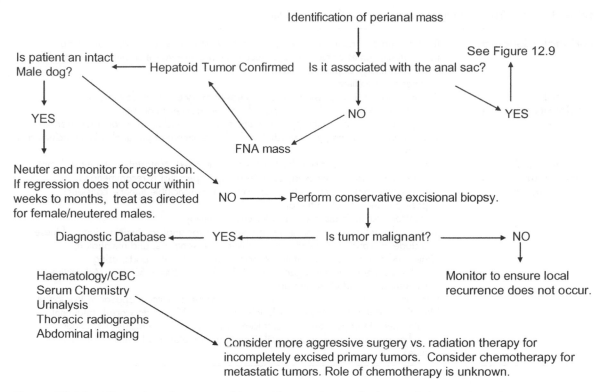

Figure 12.11. Diagnosis and treatment of hepatoid tumors (perianal adenoma/adenocarcinoma).

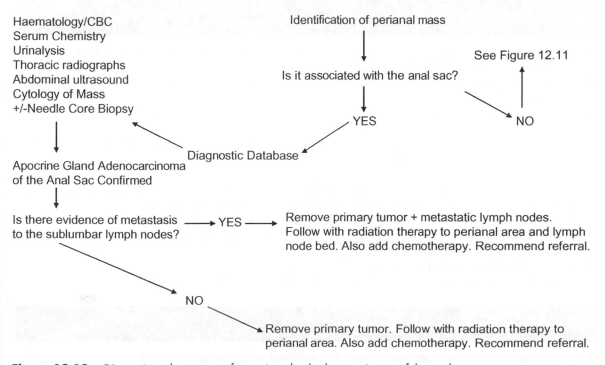

Figure 12.12. Diagnosis and treatment of apocrine gland adenocarcinoma of the anal sac.

Table 12.13. Treatment regimes and prognosis for perianal tumors

Perianal adenoma	Recommend castration for intact male dogs. Most tumors will regress over time. For neutered males or female dogs, recommend conservative surgical excision with histopathology of perianal mass. Prognosis is excellent.
Perianal adenocarcinoma	Recommend surgical excision for tumors easily excised with wide margins. However, even with surgical treatment, local recurrence is common. Postoperative radiation therapy may help reduce the likelihood of local recurrence. The role of chemotherapy and radiation in the treatment of perianal adenocarcinoma is unknown.
Apocrine gland adenocarcinoma of the anal sac	Recommend surgical excision for tumors easily excised. Metastatic sublumbar lymph nodes may also be removed, but referral to a specialist is recommended. For narrowly excised, incompletely excised or nonresectable tumors, consider postoperative radiation therapy. To control metastatic disease, consider chemotherapy. Various chemotherapeutic drugs have been used for anal sac tumors. Some of these include cisplatin, carboplatin, doxorubicin, mitoxantrone, and melphalan. Older studies reported MST of 6–12 months. More recent reports, using multimodality treatment suggest that MST is longer: 544–956 days. Adjunctive radiotherapy and chemotheraphy. Dogs treated with surgery as a part of their treatment protocol appear to live longer Negative prognostic indicators include tumor size ($>10 \text{ cm}^3$ do worse), treatment with chemotherapy alone, hypercalcemia, and pulmonary metastasis. Older studies also suggest that dogs with lymph node metastasis have shorter survival times.

Hepatobiliary Tumors

- Primary hepatobiliary tumors are more common in cats; metastatic hepatobiliary tumors are more common in dogs (Table 12.14, Figure 12.13).
- Of the primary hepatobiliary tumors, malignant tumors are more common in dogs and benign tumors are more common in cats.
- Primary malignant hepatobiliary tumors in dogs and cats include hepatocellular carcinoma, biliary carcinoma, neuroendocrine tumor, and sarcoma.
- Hepatocellular carcinoma is the most common primary hepatobiliary tumor in dogs. Biliary cystadenoma is the most common primary hepatobiliary tumor in cats.
- Hepatobiliary tumors are also characterized based on morphology. Massive tumors are large, solitary masses in a single lobe. Nodular tumors are multifocal and found in several lobes. Diffuse tumors typically involve all lobes and may result in complete effacement of the hepatic parenchyma.
- Clinical signs include weight loss, inappetence, vomiting, polyuria-polydipsia, and possibly ascites. Animals with extensive disease may also present with icterus and signs of hepatoencephalopathy.
- Typically, surgery is the treatment of choice (Table 12.15).
- The roles of radiation and chemotherapy are unknown.
- Biologic behavior and prognosis are dependent on morphology and histologic type.

Exocrine Pancreatic Tumors

- Exocrine pancreatic tumors are rare in dogs. The incidence is slightly higher in cats.
- Adenocarcinoma is the most common histologic type. Benign exocrine pancreatic masses include adenomas and pseudocysts.

- Surgical resection is the treatment of choice. However, many animals have evidence of metastatic disease at the time of diagnosis. In these cases, surgery should be performed only for palliative reasons.
- The role of chemotherapy is unknown.
- Pancreatic tumors are locally invasive, and the metastatic rate is very high. Common metastatic sites include regional lymph nodes, liver, and peritoneal cavity.

Table 12.14.   Hepatobiliary tumors

Histologic Type	Features
Hepatocellular carcinoma (HCC)	Most common primary hepatobiliary tumor in dogs. Of malignant hepatobiliary tumors in cats, HCC is the second most common. Paraneoplastic hypoglycemia has been reported. May be massive, nodular, or diffuse. Metastatic rate is dependent upon morphology and is low for massive HCC (0–37%) but high for nodular and diffuse HCC (93–100%). Common sites of metastasis: regional lymph nodes, peritoneum, and lungs.
Hepatocellular adenoma (hepatoma)	Frequently an incidental finding. More common in cats than in dogs. Benign tumor. Remove if problematic. Prognosis is good.
Biliary carcinoma (BC)	Second most common primary hepatobiliary tumor in dogs. Of malignant hepatobiliary tumors in cats, BC is the most common. Intrahepatic BC appears to be more common in dogs, whereas extrahepatic BC is more common in cats. May be massive, nodular, or diffuse. Very aggressive biologic behavior with a high metastatic rate (70–88%). Common sites of metastasis: regional lymph nodes, peritoneum, and lungs.
Biliary cystadenoma	Frequently an incidental finding. Common in cats. Benign tumor. Remove if problematic. Prognosis is good.
Neuroendocrine Tumor (Carcinoid)	Rare in dogs and cats. Often is locally aggressive with nodular or diffuse morphology. Metastatic rate is high (~93%). Common sites of metastasis: regional lymph nodes, peritoneum, and lungs.
Sarcoma	Rare in dogs and cats. Common primary hepatic sarcomas include hemangiosarcoma, leiomyosarcoma, histiocytic sarcoma, and fibrosarcoma. Often is locally aggressive with nodular or massive morphology. Very aggressive biologic behavior with a high metastatic rate (86–100%). Common sites of metastasis: spleen and lungs.

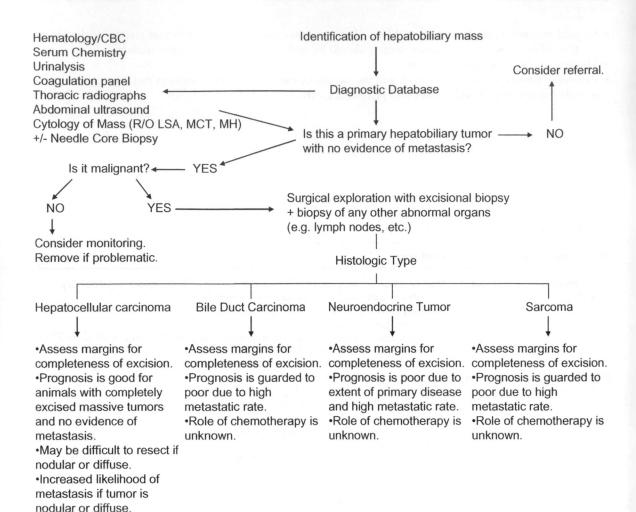

Figure 12.13. Diagnosis and treatment of hepatobiliary tumors.

Table 12.15. Treatment regimes and prognosis for hepatobiliary tumors

HCC	Recommend surgical excision for massive tumors easily excised with liver lobectomy.
	With surgical treatment, prognosis for massive HCC is good. Local recurrence and metastatic rates are generally low.
	In one study of dogs with massive HCC treated with surgery, MST was not reached (>1460 days), whereas MST for dogs treated conservatively was 270 days. Prognostic factors include surgery as part the treatment protocol, which side of liver involvement (dogs with right-sided tumors do worse perioperatively), alanine transferase (ALT) and aspartate transferase (AST) activity, and ratios of alanine phosphatase (ALP) to AST and ALT to AST.
	Nodular and diffuse HCC are typically nonresectable due to extent to disease.
	The role of chemotherapy and radiation in the treatment of HCC is unknown.
BC	Recommend surgical excision for massive tumors easily excised with liver lobectomy.
	However, even with surgical treatment, prognosis is guarded to poor. Local recurrence and metastatic rates are generally high, and survival times are short.
	Nodular and diffuse BC are typically nonresectable due to extent to disease.
	The role of chemotherapy and radiation in the treatment of BC is unknown.
Neuroendocrine tumor	Recommend surgical excision for tumors easily excised with liver lobectomy. However, the majority are nonresectable due to extent of disease.
	Prognosis is poor because this disease is highly metastatic. Survival times are short.
	The role of chemotherapy and radiation in the treatment of neuroendocrine tumors is unknown.
Sarcoma	Recommend surgical excision for massive tumors easily excised with liver lobectomy.
	However, even with surgical treatment, prognosis is guarded to poor. Local recurrence and metastatic rates are generally high, and survival times are short.
	The role of chemotherapy and radiation in the treatment of hepatobiliary sarcomas is unknown. See Chapter 5 for discussion of chemotherapy protocols for other types of soft-tissue sarcomas.

13
TUMORS OF THE RESPIRATORY SYSTEM

Michelle M. Turek

This section describes tumors of the upper and lower respiratory tract in dogs and cats. Tumors of the nasal cavity and sinuses, larynx, trachea, and lung will be discussed.

Nasosinal Tumors in Dogs

Key Points
- Tumors arise from the nasal cavity and/or paranasal sinuses and are almost always malignant.
- Older dogs are most commonly affected, although dogs as young as 1 year have been reported.
- Medium- and large-breed dogs are predisposed.
- The most common malignant tumor types are carcinoma, including adenocarcinoma, and sarcoma, including fibrosarcoma, chondrosarcoma, and osteosarcoma.
- Less common malignant tumors include lymphoma, mast cell tumor, olfactory neuroblastoma, and others.
- Benign tumors rarely occur but can include polyps and fibromas.
- Malignant tumors are locally aggressive, often causing destruction of bone. Tumors can extend beyond the cribiform plate into the calvarium.
- The rate of regional and distant metastasis is low at the time of diagnosis. Most common sites of metastasis include lymph node and lungs.
- Therapy is aimed at local tumor control or palliation of clinical signs.
- Paraneoplastic syndromes associated with nasal tumors are rare. Erythrocytosis and hypercalcemia have been reported.
- Environmental factors, including tobacco smoke and indoor exposure to fossil fuel combustion products, may be related to tumor development.

Clinical Signs

- Clinical signs are local and attributable to the presence of the primary tumor (Table 13.1).
- Clinical signs of neoplasia can mimic those of nonmalignant diseases (see list of differential diagnoses below).
- Clinical signs of neoplasia can temporarily improve with antibiotics, nonsteroidal antiinflammatory drugs, or steroids. It is important not to rule out neoplasia based solely on response to such treatments as misdiagnosis can occur.

Differential Diagnosis for Dogs with Clinical Signs Relating to the Nasal Cavity and Nasal Sinuses

- Neoplasia (see Table 13.2.)
- Fungal rhinitis (aspergillosis, blastomycosis, or sporotrichosis)

Table 13.1. Clinical signs of nasosinal tumors (Figure 13.1)

Unilateral or bilateral nasal discharge: mucoid, purulent, hemorrhagic, or any
    combination thereof
Epistaxis
Nasal congestion or stertorous breathing
Sneezing
Facial deformity due to subcutaneous extension of tumor
Epiphora
Exophthalmus
Neurologic signs including seizures, behavior change, and obtundation due to
    direct tumor extension into the calvarium
Halitosis
Oral mass due to tumor extension into the oral cavity

Table 13.2. Histologic classification of nasosinal neoplasia

Nasosinal Neoplasia in Dogs

Malignant	Benign*
Carcinoma[†], adenocarcinoma[†]	Polyp
Sarcoma:[†] fibro-, chondro- or osteosarcoma	Fibroma
Lymphoma*	Rathke's clefts cyst
Mast cell tumor*	Other
Olfactory neuroblastoma*	
Other*	

[†] Most common.
*Rare.

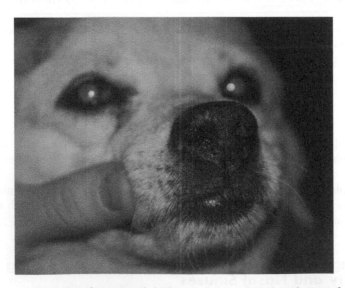

Figure 13.1. Epistaxis and/or hemorrhagic nasal discharge are common clinical signs of nasosinal tumors. In this patient with nasal carcinoma, the nostril is plugged by a blood clot resulting from epistaxis and crusted hemorrhagic nasal discharge.

- Bacterial rhinitis
- Immune-mediated lymphoplasmacytic rhinitis
- Coagulopathies
- Hypertension
- Foreign body
- Trauma
- Embryonic vestige (Rathke's clefts cyst)

Diagnosis

- If epistaxis is the only nasal sign, coagulation parameters (PT, PTT) and platelet count should be evaluated to rule out a primary coagulopathy (Figure 13.2).
- In almost all cases of nasosinal neoplasia, a mass lesion is present in the nasal cavity.
- Imaging is necessary to localize the lesion and determine its extent:
  - Advanced imaging, including computed tomography (CT) or magnetic resonance imaging (MRI), is more sensitive than radiography.
- Histopathology is required for definitive diagnosis.
- Nasal biopsy techniques include noninvasive and invasive methods (see Table 13.3).
- To avoid misdiagnosis, it is important to keep in mind that nasal signs caused by a tumor may improve temporarily with the use of antibiotics, nonsteroidal antiinflammatory drugs, or steroids.

Clinical Stage

- Tumor stage is a measure of the extent of cancer in the body (Table 13.4):
  - Size and invasiveness of primary tumor
  - Presence or not of regional lymph node metastasis
  - Presence or not of distant metastasis including pulmonary metastasis
- Determination of tumor stage is important for therapeutic planning and to predict prognosis (Table 13.5).
- **Advanced local disease** is common at the time of diagnosis.
- Regional and distant **metastasis is rare** at the time of diagnosis.
  - Lymphatic flow from the nasal cavity is filtered through the mandibular lymph nodes (regional lymph nodes).

Table 13.3. Nasal biopsy techniques

Noninvasive Nasal Biopsy Techniques	Invasive Nasal Biopsy Techniques
Nasal flushing Blind transnostril biopsy*,** Endoscopy-guided fiberoptic biopsy* Fine needle aspiration or biopsy of facial deformities	Surgical biopsy via rhinotomy

*Coagulation parameters should be assessed prior to transnostril biopsy as bleeding from the biopsy site is expected.
**Blind transnostril biopsy instruments should not be introduced further than the medial canthus of the eye to avoid penetration of the cribiform plate.

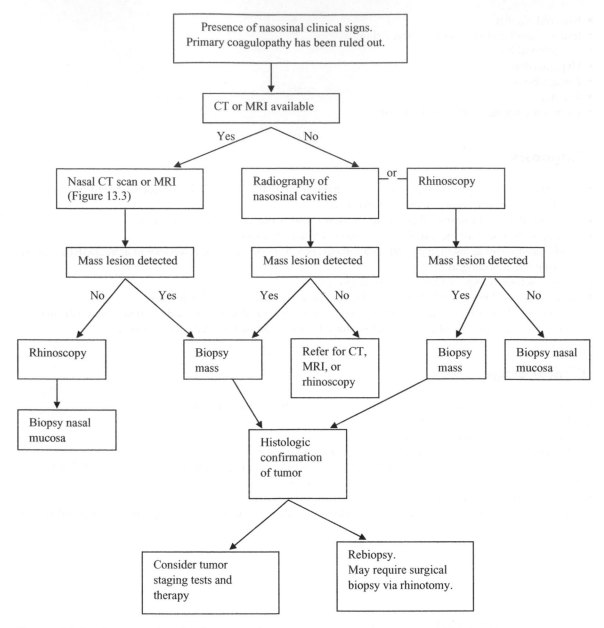

Figure 13.2. Diagnostic algorithm for nasosinal tumors.

Treatment and Prognosis

- Since the rate of metastasis is low at the time of diagnosis, local therapy is indicated.
- Radiation therapy is the treatment of choice.
- Surgery (rhinotomy) alone results in rapid tumor regrowth.
- There are two general approaches to therapy:
  - Tumor control with extended survival (definitive therapy)
  - **OR**

Table 13.4. Clinical staging of tumor

Tumor Stage Criteria	Diagnostic Test Used	Risk of Advanced Disease at Diagnosis
Size and extent of primary tumor	Advanced imaging, including CT or MRI (Figure 13.3)	High risk of locally advanced disease, including (Figure 13.4) • Bilateral nasal cavity involvement • Bone destruction, including turbinates and bones of the face • Subcutaneous tumor extension • Tumor extension beyond the cribiform plate
Lymph node status	Fine needle aspirate or biopsy of regional lymph node	Low risk of metastasis
Presence of distant metastasis	Three-view thoracic radiographs Other tests dictated by clinical signs	Low risk of metastasis

Table 13.5. Prognostic implications of clinical stage

Stage-Related Prognostic Indicator	Clinical Implication
Local tumor extension beyond the cribiform plate into the calvarium	Less effective treatment of parts of tumor that abut the brain Decreased median survival time
Lymph node or distant metastasis	Aggressive local therapy to the primary tumor site is not recommended due to presence of metastasis. Goal of therapy becomes palliation rather than local tumor control. Decreased median survival time

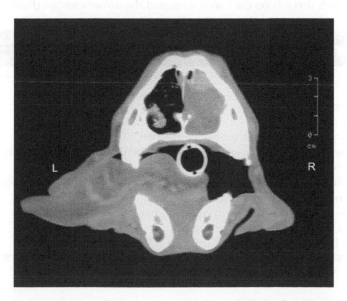

Figure 13.3. Computed tomography confirms the presence of a unilateral soft-tissue attenuating mass in the right nasal cavity. Not limited by tissue superimposition as with plain radiography, advanced imaging such as CT or MRI allows for accurate assessment of extent of disease and integrity of the cribiform plate and may be used for computerized radiation treatment planning.

243

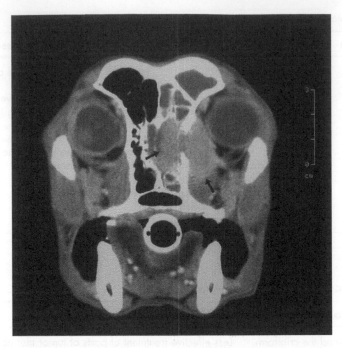

Figure 13.4. Advanced local disease is common at the time of diagnosis of nasosinal tumors. In this case, CT imaging reveals aggressive changes that would not be detectable by physical examination or by radiography. The tumor is causing destruction of the frontal bone and the cribiform plate allowing tumor extension into the retro-orbital space and the cranial vault.

- Temporary alleviation of clinical signs and short-term improvement of quality of life with no expectation of tumor control (palliative therapy)
- The therapeutic approach depends on the tumor stage and the owner's wishes (Figure 13.5, Table 13.6).

Nasosinal Tumors in Cats

Key Points
- Less common than in the dog.
- Older cats are most often affected.
- Malignant tumors are more common than benign tumors.
- Tumors are **locally aggressive,** often causing destruction of bone. Tumors can extend beyond the cribiform plate into the calvarium.
- Most common tumor type is **lymphoma,** followed by **carcinoma and adenocarcinoma.**
- Rhinitis can mimic neoplasia in clinical signs and imaging findings.
- Risk of metastasis is moderate to high for lymphoma, but low for carcinoma.
- Lack of clinical data regarding efficacy of treatment.
- Cats with nasosinal lymphoma should be tested for FeLV and FIV.

Clinical Signs

- Clinical signs of neoplasia can mimic those of nonmalignant diseases.
- Clinical signs of neoplasia can temporarily improve with antibiotics or steroids. It is important not to rule out neoplasia based solely on response to such treatments as misdiagnosis can occur.
- Clinical signs are related to the presence of the primary tumor.

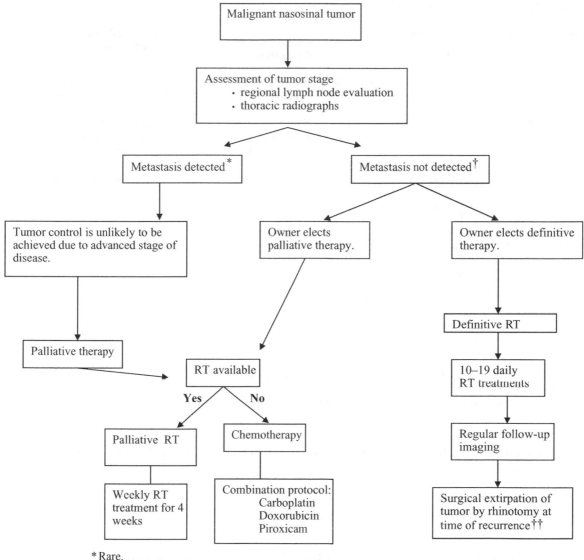

Figure 13.5. Treatment algorithm for canine nasosinal tumors.

Clinical Signs of Nasosinal Tumors

- Unilateral or bilateral nasal discharge: mucoid, purulent, hemorrhagic, or any combination thereof
- Epistaxis
- Nasal congestion or stertorous breathing
- Sneezing
- Facial deformity due to subcutaneous extension of tumor
- Epiphora
- Exophthalmos

Table 13.6. A closer look at treatment options and prognosis

Type of therapy	Radiotherapy		Chemotherapy[†] Palliative
	Definitive	**Palliative**	
Schedule	**Daily** treatment for 10–19 days	**Weekly** treatment for 4 weeks	Alternating carboplatin and doxorubicin IV q3 weeks Daily piroxicam p.o.
Possible side effects	Oral mucositis Moist desquamation* Conjunctivitis* Rhinitis* Keratoconjunctivitis sicca (KCS) Hair loss Progressive vision loss in eye in RT field[†]	Hair loss Progressive vision loss in eye in RT field[†]	Gastrointestinal effects*: vomiting, diarrhea, inappetence Myelosuppression* Hair loss in susceptible breeds*
Median survival time	12–19 months with RT alone Up to 3+ years if RT is followed by surgery Less if tumor extends beyond the cribiform plate at time of diagnosis	3–9 months	6–9 months

* Self-limiting.
[†] Caution should be used in dogs with renal insufficiency (carboplatin, piroxicam) and decreased cardiac contractility or arrythmia (doxorubicin).
[†] Vision loss is due to cataract formation or retinal changes.

- Neurologic signs, including seizures, behavior change, and obtundation due to direct tumor extension into the calvarium
- Halitosis
- Missing teeth
- Oral mass due to tumor extension into the oral cavity

Differential Diagnosis for Cats with Clinical Signs Relating to the Nasal Cavity and Nasal Sinuses

- Neoplasia (see Table 13.7)
- Immune-mediated lymphoplasmacytic rhinitis
- Infectious rhinitis
- Nasopharyngeal stenosis
- Foreign body
- Trauma

Diagnosis

- Imaging is necessary to localize the lesion and determine its extent.
- Both neoplasia and rhinitis can be associated with aggressive radiographic or CT changes:
  - Changes suggestive of, but not diagnostic for, neoplasia include unilateral changes (turbinate or bone erosion, missing teeth, facial deformity) and displacement of midline structures.

Table 13.7. Histologic classification of neoplasia of the nasal cavities and sinuses

Malignant	Benign
Lymphoma[†]	Polyp[†]
Carcinoma[†], adenocarcinoma[†]	Fibroma[*]
Sarcoma:[*] fibro-, chondro-, or osteosarcoma	Hemangioma[*]
Mast cell tumor[*]	Chrondroma[*]
Melanoma[*]	Other[*]
Olfactory neuroblastoma[*]	
Plasma Cell Tumor[*]	

[†] Most common.
[‡] Common.
[*] Rare.

Table 13.8. Clinical staging of tumor

Tumor Stage Criteria	Diagnostic Test Used	Risk of Advanced Disease at Diagnosis
Size and extent of primary tumor	Advanced imaging, including CT or MRI	High risk of locally aggressive disease, including • Bilateral nasal cavity involvement • Bone destruction, including turbinates and bones of the face • Subcutaneous tumor extension • Tumor extension beyond the cribiform plate • Displacement of midline structures
Lymph node status	Fine needle aspirate or biopsy of regional lymph node	Moderate risk of lymph node metastasis
Presence of distant metastasis	Three-view thoracic radiographs (all tumor types) Abdominal ultrasound (lymphoma) Bone marrow aspirate (lymphoma)	Low risk of distant metastasis for other tumor types Low to moderate risk of distant metastasis for lymphoma

- Histopathology is required for definitive diagnosis.
- Nasal biopsy techniques include noninvasive and invasive methods (see Table 13.2).
- To avoid misdiagnosis, it is important to keep in mind that nasal signs caused by a tumor may improve temporarily with the use of antibiotics, nonsteroidal antiinflammatory drugs, or steroids.
- See Figure 13.1 for the diagnosis algorithm.

Clinical Stage

- Tumor stage is a measure of the extent of cancer in the body (Table 13.8):
  - Size and invasiveness of primary tumor
  - Presence or not of regional lymph node metastasis
  - Presence or not of distant metastasis, including pulmonary metastasis
- Determination of tumor stage is important for therapeutic planning and to predict prognosis.
- **Advanced local disease** is common at the time of diagnosis.
- Metastasis to regional lymph nodes is more common than in the dog at the time of diagnosis.
  - Lymphatic flow from the nasal cavity is filtered through the mandibular lymph nodes (regional lymph nodes).

Table 13.9. Therapeutic approaches

Therapeutic Approach	Overall Objective of Therapy	Advantages	Disadvantages
Definitive	Tumor is controlled with resolution of clinical signs. Life expectancy is prolonged compared to no therapy or palliative therapy alone.	Goal is tumor control and maximally extended life expectancy.	Therapy is time-intensive. Therapy is expensive. Side effects are expected.
Palliative	Temporary improvement of clinical signs resulting in improved quality of life. Tumor control is not expected. Life expectancy may not be longer than with no therapy.	Temporary improvement of clinical signs and quality of life. Less intensive therapy. Less expensive. Fewer to no side effects.	Tumor control is not achieved so life expectancy is not maximally prolonged.

- Due to the potential for visceral involvement associated with lymphoma of any form in the cat, staging tests for that tumor type include abdominal ultrasound and bone marrow aspiration in addition to lymph node evaluation and thoracic radiography:
  - Risk of visceral involvement at the time of diagnosis of nasal lymphoma is low to moderate.

Treatment

- As in dogs, there are two general approaches to therapy (Table 13.9):
  - Tumor control with extended survival (definitive therapy)
  - OR
  - Temporary alleviation of clinical signs and short-term improvement of quality of life with no expectation of tumor control (palliative therapy)
- The therapeutic approach depends on the tumor stage and the owner's wishes.
- Radiotherapy is the treatment of choice for nasosinal tumors:
  - The efficacy of adjuvant chemotherapy has not been investigated
- Lymphoma is both chemo- and radiosensitive. Either treatment modality, or both, may be considered for cats with nasal lymphoma. Treatment of choice depends on the clinical stage of the disease (Figure 13.6):
  - For focal, nonmetastatic lymphoma, radiotherapy is the treatment of choice. Adjuvant chemotherapy may improve tumor control and survival.

Prognosis

- Due to a lack of available clinical data, the prognosis associated with nasal tumors is cats is not clearly defined.
  - Median survival time for malignant nonlymphoid tumors treated with definitive radiation has been suggested to be 1 year or longer.
  - Palliative radiation of malignant nonlymphoid tumors may afford favorable survival time.
  - Median survival time for cats with nasal lymphoma treated with radiation and chemotherapy is reported between 2 and 3 years.
- FeLV or FIV infection may be a negative prognostic indicator for cats with nasosinal lymphoma.

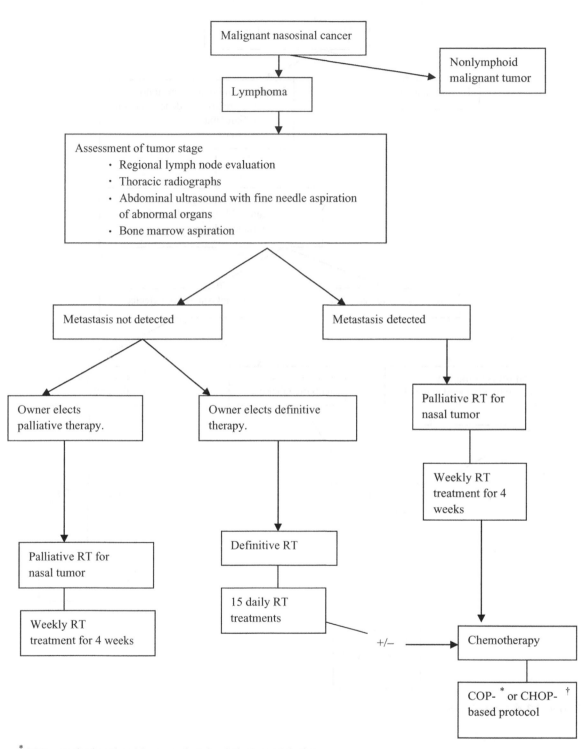

* COP = cyclophosphamide, oncovin (vincristine), prednisolone.

† CHOP = cyclophosphamide, hydroxydaunorubicin (doxorubicin), oncovin (vincristine), prednisolone.

Figure 13.6. Treatment algorithm for cats with nasosinal tumors.

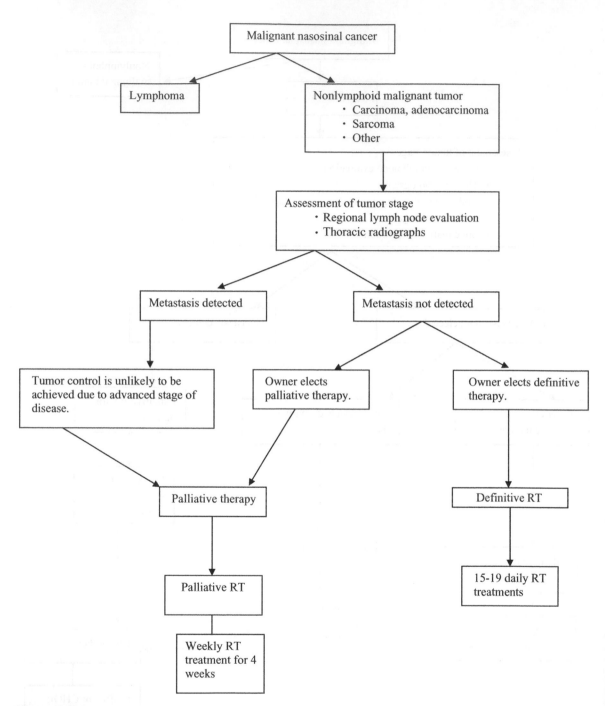

Figure 13.6. *Continued*

Laryngeal Tumors in Dogs

Key Points
- These tumors are rare.
- Malignant tumors are more common than benign ones, and occur in middle-aged to older dogs.
- Malignant tumors are locally invasive and are associated with a moderate risk of metastasis.
- While surgery is the treatment of choice for most tumors if there is no evidence of metastasis, malignant tumors are often nonresectable due to their invasive nature:
  - Incomplete excision is frequently followed by tumor recurrence.
  - Radical excision by complete laryngectomy with permanent tracheostomy has been reported but risk of complications is high.
- The role of chemotherapy and radiation therapy has not been investigated. These modalities may be useful in the adjuvant setting if the primary tumor is incompletely excised, or for radioresponsive and chemoresponsive tumors such as lymphoma, mast cell tumor, and plasma cell tumor.
- Benign tumors may be resectable and do not metastasize.

Clinical Signs of Laryngeal Tumors

- Progressive voice (bark) change or loss of voice
- Snoring or noisy breathing
- Dyspnea
- Exercise intolerance
- Hemoptysis
- Dysphagia
- Coughing
- Neck mass
- Clinical signs can overlap with those associated with tracheal tumors.

Differential Diagnosis for Dogs with Clinical Signs Attributable to an Upper Respiratory Obstruction

- Laryngeal neoplasia (see Table 13.10)
- Laryngitis
  - Lesions can be proliferative and can appear as masses.
- Abcess
- Polyp
- Foreign body
- Trauma
- Tracheal obstruction (see the section "Tracheal Tumors in Dogs and Cats")

Diagnosis

- Histopathology is needed to differentiate inflammatory lesions from malignant or benign tumors.
- Nonresectable masses should be definitively diagnosed as inflammatory lesions may be responsive to glucocorticoids and some malignant tumors (lymphoma, mast cell tumor, plasma cell tumor) may respond to radiotherapy and/or chemotherapy.
- Tumor staging involves evaluation of the regional lymph nodes and lungs for metastasis. Abdominal organs and bone marrow should be evaluated in cases of lymphoma.

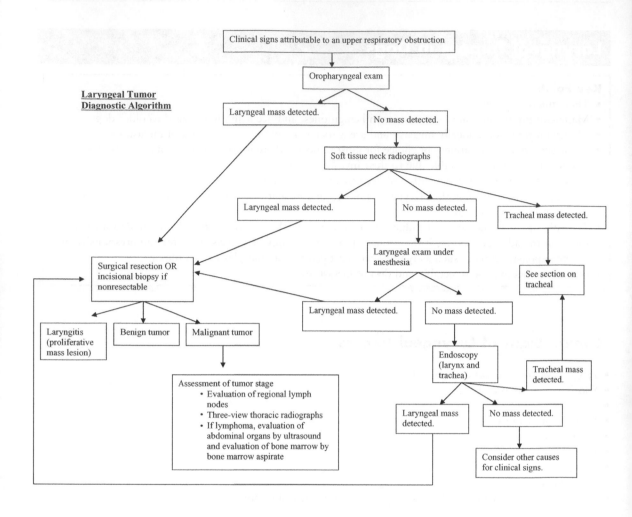

Laryngeal Tumor Diagnostic Algorithm

Clinical signs attributable to an upper respiratory obstruction

Oropharyngeal exam

Laryngeal mass detected.

No mass detected.

Soft tissue neck radiographs

Laryngeal mass detected.

No mass detected.

Tracheal mass detected.

Laryngeal exam under anesthesia

See section on tracheal

Surgical resection OR incisional biopsy if nonresectable

Laryngeal mass detected.

No mass detected.

Laryngitis (proliferative mass lesion)

Benign tumor

Malignant tumor

Endoscopy (larynx and trachea)

Tracheal mass detected.

Assessment of tumor stage
- Evaluation of regional lymph nodes
- Three-view thoracic radiographs
- If lymphoma, evaluation of abdominal organs by ultrasound and evaluation of bone marrow by bone marrow aspirate

Laryngeal mass detected.

No mass detected.

Consider other causes for clinical signs.

Table 13.10. Histologic classification of laryngeal neoplasia

Laryngeal Neoplasia in Dogs

Malignant*	Benign
Squamous cell carcinoma	Laryngitis (mass)
Adenocarcinoma	Rhabdomyoma†
Poorly differentiated carcinoma	Oncocytoma†
Osteosarcoma	Lipoma
Fibrosarcoma	Fibropapilloma
Chondrosarcoma	
Lymphoma	
Mast cell tumor	
Plasma cell tumor	
Melanoma	

*Malignant tumors are more common than benign tumors. Among malignant tumors, no tumor type predominates.
†Rhabdomyoma arises from striated muscle cells. Oncocytoma arises from epithelial cells called *oncocytes*. These tumors can be difficult to differentiate histologically due to the presence of granular eosinophilic cytoplasm in the cells of both tumors. Immunohistochemistry can be used to differentiate the two.

Treatment and Prognosis

- In cases of respiratory distress, tracheostomy should be performed to relieve the upper airway obstruction caused by the tumor.
- Surgery is the treatment of choice:
  - Resectable benign tumors can be cured with surgical excision.
  - Malignant tumors are often not completely excisable due to their invasive nature. Debulking is temporarily palliative and frequently results in tumor recurrence.
  - Radical laryngectomy with permanent tracheostomy can result in complete excision but has limited use in veterinary medicine due to high risk of complications.
  - The efficacy of radiation and/or chemotherapy has not been investigated.
- Some tumor types may be radioresponsive or chemoresponsive. These treatment modalities should be considered for these tumor types:
  - Lymphoma, mast cell tumor, plasma cell tumor
- Prognosis is usually good for resectable benign tumors after surgical excision.
- Prognosis for malignant tumors is variable and depends on the resectability of the mass. Advanced, nonresectable, and incompletely excised malignant tumors, as well as those associated with metastasis, are considered to have a poor prognosis.

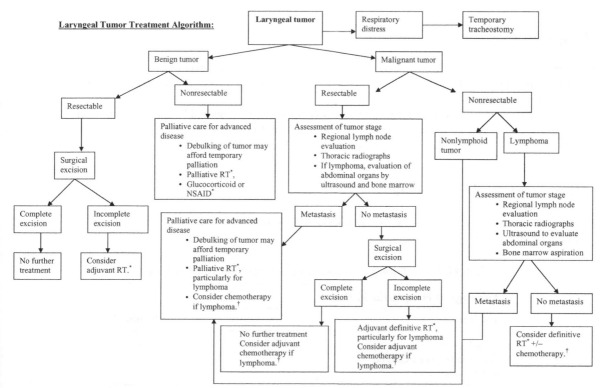

*Efficacy has not been investigated.
†COP- or CHOP-based protocol: cyclophosphamide, hydroxydaunorubicin (doxorubicin), Oncovin (vincristine), prednisolone.
RT = radiotherapy.
NSAID = nonsteroidal antiinflammatory drug.

Laryngeal Tumors in Cats

Key Points
- These tumors are rare.
- Almost all tumors are malignant.
- Lymphoma is the most common tumor. Squamous cell carcinoma and adenocarcinoma have also been reported.
- While surgery is the treatment of choice, radiation and chemotherapy are also treatment options for lymphoma since it is radioresponsive and chemoresponsive.
- Cats with laryngeal lymphoma should be tested for FeLV and FIV.

Clinical Signs

- Signs are similar to those in the dog.
- Nonspecific signs including anorexia, weight loss, vomiting, and lethargy can occur.

Differential Diagnosis

- Signs are similar to those in the dog.
- Neoplasia is the most common diagnosis (see Table 13.11).
- Lymphoma is the most common tumor type.

Diagnosis

- Histopathology is needed for definitive diagnosis and to identify tumor type.
- Tumor staging for nonlymphoid tumors includes evaluation of regional lymph nodes and lungs for metastasis.
- Tumor staging for laryngeal lymphoma involves evaluation of the regional lymph nodes, thoracic cavity (lungs, lymph nodes), abdominal organs, and bone marrow for metastasis.
- Cats with laryngeal lymphoma should be tested for FeLV and FIV.

Treatment and Prognosis

- In cases of respiratory distress, tracheostomy should be performed to relieve the upper airway obstruction caused by the tumor.

Table 13.11. Histologic classification of laryngeal neoplasia in the cat

Laryngeal Neoplasia in Cats	
Malignant	**Benign**[†]
Lymphoma*	Cysts
Squamous cell carcinoma	
Adenocarcinoma	

*The most common tumor type.
[†] Rare.

- Surgery is the treatment of choice:
  - Malignant tumors are often not completely excisable due to their invasive nature.
- Lymphoma is radioresponsive and chemoresponsive. These treatment modalities should be considered for this tumor type in both the gross-disease and adjuvant settings.
- Limited clinical information is available on the efficacy of therapy, but prognosis is considered guarded to poor for nonresectable or incompletely excised nonlymphoid tumors or tumors associated with metastasis. Laryngeal lymphoma may have a more favorable outcome.
- FeLV or FIV infection may be a negative prognostic indicator for cats with laryngeal lymphoma.
- Benign lesions (rare) can be cured if they are amenable to surgical resection.

Tracheal Tumors in Dogs and Cats

Key Points
- Primary tracheal tumors are rare in dogs and cats.
- Malignant tumors are more common than benign neoplasms and occur in middle aged to older animals.
- Young dogs can develop benign tumors composed of bone and cartilage that grow at the same rate as the skeleton.
- Surgical excision is the treatment of choice.
- The efficacy of radiotherapy and chemotherapy has not been defined. These modalities have a role in treatment of lymphoma, which is radioresponsive and chemosensitive.
- Risk of metastasis associated with malignant tumors is low to moderate.
- Cats with tracheal lymphoma should be tested for FeLV and FIV.

Clinical Signs of Tracheal Tumors

- Snoring, noisy breathing, wheezing
- Dyspnea
- Exercise intolerance
- Neck extension
- Collapse
- Hemoptysis
- Coughing
- Neck mass
- In cats, nonspecific signs including anorexia, weight loss, vomiting, and lethargy can occur
- Clinical signs can overlap with those associated with laryngeal tumors.

Differential Diagnosis for Dogs with Clinical Signs Attributable to an Upper Respiratory Obstruction

- Neoplasia (see Table 13.12)
- Polyp
- Collapsing trachea
- Foreign body
- Abcess
- Laryngeal obstruction (see the sections "Laryngeal Tumors in Dogs" and "Laryngeal Tumors in Cats")

Table 13.12. Histopathologic classification of tracheal neoplasia

| | Tracheal Neoplasia | |
	Malignant	**Benign**
Dog	Carcinoma, adenocarcinoma, squamous cell carcinoma[†] Lymphoma Mast cell tumor Plasma cell tumor Osteosarcoma	Osteochondral dysplasia or osteochondroma[*] Leiomyoma
Cat	Carcinoma[†] Lymphoma[†]	Polyp

[*]Benign tumors composed of cartilage and bone (cartilage-capped bone spurs) associated with skeletal growth in the young dog.
[†]Most common among these rare tumors.

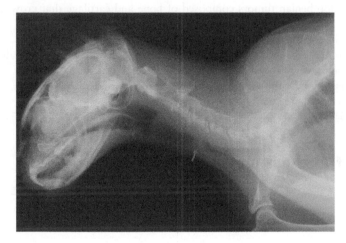

Figure 13.7. In this cat with progressive dyspnea and exercise intolerance, cervical soft-tissue radiographs reveal a mass effect within the cervical tracheal lumen. Histopathology after surgical resection confirmed tracheal carcinoma.

Diagnosis

- Histopathology is required for a definitive diagnosis:
  - Definitive diagnosis is important as noninvasive treatment options, including radiotherapy and chemotherapy, may be considered for radioresponsive and chemoresponsive tumors such as lymphoma.
- Tumor localization is determined by radiography, tracheoscopy, or CT (Figure 13.7):
  - CT is the most sensitive to assess the extent and invasiveness of the tumor and the size of regional peritracheal lymph nodes.
- Tumor staging involves evaluation of the regional lymph nodes and lungs for metastasis. Abdominal organs and bone marrow should be evaluated in cases of lymphoma.

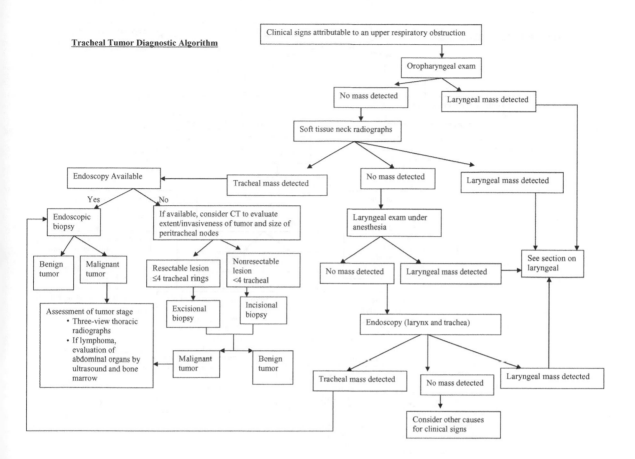

Tracheal Tumor Diagnostic Algorithm

Treatment

- In cases of respiratory distress caused by proximal tracheal tumors, tracheostomy should be performed distally to the tumor to relieve the upper airway obstruction.
- Surgery is the treatment of choice for benign and malignant tumors.
  - Up to 4 tracheal rings can be removed with closure by anastomosis.
- Lymphoma is radioresponsive and chemoresponsive. These treatment modalities should be considered for this tumor type in both the adjuvant and gross disease settings, but their clinical benefit is not well defined.
- The efficacy of radiotherapy and chemotherapy for nonlymphoid tumors has not been investigated.

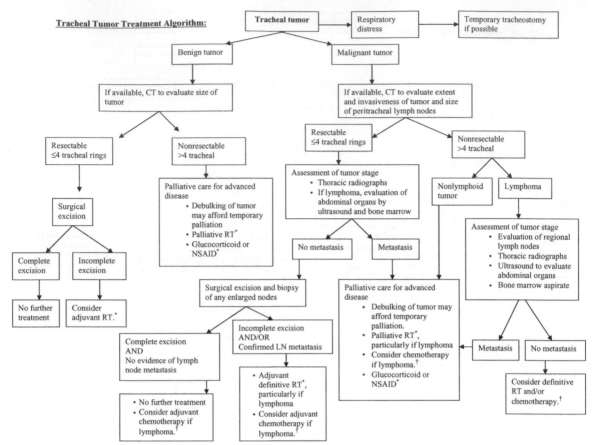

Tracheal Tumor Treatment Algorithm:

*Efficacy has not been investigated.
†COP- or CHOP-based protocol: cyclophosphamide, hydroxydaunorubicin (doxorubicin), Oncovin (vincristine), prednisolone.
RT = radiotherapy.
NSAID = nonsteroidal antiinflammatory drug.
LN = lymph node

Prognosis

- Complete excision of resectable tumors may result in a favorable prognosis.
- Incomplete excision of malignant tumors frequently results in tumor recurrence.
- The efficacy of radiotherapy and chemotherapy for nonlymphoid tumors in the gross-disease or adjuvant settings has not been investigated.
- Prognosis is considered guarded to poor for nonresectable or incompletely excised nonlymphoid tumors, as well as for tumors with metastasis.
- Prognosis associated with tracheal lymphoma may be more favorable even for nonresectable tumors due to treatment options, including radiotherapy and chemotherapy.
- In cats with tracheal lymphoma, FeLV or FIV infection may be a negative prognostic indicator.
- Benign lesions can be cured if they are amenable to surgical resection.

Lung Tumors in Dogs

Key Points
- Pulmonary neoplasia is either primary or metastatic.
- Metastatic neoplasia is more common than primary lung cancer. The lungs are the most common site of distant metastasis for most cancers.
- Middle to older animals are most commonly affected.
- Most primary lung tumors are malignant, with epithelial tumors (carcinoma) predominating.
- Rate of metastasis of primary tumors is moderate at the time of diagnosis and high late in the course of the disease:
  - Sites of metastasis include regional lymph nodes, lung, and bone.
- Surgery is the treatment of choice for nonmetastatic, resectable primary lung tumors.
- Prognosis associated with primary lung tumors is most favorable for well-differentiated tumors without metastasis and without clinical signs.
- Primary tumors detected incidentally are associated with the best prognosis.
- Prognosis associated with pulmonary metastatic disease is often poor unless effective chemotherapy treatments exist.
- Hypertrophic osteopathy is the most common paraneoplastic syndrome associated with pulmonary neoplasia.

Clinical Signs

- Clinical signs of pulmonary neoplasia (Table 13.13, Figure 13.8) include those attributable to the presence of the tumor(s), nonspecific signs, and signs related to paraneoplastic syndromes (hypertrophic osteopathy, see Table 13.14).
- Clinical signs have often been present for weeks to months.
- Clinical signs can develop acutely secondary to tumor-related pneumothorax, hemothorax, or pleural effusion.

Diagnosis

- Thoracic radiography is the first step in the diagnostic process:
  - Three-view radiographs including two lateral and one dorsoventral or ventrodorsal views are preferred.

Table 13.13. Clinical signs of pulmonary neoplasia

Signs attributable to the presence of the primary tumor	Cough
	Dyspnea
	Tachypnea
	Exercise intolerance
	Hemoptysis
	Wheezing
	Lameness
Nonspecific clinical signs	Lethargy
	Anorexia
	Weight loss
Signs related to hypertrophic osteopathy	Nonpitting, warm swelling of distal limbs
	Progressive lameness and reluctance to walk

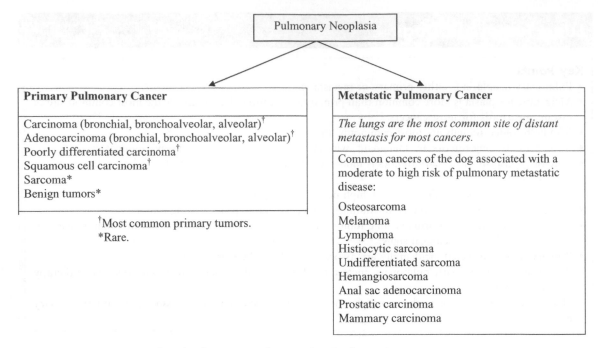

Figure 13.8. Diagnostic algorithm for canine pulmonary lymphoid granulomatosis.

Table 13.14. Paraneoplastic Syndrome; hypertrophic osteopathy

Definition	Periosteal new bone formation developing from the distal end of long bones
	Most commonly associated with intrathoracic disease, including neoplasia
Mechanism	Unclear
Clinical signs	Nonpitting warm swelling of distal limbs
	Progressive lameness and reluctance to walk
Diagnosis	1. Radiography of affected limbs (Figure 13.9)
	• Symmetric periosteal new bone formation along long bones, metacarpi/tarsi, digits that is more predominant distally
	• Soft-tissue swelling
	• Other bones, including pelvis, can be affected
	2. Thoracic radiographs to identify cause (Figure 13.10)
Treatment	Removal of underlying cause
	Pain management if removal of underlying cause is not possible
Prognosis	Good if underlying cause is removed:
	• Rapid regression of clinical signs
	• Slowly progressive regression of new bone formation
	• Poor if underlying cause is not removed due to progressive disabling discomfort.

- Histology or cytology is required for a definitive diagnosis of primary neoplasia.
- Tumor staging involves determining the size of the primary tumor and the presence or absence of regional lymph node metastasis (tracheobronchial and less commonly sternal nodes) or distant metastasis (lung, bone) (see Figure 13.11).
- Advanced imaging using computed tomography (CT) is the most sensitive method to evaluate tracheobronchial lymph node size and the lungs for metastasis.
- Diagnosis of diffuse pulmonary metastasis is often presumed based on radiographic findings and a concurrent or previous diagnosis of a tumor with metastatic potential.

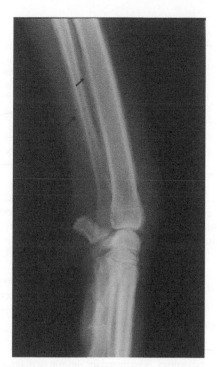

Figure 13.9. Radiographs reveal smooth, laminated periosteal new bone formation along the radius, ulna, and metacarpal bones associated with soft-tissue swelling and lameness. These findings are consistent with a diagnosis of hypertrophic osteopathy. Thoracic radiographs were performed (Figure 13.10).

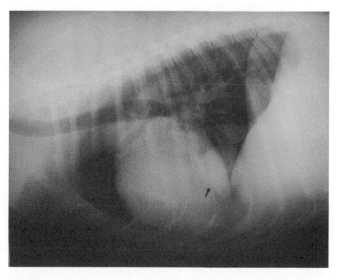

Figure 13.10. Thoracic radiographs show the presence of a large (3–5 cm) solitary pulmonary mass located in the cranial aspect of the right caudal lung lobe. Hypertrophic osteopathy is commonly associated with intrathoracic pathology. The soft-tissue swelling and lameness resolved in this patient shortly after the pulmonary sarcoma was surgically excised.

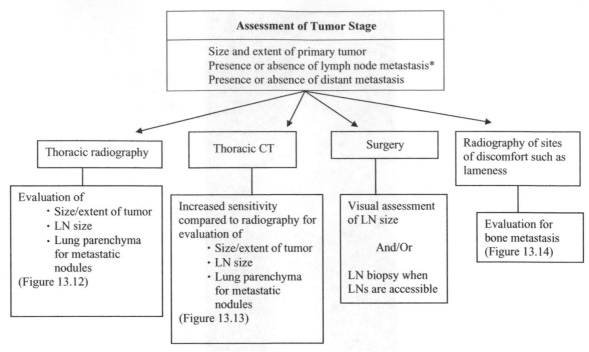

Figure 13.11. Tumor staging algorithm.

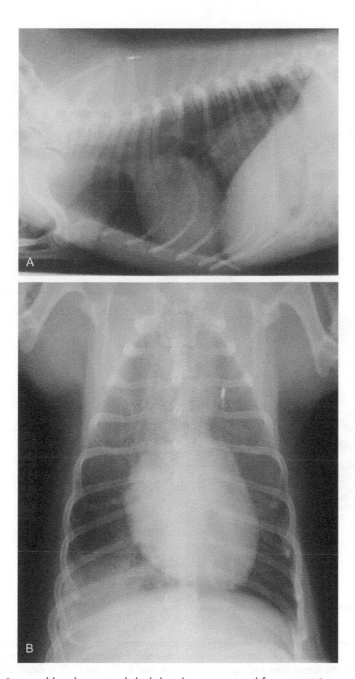

Figure 13.12. This 9-year-old male neutered dachshund was presented for progressive cough over several weeks' duration. Thoracic radiographs show a mass effect in the right caudal lung lobe region. Although primary tumor is most likely, granuloma or abscess cannot be ruled out based on radiographic findings alone. Based on the location of the mass effect on the left side on B, diaphragmatic hernia is considered much less likely. Bronchoalveolar carcinoma was confirmed histologically in this case.

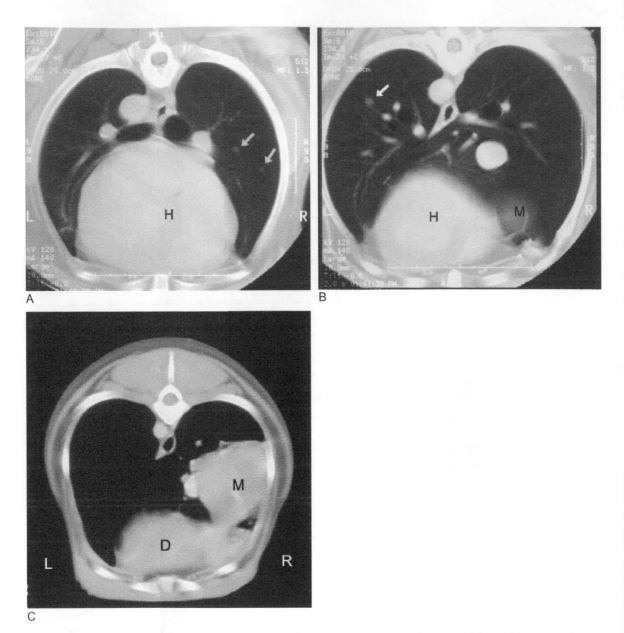

Figure 13.13. CT offers higher imaging sensitivity than radiography. The soft-tissue nodules visible in A and B are consistent with metastatic disease and are not detectable on thoracic radiographs taken of the same patient. C shows, by computed tomography, the tumor seen radiographically in A and B. H = heart; D = diaphragm; M = mass.

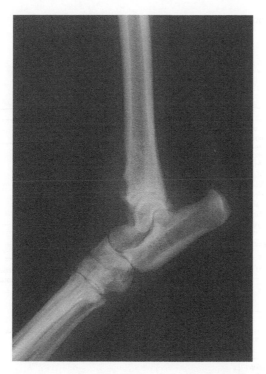

Figure 13.14. A 12-year-old mixed breed dog with a history of pulmonary carcinoma is presented for lameness on a pelvic limb. Physical exam reveals soft-tissue swelling surrounding the tarsocrural joint, as seen here radiographically. Multiple small lytic foci are visible in the distal and medial aspect of the tibia. Metastatic carcinoma was confirmed histologically.

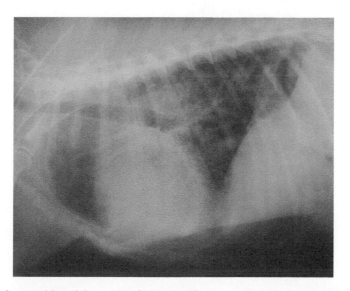

Figure 13.15. The left cranial lung lobe is opacified with soft tissue suggesting the presence of a lung lobe mass. A severe unstructured interstitial pattern is present throughout the lung suggestive of interstitial metastasis, and several poorly defined nodules are seen multifocally.

Canine lung tumor diagnostic algorithm:

```
                    ┌─────────────────────────────────────────────────┐
                    │ Clinical signs referable to the lower respiratory tract │
                    └─────────────────────────────────────────────────┘
                                        │
                    ┌─────────────────────────────────────┐
                    │     Three-view thoracic radiographs   │
                    └─────────────────────────────────────┘
```

Solitary pulmonary nodule (Figures 13.10, 13.12, 13.15)	Diffuse unstructured interstitial or bronchointerstitial pattern (Figure 13.16)	Pleural effusion (Figure 13.17)	Diffuse nodular pulmonary pattern
Differential diagnoses: • Primary pulmonary tumor • Metastatic nodule • Granuloma • Abcess • Cyst	Differential diagnoses: • Primary pulmonary cancer • Metastatic cancer • Viral pneumonia • Heartworm disease • Parasitic pneumonia • Acute respiratory distress syndrome	Differential diagnoses: • Malignant effusion • Hemothorax • Chylothorax • Pyothorax • Hydrothorax due to heart failure or low oncotic pressure	Differential diagnoses: • Metastatic cancer • Granulomatous/fungal disease • Pulmonary lymphomatoid granulomatosis • Embolic pneumonia

No lameness or other indication of bone pain

Lameness or other indication of bone pain

No lameness or other indication of bone pain

No lameness or other indication of bone pain

Lameness or other indication of bone pain

No lameness or other indication of bone pain

Radiography of affected area

Continued on page 267

Continued on page 267

Continued on page 268

Osteolytic lesion consistent with metastasis

Consider biopsy of bone lesions to confirm diagnosis.

LN= lymph node; CT= computed tomography; FNA= fine needle aspiration; PE= physical examination; US= ultrasound

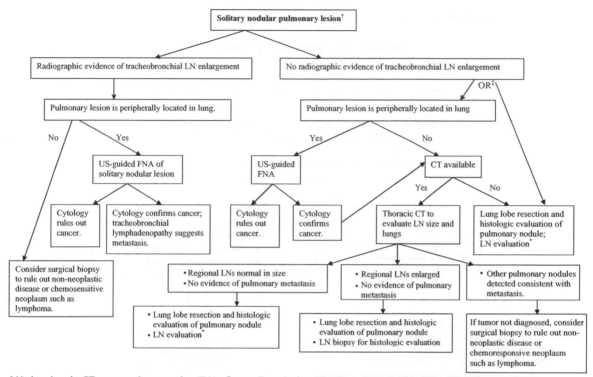

LN= lymph node; CT= computed tomography; FNA= fine needle aspiration; PE= physical examination; US= ultrasound

[†]Algorithm assumes that the likelihood that the solitary pulmonary nodule represents metastatic disease from another nonpulmonary primary tumor is low based on the lack of a previous history of cancer as well as lack of evidence of a nonpulmonary tumor on PE, abdominal US, and other diagnostic tests.

[‡]While surgery can be pursued immediately (combining diagnosis and treatment), preoperative confirmation of diagnosis and tumor staging by CT is preferable.

*Histologic assessment is preferred to rule out LN metastasis if LNs are accessible for biopsy.

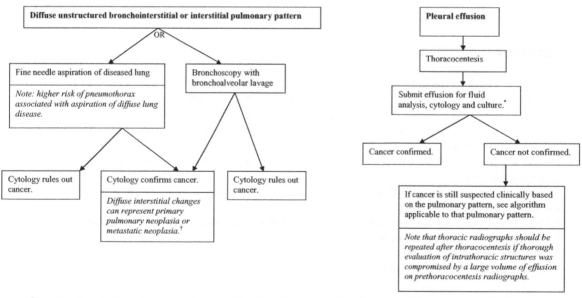

[†]A previous diagnosis of cancer or presence of a nonpulmonary primary tumor suggests that pulmonary neoplasia may represent metastatic disease.

*Physicochemical characteristics, including specific gravity, total protein, and cell count, of malignant effusion can mimic non-neoplastic effusions. The presence confirms intrathoracic neoplasia. The absence of neoplastic cells does not rule out neoplasia.

LN= lymph node; CT= computed tomography; FNA= fine needle aspiration; PE= physical examination; US= ultrasound

Canine lung tumor diagnostic algorithm:

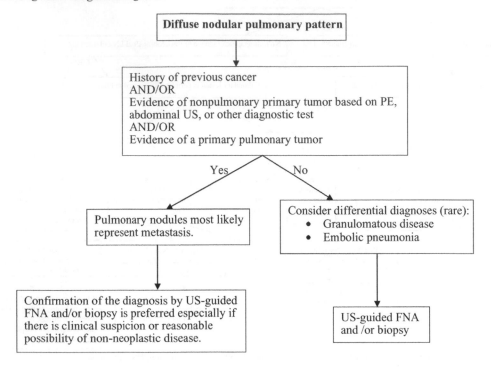

LN = lymph node; CT = computed tomography; FNA = fine needle aspiration; PE = physical examination; US = ultrasound

Treatment

- Treatment is based on clinical stage of disease.
- Surgical excision is the treatment of choice for solitary lung tumors with no distant metastasis.
- Chemotherapy has low to modest activity against primary lung cancer.
- Chemotherapy may be considered for nonresectable or incompletely excised primary tumors as well as tumors with metastasis.
- Platinum drugs (cisplatin, carboplatin) and vinorelbine have been reported for primary tumors of epithelial origin (carcinomas).
- Chemotherapy may be considered for pulmonary metastatic disease secondary to chemosensitive cancers elsewhere in the body such as:
  - CHOP-based protocol for lymphoma (CHOP: cyclophosphamide, hydroxydaunorubicin (doxorubicin), Oncovin (vincristine), prednisolone)
  - CCNU for histiocytic sarcoma
  - Platinum drugs for osteosarcoma

Treatment algorithm for canine lung tumors:

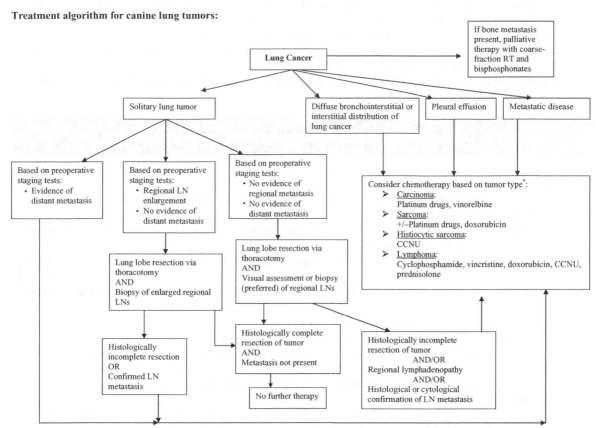

*Efficacy is considered minimal to modest, except for lymphoma, which is chemosensitive. Tumor response may be more favorable for epithelial tumors (carcinomas) than for mesenchymal tumors (sarcomas). A short-lived partial or complete remission is possible for histiocytic sarcoma. Limited clinical information is available regarding efficacy of chemotherapy for nonlymphoid lung cancer.

Table 13.15. Prognostic indicators for dogs with resectable lung tumors

	Positive Indicators	Negative Indicators
Tumor type	Adenocarcinoma Papillary carcinoma	Squamous cell carcinoma (usually diffuse)
Histologic grade	Well-differentiated tumors Low-grade tumors	Poorly differentiated tumors High-grade tumors
Tumor size	<5 cm diameter	>5 cm diameter
Tumor location	Located peripherally in the lung	Located centrally or in the perihilar region Pleural effusion
Presence of clinical signs at diagnosis	No clinical signs Incidental finding	Presence of clinical signs
Size of regional lymph nodes (radiographically, by CT, or grossly)	Not detectably enlarged	Detectably enlarged
Lymph node status or presence of distant metastasis	No metastasis	Metastasis
MEDIAN SURVIVAL TIME	*>1 year* *>2 years in some cases*	*1–8 months*

Prognosis

- Overall median survival time for dogs with resectable primary lung tumors is approximately 1 year after surgery. Clinical and histologic variables are predictive for outcome (Table 13.15).
- Median survival time for dogs with unresectable primary tumors is several weeks to a few months.
- The benefit of chemotherapy for primary lung tumors in the adjuvant or gross disease setting is unclear but is considered to be low to modest.
- Median survival time for dogs with metastatic cancer in the lungs is generally poor. Lymphoma may be an exception if chemotherapy is used.

Pulmonary Lymphomatoid Granulomatosis in the Dog

Key Points
- Pulmonary lymphomatoid granulomatosis (PLG) is an uncommon infiltrative pulmonary disease that clinically mimics neoplasia.
- PLG is characterized by cellular infiltrates of atypical lymphohistiocytic cells and normal inflammatory cells that center around and destroy blood vessels.
- Etiology is unknown. It may be preneoplastic, allergic, or immune-mediated. Some consider it an atypical form of lymphoma.
- Extrapulmonary involvement includes skin, lymph nodes, visceral organs, and the central nervous system.
- Dogs present for respiratory and/or nonrespiratory signs.
- Treatment includes immunosuppressive therapy and chemotherapy.
- Response to treatment is variable. Some patients' experience excellent, durable responses to therapy while others do not.
- Prognosis is influenced by response to therapy. Long-term survival has been reported in dogs that experience a complete remission.

Table 13.16. Clinical signs of pulmonary lymphomatoid granulomatosis

Signs attributable to the presence of the pulmonary infiltrates	Cough
	Hemoptysis
	Wheezing
Nonspecific clinical signs	Lethargy
	Anorexia
	Weight loss

Clinical Signs

- Similar to clinical signs of lung cancer (Table 13.16).
- Dogs can present for nonrespiratory signs including weight loss, weakness, and lethargy.

Diagnosis (Figures 13.16 and 13.17)

- Diagnosis involves thoracic radiography and biopsy of the pulmonary lesions (Figure 13.18).
- Thoracic radiographs show large pulmonary masses or lobar consolidation. Tracheobronchial lymphadenopathy can also occur (Figure 13.19).
- Tissue biopsy is necessary as fine needle aspiration cytology is often nondiagnostic revealing nonspecific eosinophilic or neutrophilic inflammation.
- Histologic findings include angiocentric and angiodestructive infiltration of pulmonary parenchyma by large lymphoreticular and plasmacytoid cells along with normal lymphocytes, eosinophils, and plasma cells. Infiltrate is centered around arteries and veins.
- Complete blood count may reveal basophilia and leukocytosis.

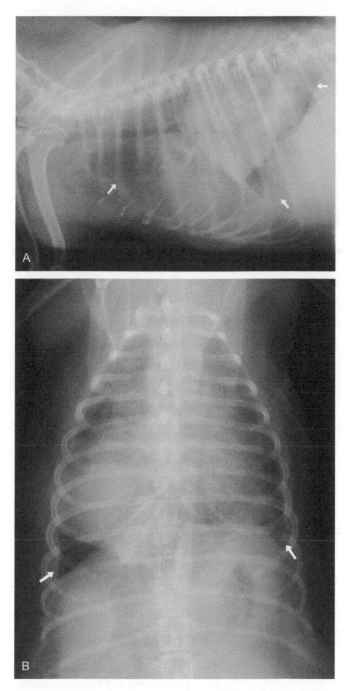

Figure 13.16. In addition to a right caudal pulmonary mass and mild diffuse bronchointerstitial pattern in this dog with pulmonary carcinoma, pleural effusion is also present (arrows). There is retraction of the pleural surface of lung away from the pleural surface of the thoracic wall, and the space between lung and thoracic walls is of soft-tissue opacity. The margins of the lungs are scalloped and there is blunting of the costophrenic sulci.

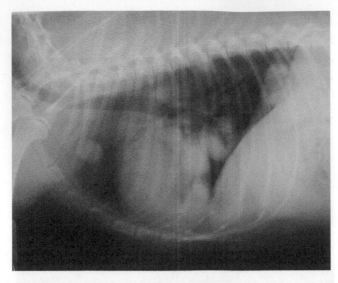

Figure 13.17. Multiple pulmonary soft-tissue nodules of varying size are seen in this dog with metastatic anal sac adenocarcinoma.

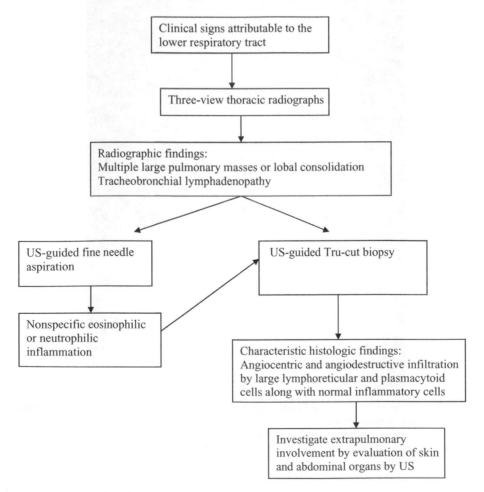

Figure 13.18. Diagnosis algorithm.

Differential Diagnosis

- Malignant neoplasia
  - Primary pulmonary cancer with metastasis
  - Metastasis from a nonpulmonary primary tumor such as histiocytic sarcoma/malignant histiocytosis
  - Lymphoma
  - Granulomatous/fungal disease
  - Heartworm granulomas

Treatment

- PLG is treated medically. This is not considered a surgical disease.
- Treatment consists of immunosuppressive drugs and cytotoxic chemotherapy:
  - Prednisolone
  - Cytoxan
  - Vincristine
  - Doxorubicin

Prognosis

- Prognosis is influenced by response to therapy. Long-term survival has been reported in dogs that experience a complete remission.
- Prognosis is guarded for those dogs in which PLG does not respond to treatment.
- Lymphoid neoplasia (lymphoma, leukemia) develops in some dogs after a diagnosis of PLG.

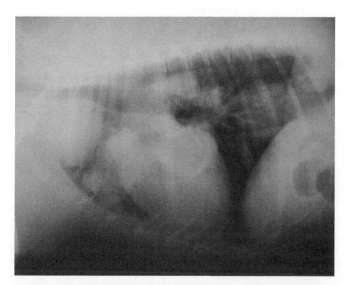

Figure 13.19. Pulmonary lymphomatoid granulomatosis in a Golden Retriever, shown by areas of alveolar consolidation in the peripheral, ventral regions of the right caudal, middle, and cranial lung lobe. There is enlargement of perihilar lymph nodes and narrowing of the caudal trachea by the mediastinal mass (lymph node).

Lung Tumors in Cats

Key Points

- Pulmonary neoplasia is either primary or metastatic.
- Metastatic neoplasia is more common than primary lung cancer. The lungs are the most common site of distant metastasis for most cancers.
- Primary lung cancer is less common in the cat than in the dog.
- Older animals are most commonly affected.
- Almost all primary lung tumors are malignant, with epithelial tumors (carcinoma) predominating.
- Rate of metastasis of primary tumors is moderate to high at the time of diagnosis unless tumors are detected incidentally.
- Sites of metastasis include regional lymph nodes, lung, and bone.
- Metastasis of pulmonary epithelial tumors can occur to multiple digits (lung-digit syndrome).
- Surgery is the treatment of choice for nonmetastatic resectable primary lung tumors.
- Tumors detected incidentally are associated with the best prognosis.
- Histologic grade is predictive of outcome (Figure 13.20).
- Prognosis associated with pulmonary metastatic disease is generally poor.

Clinical Signs

- Clinical signs have often been present for weeks to months.
- Clinical signs can develop acutely secondary to tumor-related pneumothorax, hemothorax, or pleural effusion (Table 13.17).

Table 13.17. Clinical Signs of Pulmonary Neoplasia

Signs attributable to the presence of the primary tumor	Cough
	Dyspnea
	Tachypnea
	Exercise intolerance
	Hemoptysis
	Wheezing
	Lameness
Nonspecific clinical signs	Lethargy
	Anorexia
	Weight loss
Lung-digit syndrome	Progressive lameness
	Soft-tissue swelling associated with digital metastasis

Diagnosis

- Thoracic radiography is the first step in the diagnostic process:
  - Three-view radiographs including two lateral and one dorsoventral or ventrodorsal views are preferred.
- Histology or cytology is required for a definitive diagnosis of primary neoplasia (Figure 13.21).
- Common sites of metastasis of primary lung tumors include
  - Regional lymph nodes (tracheobronchial, sternal nodes)
  - Lung
  - Bone, in particular digits
- Advanced imaging using computed tomography (CT) is the most sensitive method to evaluate regional lymph node size and the lungs for metastasis.
- Diagnosis of pulmonary metastasis is often presumed based on radiographic findings and a concurrent or previous diagnosis of a tumor with metastatic potential.

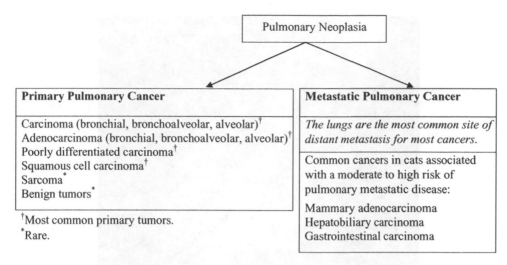

Figure 13.20. Histologic classification of pulmonary neoplasia.

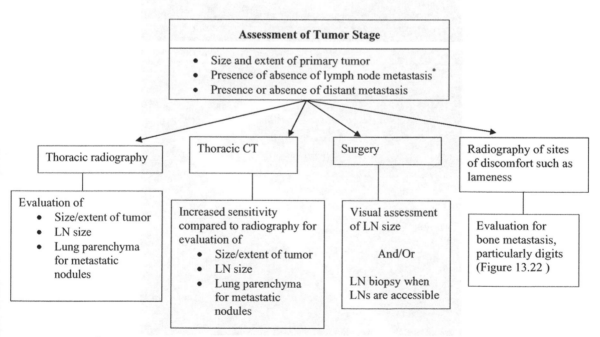

*Histology or cytology is required for definitive diagnosis of lymph node metastasis.

Figure 13.21. Tumor staging algorithm.

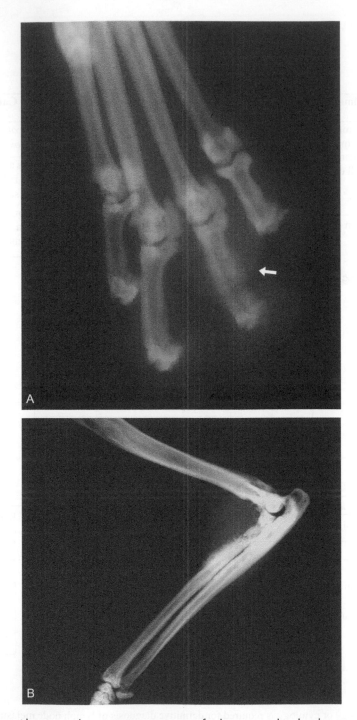

Figure 13.22. Cats with primary lung cancer may present for lameness related to bone metastasis, particularly to the digits (so called "lung-digit syndrome"). A shows an osteolytic-osteoproliferative digital lesion associated with a soft-tissue mass. B shows a similar aggressive lesion affecting the proximal radius. In both cases, histopathology confirmed metastatic carcinoma.

Feline lung tumor diagnostic algorithm:

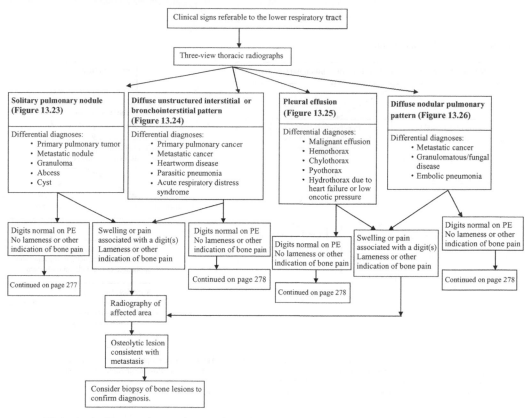

Clinical signs referable to the lower respiratory tract

Three-view thoracic radiographs

Solitary pulmonary nodule (Figure 13.23)

Differential diagnoses:
- Primary pulmonary tumor
- Metastatic nodule
- Granuloma
- Abcess
- Cyst

Diffuse unstructured interstitial or bronchointerstitial pattern (Figure 13.24)

Differential diagnoses:
- Primary pulmonary cancer
- Metastatic cancer
- Heartworm disease
- Parasitic pneumonia
- Acute respiratory distress syndrome

Pleural effusion (Figure 13.25)

Differential diagnoses:
- Malignant effusion
- Hemothorax
- Chylothorax
- Pyothorax
- Hydrothorax due to heart failure or low oncotic pressure

Diffuse nodular pulmonary pattern (Figure 13.26)

Differential diagnoses:
- Metastatic cancer
- Granulomatous/fungal disease
- Embolic pneumonia

Digits normal on PE No lameness or other indication of bone pain

Swelling or pain associated with a digit(s) Lameness or other indication of bone pain

Digits normal on PE No lameness or other indication of bone pain

Digits normal on PE No lameness or other indication of bone pain

Swelling or pain associated with a digit(s) Lameness or other indication of bone pain

Digits normal on PE No lameness or other indication of bone pain

Continued on page 277

Continued on page 278

Continued on page 278

Continued on page 278

Radiography of affected area

Osteolytic lesion consistent with metastasis

Consider biopsy of bone lesions to confirm diagnosis.

LN= lymph node; CT= computed tomography; FNA= fine needle aspiration; PE= physical examination; US= ultrasound

Feline lung tumor diagnostic algorithm:

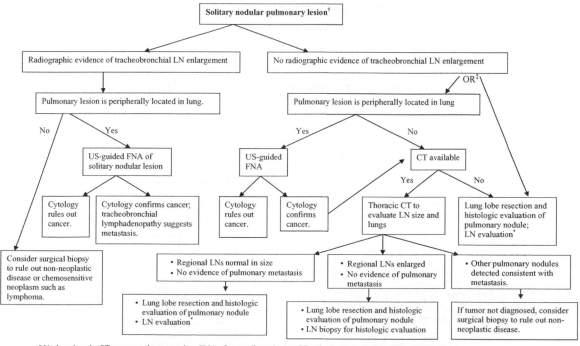

Solitary nodular pulmonary lesion[†]

Radiographic evidence of tracheobronchial LN enlargement

No radiographic evidence of tracheobronchial LN enlargement

OR[‡]

Pulmonary lesion is peripherally located in lung.

Pulmonary lesion is peripherally located in lung

No   Yes

Yes   No

CT available

Yes   No

US-guided FNA of solitary nodular lesion

US-guided FNA

Thoracic CT to evaluate LN size and lungs

Lung lobe resection and histologic evaluation of pulmonary nodule; LN evaluation[*]

Cytology rules out cancer.

Cytology confirms cancer; tracheobronchial lymphadenopathy suggests metastasis.

Cytology rules out cancer.

Cytology confirms cancer.

Consider surgical biopsy to rule out non-neoplastic disease or chemosensitive neoplasm such as lymphoma.

- Regional LNs normal in size
- No evidence of pulmonary metastasis

- Regional LNs enlarged
- No evidence of pulmonary metastasis

- Other pulmonary nodules detected consistent with metastasis.

- Lung lobe resection and histologic evaluation of pulmonary nodule
- LN evaluation[*]

- Lung lobe resection and histologic evaluation of pulmonary nodule
- LN biopsy for histologic evaluation

If tumor not diagnosed, consider surgical biopsy to rule out non-neoplastic disease.

LN= lymph node; CT= computed tomography; FNA= fine needle aspiration; PE= physical examination; US= ultrasound

[†]Algorithm assumes that the likelihood that the solitary pulmonary nodule represents metastatic disease from another nonpulmonary primary tumor is low based on the lack of a previous history of cancer as well as lack of evidence of a nonpulmonary tumor on PE, abdominal US, and other diagnostic tests.

[‡]While surgery can be pursued immediately (combining diagnosis and treatment), preoperative confirmation of diagnosis and tumor staging by CT is preferable.

Feline lung tumor diagnostic algorithm:

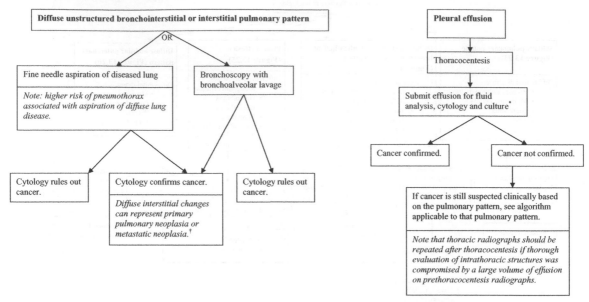

Diffuse unstructured bronchointerstitial or interstitial pulmonary pattern

OR

Fine needle aspiration of diseased lung

Note: higher risk of pneumothorax associated with aspiration of diffuse lung disease.

Bronchoscopy with bronchoalveolar lavage

Cytology rules out cancer.

Cytology confirms cancer.

Diffuse interstitial changes can represent primary pulmonary neoplasia or metastatic neoplasia.[†]

Cytology rules out cancer.

Pleural effusion

Thoracocentesis

Submit effusion for fluid analysis, cytology and culture[*]

Cancer confirmed.

Cancer not confirmed.

If cancer is still suspected clinically based on the pulmonary pattern, see algorithm applicable to that pulmonary pattern.

Note that thoracic radiographs should be repeated after thoracocentesis if thorough evaluation of intrathoracic structures was compromised by a large volume of effusion on prethoracocentesis radiographs.

[†]A previous diagnosis of cancer or presence of a nonpulmonary primary tumor suggests that pulmonary neoplasia may represent metastatic disease.
[*]Physicochemical characteristics, including specific gravity, total protein, and cell count, of malignant effusion can mimic non-neoplastic effusions. The presence confirms intrathoracic neoplasia. The absence of neoplastic cells does not rule out neoplasia.
LN= lymph node; CT= computed tomography; FNA= fine needle aspiration; PE= physical examination; US= ultrasound

Feline lung tumor diagnostic algorithm:

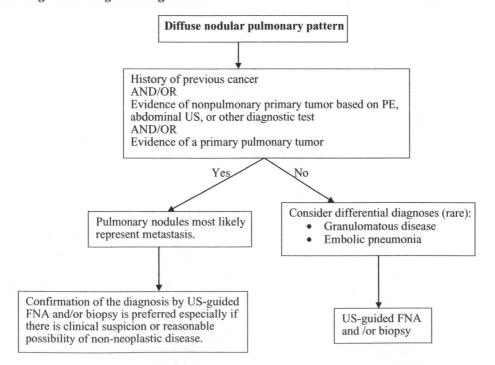

Diffuse nodular pulmonary pattern

History of previous cancer
AND/OR
Evidence of nonpulmonary primary tumor based on PE, abdominal US, or other diagnostic test
AND/OR
Evidence of a primary pulmonary tumor

Yes

No

Pulmonary nodules most likely represent metastasis.

Consider differential diagnoses (rare):
- Granulomatous disease
- Embolic pneumonia

Confirmation of the diagnosis by US-guided FNA and/or biopsy is preferred especially if there is clinical suspicion or reasonable possibility of non-neoplastic disease.

US-guided FNA and /or biopsy

LN = lymph node; CT = computed tomography; FNA = fine needle aspiration; PE = physical examination; US = ultrasound

Treatment

- Treatment is based on clinical stage of disease.
- Surgical excision is the treatment of choice for solitary lung tumors with no metastasis.
- The efficacy of chemotherapy in the adjuvant or gross disease setting is not defined.

Feline lung tumor treatment algorithm:

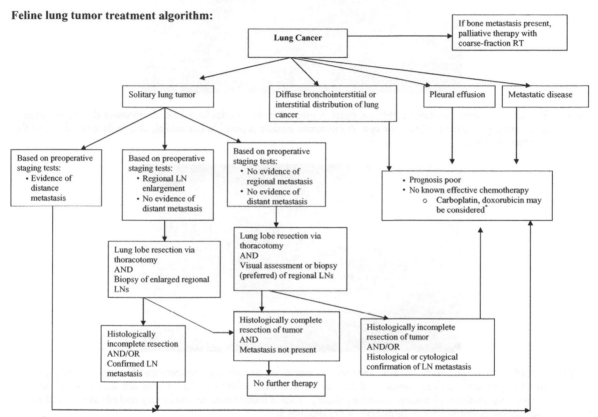

*Efficacy is considered minimal. Tumor response may be more favorable for epithelial tumors (carcinomas) than for mesenchymal tumors (sarcomas). Limited clinical information is available regarding efficacy of chemotherapy for feline lung cancer.

Prognosis

- Overall median survival time for cats with resectable primary lung tumors is approximately 4 months after surgery; however, individual cats can survive 2–3 years or longer:
  - Histologic grade is prognostic (Table 13.18).
- Poorly differentiated tumors are associated with an unfavorable prognosis.
  - Prognosis for cats with nonresectable lung cancer or metastasis is generally poor.
  - The benefit of chemotherapy in the adjuvant or gross disease setting for primary pulmonary or metastatic disease is unclear and considered minimal.

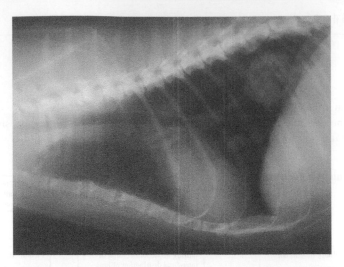

Figure 13.23. A large, cavitated soft-tissue mass is present in the caudal lung field. Differential diagnoses include primary lung tumor, granuloma, abcess, or cyst. A metastatic nodule is possible but unlikely due to its large size and the absence of other nodules.

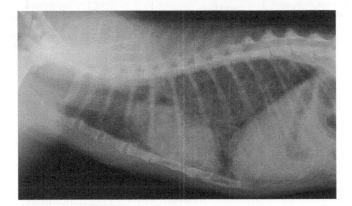

Figure 13.24. A 14-year-old domestic shorthair presents for progressive inappetence. No respiratory signs are present. Radiographs show diffuse unstructured pulmonary interstitial infiltrates. The findings are suggestive of disseminated neoplasia. No evidence of a nonpulmonary primary tumor is found based on the history and physical examination. Further investigation is needed for confirmation of the diagnosis.

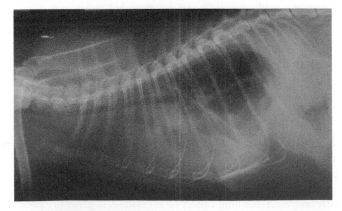

Figure 13.25. A large volume of pleural fluid is seen with rounding of lung margins and soft tissue opacity between the thoracic wall and the lung. The cardiac silhouette is obscured due to the presence of pleural fluid. Differential diagnoses include malignant effusion, hemothorax, chylothorax, pyothorax, and hydrothorax. Thoracocentesis should be performed for diagnostic and therapeutic purposes. A fluid analysis and cytology should be performed on the pleural fluid.

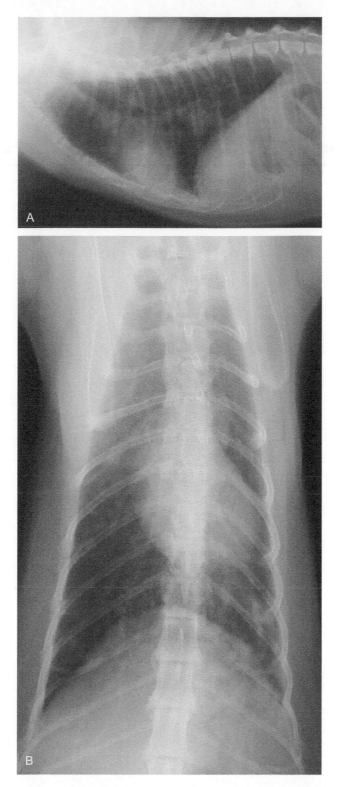

Figure 13.26. There are diffuse small nodular opacities in the lungs. There is an ill-defined but probably cavitary mass in the left caudal lung lobe. These findings are suspicious for a primary lung tumor in the left caudal lung lobe and metastatic spread to the remainder of the lung fields. A cytologic or histologic diagnosis is needed for confirmation.

Table 13.18. Prognostic indicator for cats with resectable lung tumors

	Positive Indicator	Negative Indicator
Histologic grade	Well differentiated tumor Moderately differentiated tumor	Poorly differentiated tumor
MEDIAN SURVIVAL TIME	2 years	2.5 months

14
ENDOCRINE TUMORS

David J. Argyle and Laura Blackwood

Key Points
- There are common clinical syndromes in small animal practice (Table 14.1).
- Endocrine tissue is subjected to positive and negative stimuli from hormones, maintaining normal homeostasis.
- Endocrine tissue can become hyperplastic when subjected to excessive trophic factors.
- In contrast, adenomas or adenocarcinomas grow independently of any trophic factors.

Table 14.1. Tumors of the endocrine system and their associated syndromes

Gland	Tumor Types	Syndrome

Pituitary	**Primary tumors of the adenohypohysis or neurohypophysis**
	 • Corticotroph cells
	 • Somatotroph cells
	 Secondary tumor, e.g.:
	 • Lymphoma
	 • Melanoma
	 Extension of an adjacent tumor, e.g.:
	 • Meningioma
	 • Glioma
		Functional tumors
		 • Endocrinopathy associated with hormone secretion
		 • Hyperadrenocorticism (Cushing's syndrome)
		 • Acromegaly (feline less rare)
		 • ±Neurological signs
		 Nonfunctional tumors
		 • Neurological signs associated with space-occupying lesions:
		   ◦ Behavior
		   ◦ Gait
		   ◦ Cranial nerve deficits
		 Compression and destruction of normal pituitary tissue:
		   ◦ Panhypopituitarism or selective hypopituitarism
		   ◦ Hypothyroidism, hypoadrenocorticism, central diabetes insipidus

Adrenal	**Adrenocortical tumors:** • Functional glucocorticoid secreting • Functional aldosterone secreting **Adrenal medullary tumors:** • Pheochromocytoma	Hyperadrenocorticism (Cushing's syndrome) Hyperaldosteronism (Conn's syndrome) Episodic collapse, hypertension
Thyroid	Canine thyroid adenoma or carcinoma Feline functional tumor	Space-occupying lesion ± metastasis Hyperthyroidism
Parathyroid	Adenoma/carcinoma	Hyperparathyroidism and associated hypercalcemia
Pancreas	Insulinoma Gastrinoma	Hypoglycemia ± Paraneoplastic neuropathy Zollinger-Ellison Syndrome

Pituitary and Adrenal (Functional Glucocorticoid-Secreting) Tumors

- Primary or secondary tumors of the pituitary can lead to neurological deficits and compression of normal pituitary tissue (leading to pan- or selective hypopituitarism), or they can be functional and give rise to hyperadrenocorticism (Figures 14.1–14.5).
- 80–85% of canine hyperadrenocorticism cases arise because of a chromophobe (corticotroph) tumor in the pars distalis (rarely pars intermedia) of the pituitary gland.
- The remainder of dogs with hyperadrenocorticism have an adrenal-dependent disease.
- 80% of functional adrenal tumors are adenocarcinomas.
- Tumors of the pituitary somatotroph cells cause acromegaly in cats.

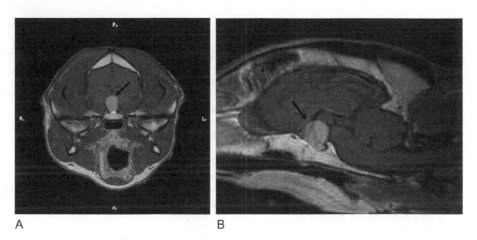

A   B

Figure 14.1.   MRI of a pituitary tumor (A and B).

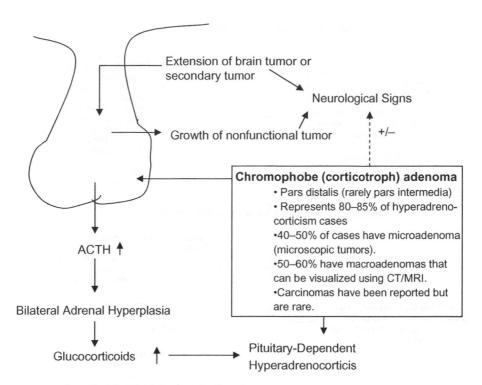

Extension of brain tumor or secondary tumor

Neurological Signs

Growth of nonfunctional tumor

+/–

Chromophobe (corticotroph) adenoma
• Pars distalis (rarely pars intermedia)
• Represents 80–85% of hyperadreno-corticism cases
•40–50% of cases have microadenoma (microscopic tumors).
•50–60% have macroadenomas that can be visualized using CT/MRI.
•Carcinomas have been reported but are rare.

ACTH ↑

Bilateral Adrenal Hyperplasia

Glucocorticoids ↑ ⟶ **Pituitary-Dependent Hyperadrenocorticis**

Figure 14.2. Neurological signs of pituitary and adrenal tumor.

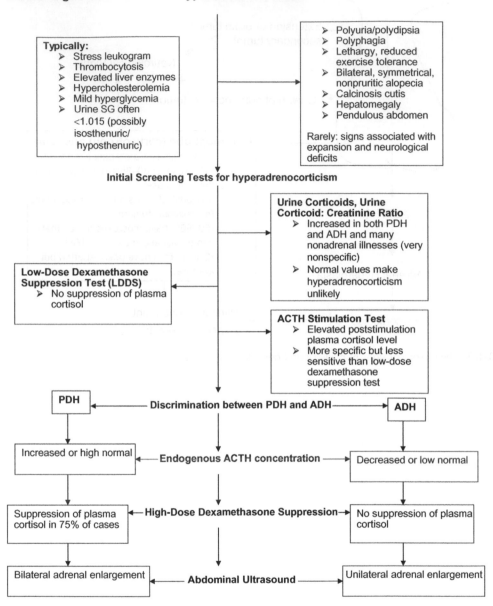

Figure 14.3. Clinical signs associated with hyperadrenocorticism.

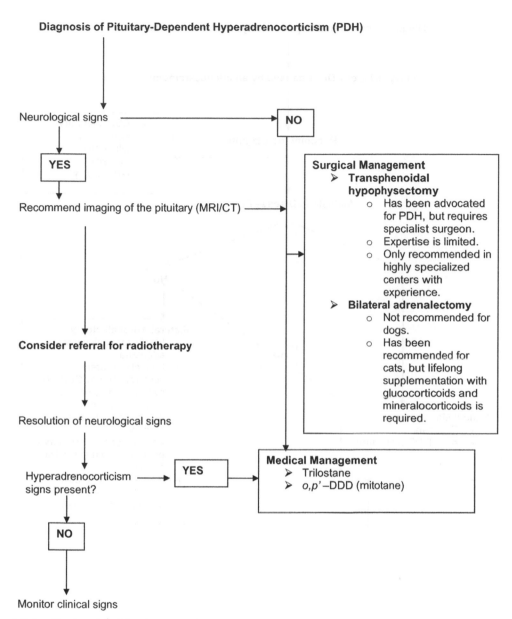

Figure 14.4. Treatment decision tree.

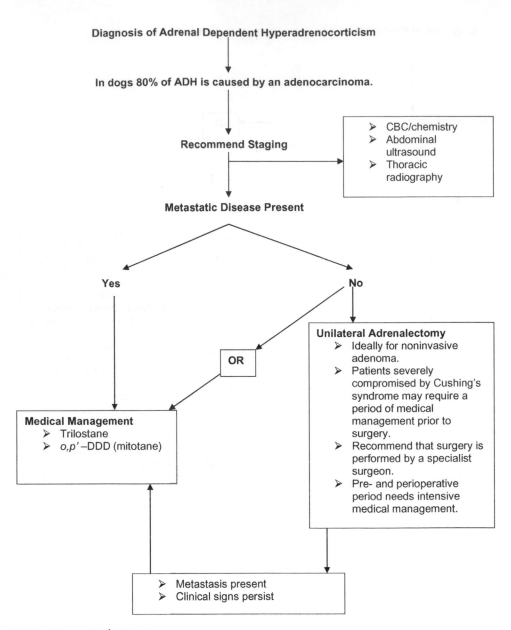

Figure 14.5. Diagnosis decision tree.

Surgical Considerations in Adrenalectomy

- If patients are severely compromised with signs associated with hyperadrenocorticism, presurgical therapy with trilostane or o, p'-DDD may be required.
- Patients that undergo surgery are at increased risk of
  - Pancreatitis
  - Iatrogenic hypoadrenocorticism (transient)
  - Hemorrhage
  - Pulmonary thromboembolism
- Dexamethasone is administered intraoperatively and postoperatively.
- An ACTH test should be performed the day after surgery and should be low.
- Glucocorticoid therapy is continued until the ACTH test results fall into the low-normal range (4–5 months postsurgery).
- Postoperative monitoring of electrolytes is imperative. Mineralocorticoid therapy may be required, but usually for a shorter period than for glucocorticoids.
- Heparin or low molecular weight heparin and plasma therapy may be required during/after surgery to reduce the risk of thromboembolism.
- Of those patients that survive surgery (estimated 20% mortality rate), 80–90% have no recurrence of clinical signs.

Medical Management of Hyperadrenocorticism

- Trilostane inhibits synthesis of steroids so reduces clinical signs but has no effect on the underlying tumor
  - Trilostane has a short half-life, so treatments must not be missed and some animals need twice-daily, rather than once-daily, treatment.
  - Monitoring is by ACTH stimulation test 4–6 hours after therapy.
- Mitotane (o, p'-DDD) is not licensed in the U.K.
- Mitotane is a cytotoxic agent that causes cell death in the adrenal zona fasciculata and zona reticularis.
  - Treatment is by initial induction and then maintenance.
  - Development of acute hypoadrenocorticism is a risk.
  - Monitor by ACTH stimulation test.
- Ketoconazole is used in some countries where trilostane is not available.
- Retinoids.
  - Early work has suggested beneficial effects in pituitary macroadenomas.

Somatotroph Tumors (Causing Acromegaly)

- Mainly cats.
- A rise in growth hormone levels (GH) with a concurrent increase in Insulin-Like Growth Factor-1 (IGF-1/Somatomedin C) levels gives rise to clinical signs (Figures 14.6, 14.7).

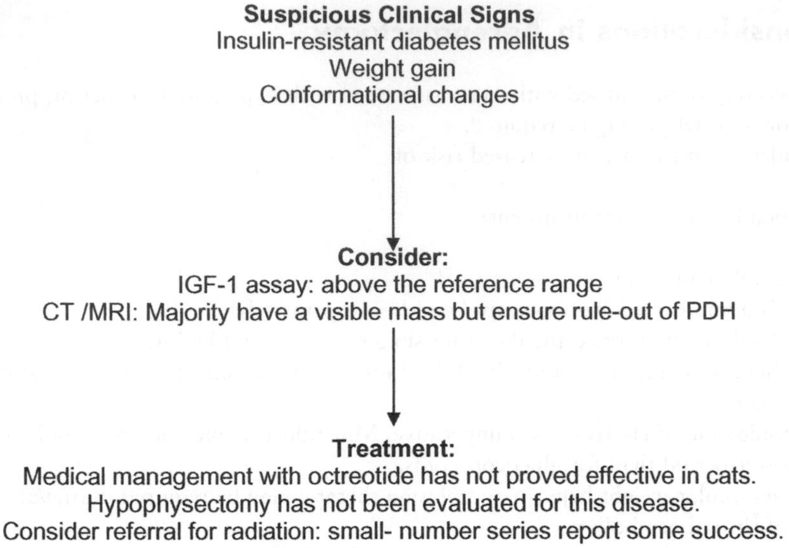

Suspicious Clinical Signs
Insulin-resistant diabetes mellitus
Weight gain
Conformational changes

Consider:
IGF-1 assay: above the reference range
CT /MRI: Majority have a visible mass but ensure rule-out of PDH

Treatment:
Medical management with octreotide has not proved effective in cats.
Hypophysectomy has not been evaluated for this disease.
Consider referral for radiation: small- number series report some success.

Figure 14.6. Somatotroph tumor decision tree.

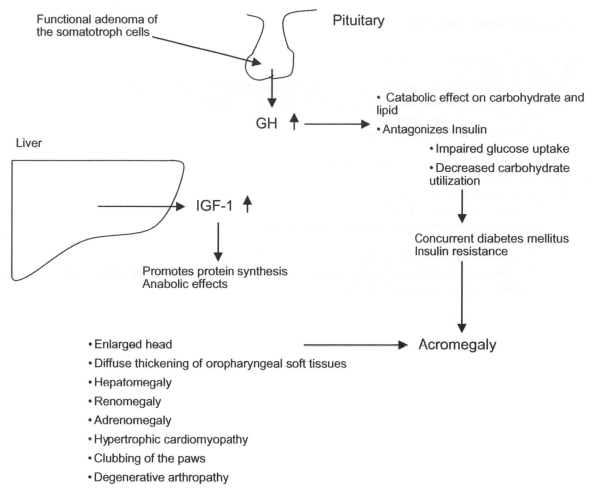

Functional adenoma of
the somatotroph cells

Pituitary

GH ↑

• Catabolic effect on carbohydrate and
lipid

• Antagonizes Insulin

• Impaired glucose uptake

• Decreased carbohydrate
utilization

Concurrent diabetes mellitus
Insulin resistance

Liver

IGF-1 ↑

Promotes protein synthesis
Anabolic effects

• Enlarged head
• Diffuse thickening of oropharyngeal soft tissues
• Hepatomegaly
• Renomegaly
• Adrenomegaly
• Hypertrophic cardiomyopathy
• Clubbing of the paws
• Degenerative arthropathy

Acromegaly

Figure 14.7. Clinical signs of somatotroph tumor.

Adrenal Gland Tumors

- Adrenal gland tumors are divided as
- **Adrenocortical tumors:**
  - Functional glucocorticoid-secreting causing hyperadrenocorticism (see previous section)
  - Functional aldosterone-secreting (very rare) causing Conn's syndrome
    - Typically episodic weakness.
    - Hypokalemia and hypernatremia.
    - Hypertension.
    - Adrenalectomy is the treatment of choice.
- **Adrenal Medullary Tumors**
  - Pheochromocytoma (Figure 14.8)
    - Arise from the chromaffin cells.
    - Secrete catecholamines (predominantly noradrenalin).
    - Rare in dogs and cats.
    - Most arise in the adrenal medulla.
    - When they arise from the extra-adrenal neural crest cells, they are known as *paragangliomas.*
  - The incidental adrenal mass (Figure 14.9)

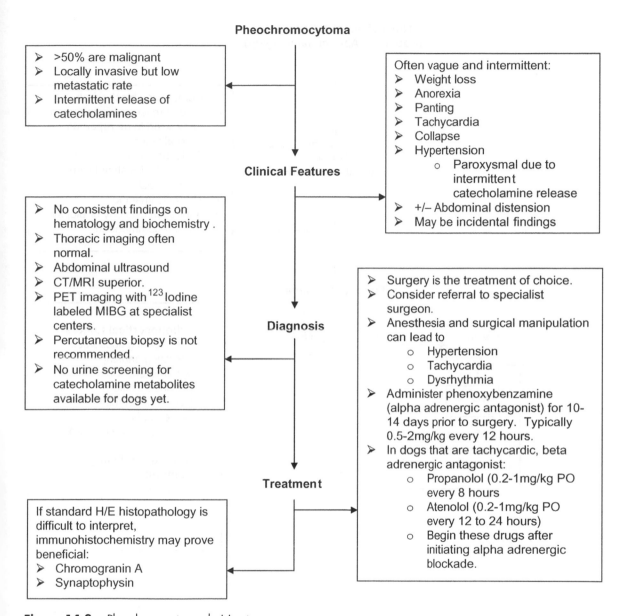

Pheochromocytoma

> - >50% are malignant
> - Locally invasive but low metastatic rate
> - Intermittent release of catecholamines

Clinical Features

Often vague and intermittent:
> - Weight loss
> - Anorexia
> - Panting
> - Tachycardia
> - Collapse
> - Hypertension
>   - Paroxysmal due to intermittent catecholamine release
> - +/– Abdominal distension
> - May be incidental findings

> - No consistent findings on hematology and biochemistry.
> - Thoracic imaging often normal.
> - Abdominal ultrasound
> - CT/MRI superior.
> - PET imaging with ^{123}Iodine labeled MIBG at specialist centers.
> - Percutaneous biopsy is not recommended.
> - No urine screening for catecholamine metabolites available for dogs yet.

Diagnosis

> - Surgery is the treatment of choice.
> - Consider referral to specialist surgeon.
> - Anesthesia and surgical manipulation can lead to
>   - Hypertension
>   - Tachycardia
>   - Dysrhythmia
> - Administer phenoxybenzamine (alpha adrenergic antagonist) for 10-14 days prior to surgery. Typically 0.5-2mg/kg every 12 hours.
> - In dogs that are tachycardic, beta adrenergic antagonist:
>   - Propanolol (0.2-1mg/kg PO every 8 hours
>   - Atenolol (0.2-1mg/kg PO every 12 to 24 hours)
>   - Begin these drugs after initiating alpha adrenergic blockade.

Treatment

If standard H/E histopathology is difficult to interpret, immunohistochemistry may prove beneficial:
> - Chromogranin A
> - Synaptophysin

Figure 14.8. Pheochromocytoma decision tree.

293

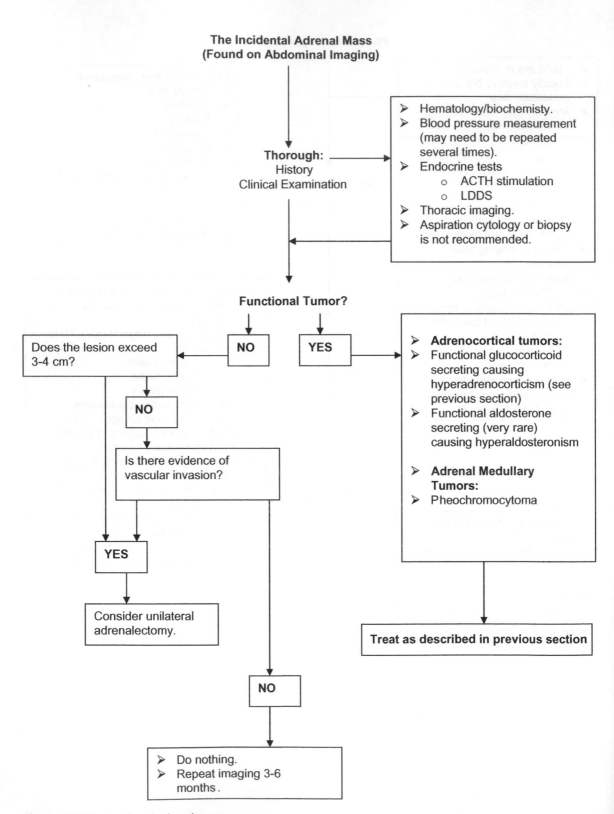

Figure 14.9. Incidental adrenal masses.

Thyroid Tumors in Dogs

Key Points
- Account for 1–4% of all tumors in dogs (Table 14.2, Figure 14.10).
- 30–50% are benign, nonfunctional adenomas.
- Adenomas are very small and are usually not detected clinically (incidental finding at necropsy).
- Most clinically detected tumors are classified as malignant.
- Age range of 9–11 years.
- In rare cases, ectopic thyroid tissue can be affected.
- 35–40% of dogs have visibly detectable metastatic disease at presentation (lymph nodes and lungs).

Key Points on Treatment
- **The treatment of choice is dictated by**
  - Size of the mass
  - Degree of invasion
  - Concurrent metastatic disease
  - Evidence of thyrotoxicosis
- **For freely movable, noninvasive tumors,** surgical excision is the treatment of choice, giving a median survival time of around 3 years.
- **Nonresectable tumors** are managed with external beam radiation:
  - May be used in the neoadjuvant setting to improve a definitive surgery
  - Can be used postoperatively to treat minimal residual disease
  - Used alone: shrinks tumors over a 6-month period giving very good local control
- **Dogs with gross metastatic disease:**
  - Metastasis (even when detected visually), takes a long time to become clinical (sometimes 1–2 years).
  - Surgery for freely mobile tumors or palliative radiotherapy for nonmobile tumors is therefore still a reasonable option without compromising patient quality of life.

Is Radioactive Iodine Ever Indicated in Canine Thyroid Tumors?

- In humans ^{131}I is often used postsurgically to treat microscopic disease. Experience in dogs is limited.
- The major limiting factor in dogs is the high dose of ^{131}I that is required, because these tumors do not accumulate iodine in the same way as functional adenomas. Most centers do not have the facilities required (health and safety) to handle such doses.

Table 14.2. Thyroid tumors in dogs

Tumor	Subclassification	Pathology
Follicular cell of origin	Papillary Follicular Compact Anaplastic	Immunohistochemically stain positive for • Thyroglobulin • Thyroid transcription factor-1
Parafollicular (C-cell carcinoma)	N/A	Immunohistochemically stain positive for • Calcitonin • Calcitonin-gene related peptide

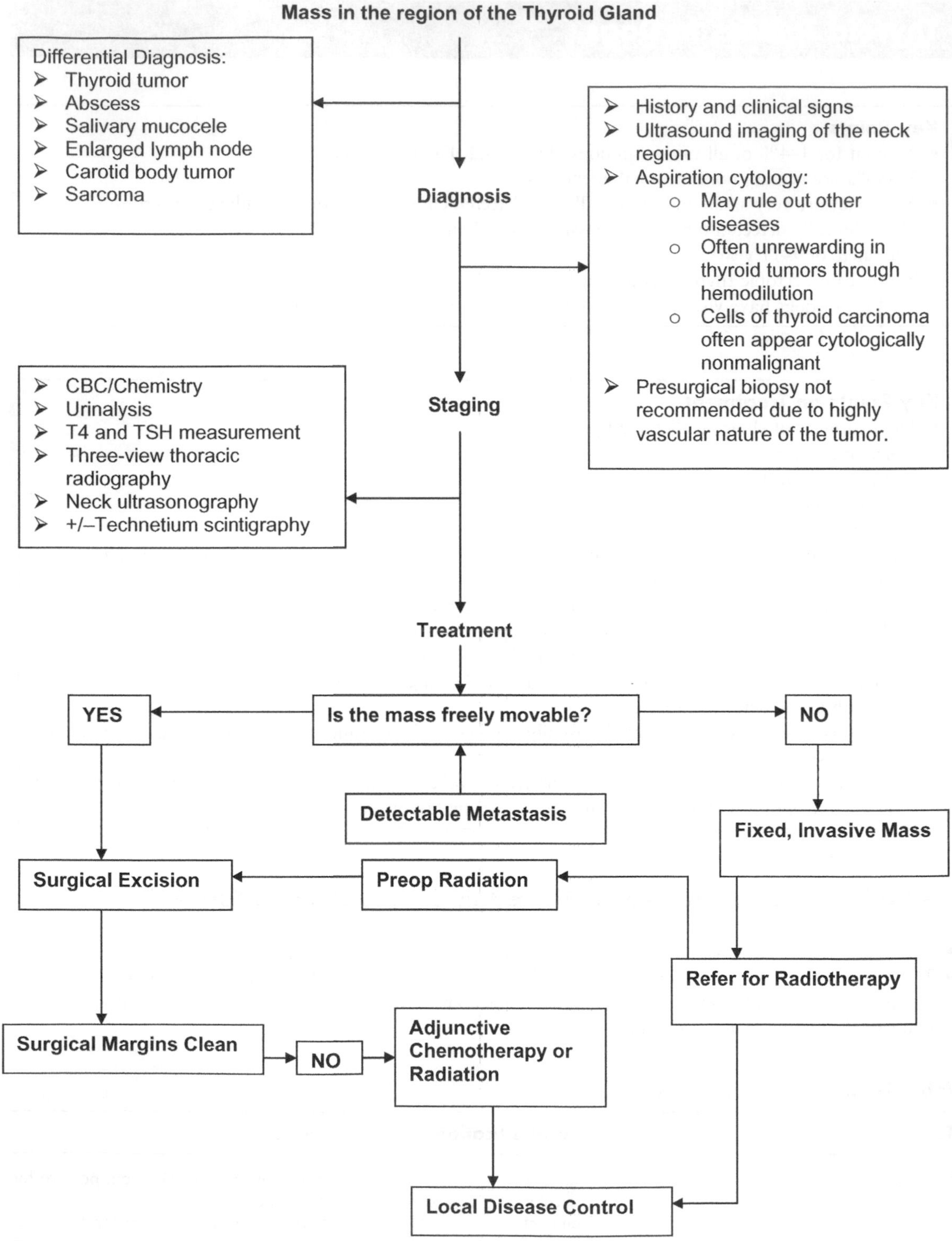

Mass in the region of the Thyroid Gland

Differential Diagnosis:
➤ Thyroid tumor
➤ Abscess
➤ Salivary mucocele
➤ Enlarged lymph node
➤ Carotid body tumor
➤ Sarcoma

Diagnosis

➤ History and clinical signs
➤ Ultrasound imaging of the neck region
➤ Aspiration cytology:
  ○ May rule out other diseases
  ○ Often unrewarding in thyroid tumors through hemodilution
  ○ Cells of thyroid carcinoma often appear cytologically nonmalignant
➤ Presurgical biopsy not recommended due to highly vascular nature of the tumor.

➤ CBC/Chemistry
➤ Urinalysis
➤ T4 and TSH measurement
➤ Three-view thoracic radiography
➤ Neck ultrasonography
➤ +/–Technetium scintigraphy

Staging

Treatment

YES ← **Is the mass freely movable?** → **NO**

Detectable Metastasis

Fixed, Invasive Mass

Surgical Excision ← **Preop Radiation** ←

Refer for Radiotherapy

Surgical Margins Clean → **NO** → **Adjunctive Chemotherapy or Radiation**

Local Disease Control

Figure 14.10. Thyroid tumor decision tree.

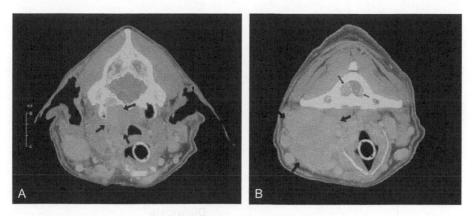

Figure 14.11.   Invasive thyroid carcinoma showing invasion of the bulla (A) and invasion of the spinal cord (B).

Is Chemotherapy Indicated in the Management of Canine Thyroid Tumors?

- Where surgery or radiotherapy is not a viable option, chemotherapy with either doxorubicin or carboplatin could be considered. However, only partial responses should be expected and it must be considered palliative only.
- Where radiation is not available, chemotherapy may be considered where surgical resection has been performed but surgical margins demonstrate microscopic disease.
- Chemotherapy can be considered where there is gross metastatic disease. However, disease progression in these cases is often slow anyway. The beneficial effects of adding in chemotherapy are unproven.
- Large tumors and bilateral tumors have been shown to have a greater metastatic potential. Consequently, adjunctive chemotherapy may be considered for tumors above 20–30 cm^3.

Feline Thyroid Tumors

Key Points
- Hyperthyroidism is the most common endocrinopathy in cats (Figures 14.12, 14.13).
- 70–75% of cases are caused by multinodular adenomatous hyperplasia.
- 20–25% are caused by solitary adenomas.
- 1–3% are caused by malignant carcinomas.

Diagnosis

- See decision tree in hypercalcemia (Chapter 2)
- Elevated PTH relative to serum calcium: i.e., if the PTH level is in the reference range or higher, in the face of hypercalcemia, this supports a diagnosis of primary hyperparathyroidism.

Treatment

- Treat any medical issues associated with hypercalcemia.
- Surgically excise the parathyroid tissue.

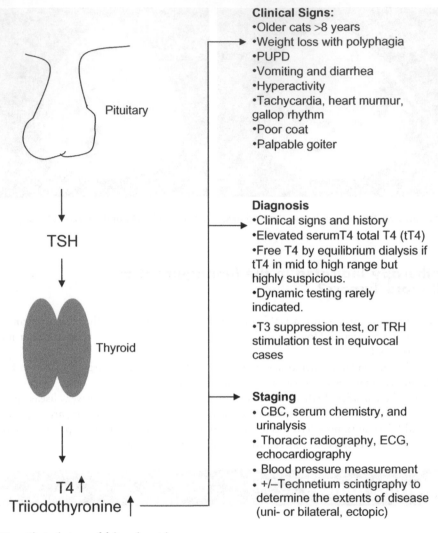

Clinical Signs:
•Older cats >8 years
•Weight loss with polyphagia
•PUPD
•Vomiting and diarrhea
•Hyperactivity
•Tachycardia, heart murmur,
gallop rhythm
•Poor coat
•Palpable goiter

Diagnosis
•Clinical signs and history
•Elevated serumT4 total T4 (tT4)
•Free T4 by equilibrium dialysis if
tT4 in mid to high range but
highly suspicious.
•Dynamic testing rarely
indicated.

•T3 suppression test, or TRH
stimulation test in equivocal
cases

Staging
• CBC, serum chemistry, and
  urinalysis
• Thoracic radiography, ECG,
  echocardiography
• Blood pressure measurement
• +/–Technetium scintigraphy to
  determine the extents of disease
  (uni- or bilateral, ectopic)

Pituitary

TSH

Thyroid

T4 ↑
Triiodothyronine ↑

Figure 14.12. Clinical signs of feline thyroid tumors.

• Three of the for glands can be removed without causing permanent hypoparathyroidism.
• Removal of all glands necessitates lifelong supplementation with calcium and vitamin D.
• Serum PTH and calcium decline over 1–7 days; calcium should be monitored carefully.
• Dogs that have severe hypercalcemia prior to therapy are at greater risk of postoperative hypocalcemia (negative feedback effects).
• Treat with vitamin D and calcium if calcium level drops below normal.
• Treatment can be tailored off, where dogs have residual parathyroid tissue.
• In cases where renal function has not been compromised, prognosis is good.

Treatment Options for Hyperthyroidism

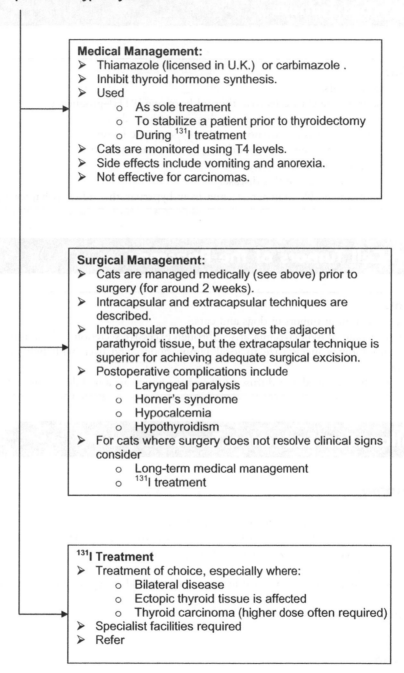

Medical Management:
- Thiamazole (licensed in U.K.) or carbimazole .
- Inhibit thyroid hormone synthesis.
- Used
    - As sole treatment
    - To stabilize a patient prior to thyroidectomy
    - During ^{131}I treatment
- Cats are monitored using T4 levels.
- Side effects include vomiting and anorexia.
- Not effective for carcinomas.

Surgical Management:
- Cats are managed medically (see above) prior to surgery (for around 2 weeks).
- Intracapsular and extracapsular techniques are described.
- Intracapsular method preserves the adjacent parathyroid tissue, but the extracapsular technique is superior for achieving adequate surgical excision.
- Postoperative complications include
    - Laryngeal paralysis
    - Horner's syndrome
    - Hypocalcemia
    - Hypothyroidism
- For cats where surgery does not resolve clinical signs consider
    - Long-term medical management
    - ^{131}I treatment

^{131}**I Treatment**
- Treatment of choice, especially where:
    - Bilateral disease
    - Ectopic thyroid tissue is affected
    - Thyroid carcinoma (higher dose often required)
- Specialist facilities required
- Refer

Figure 14.13. Treatment options.

Parathyroid Tumors

Key Points
- Rare in dogs and cats.
- Tumors arise from the chief cells (parathyroid hormone [PTH]–producing).
- They produce a syndrome associated with hyperparathyroidism.
- Tumors can be adenomas or carcinomas (also hyperplastic lesions).
- Masses are not palpable and may be difficult to see on ultrasound.
- CT/MRI may give greater sensitivity.
- Metastasis is not a feature of this disease.
- Clinical signs are referable to hypercalcemia from hyperparathyroidism (Chapter 2).

Islet β-Cell Tumors of the Pancreas

Key Points
- These are uncommon tumors in dogs and cats.
- Clinical syndrome of hypoglycemia arises through excessive secretion of insulin (Figure 14.14).
- 50% of insulinomas metastasize to local lymph nodes, and liver, with pulmonary metastasis being uncommon.
- A tumor can be identified as a diffuse tumor of the pancreas, a nodule, or multiple nodules.

Miscellaneous Endocrine Tumors

Gastrinoma

- This is a rare neuroendocrine tumor of the pancreas.
- The triad of non–beta-cell neuroendocrine tumor of the pancreas, hypergastrinemia, and gastrointestinal ulceration is referred to as the Zollinger-Ellison syndrome.
- Tumors are highly metastatic.
- Surgery may be indicated with medical management using H_2 receptor antagonists or, better, proton pump inhibitors.
- Survival times are less than 8 months.

APUDomas

- These are tumors that arise in Amine Uptake Precursor and Decarboxylation (APUD) cells
- These tumors include
  - Insulinomas
  - Pheochromocytomas
  - Parathyroid tumors
  - Medullary thyroid tumors
  - Gastrinomas
  - Glucagonomas (cause superficial necrolytic dermatitis)
  - Carcinoids

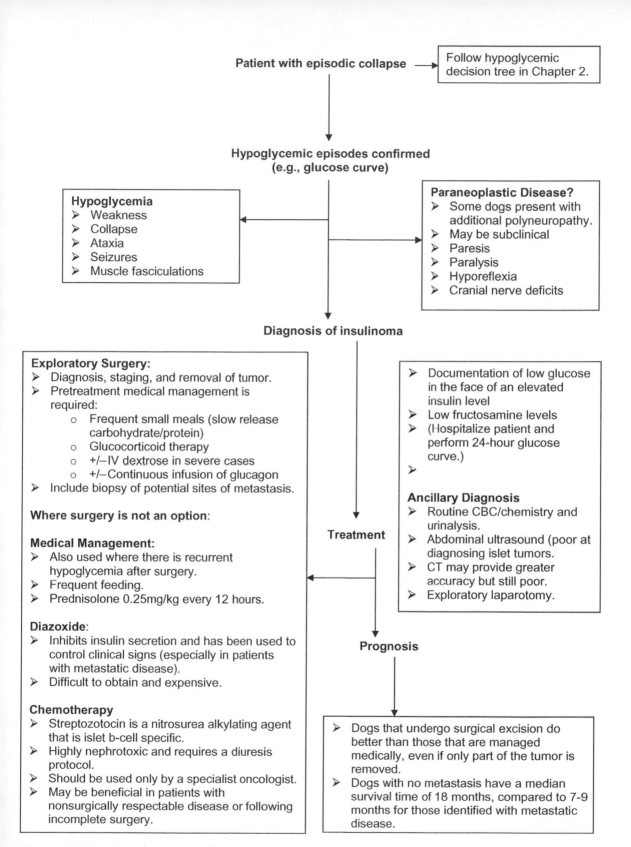

Figure 14.14. Hypoglycemic episode.

15
TUMORS OF THE URINARY SYSTEM

David J. Argyle and Alison Hayes

This section describes the main clinical and pathological features of urinary system tumors in dogs and cats. It includes tumors of the kidney ureters, bladder, and urethra.

Key Points
- Tumors of the urinary tract may occur in the upper urinary tract, which comprises the kidneys and ureters, or in the lower urinary tract comprising the bladder and urethra.
- The presenting signs and signalment differ between the upper and lower tract tumors.
- Tumors originating in one compartment rarely spread to the other.
- Tumors of the upper urinary tract are uncommon and may be clinically silent.
- Tumors of the lower urinary tract are more common, and the associated dysfunction is readily detected clinically.
- Tumors may originate in more that one locus along the lower urinary tract at similar time points due to field carcinogenesis.
- Tumors of the lower urinary tract can originate in either the epithelial or supporting connective tissues or stromal layers.
- The most common tumors are of primary, epithelial origin and are most often malignant.
- In addition to transitional cell carcinoma (TCC), other epithelial tumors include squamous cell carcinoma, adenocarcinoma, and undifferentiated carcinoma, as well as papillomas and adenomas.
- Bladder tumors of mesenchymal origin arising in the connecting tissues or supporting stroma also comprise both benign and malignant tumors. These include leiomysarcoma and leiomyoma; fibrosarcoma and fibroma; hemangiosarcoma and hemangioma; plus rhabdomyosarcoma and other, undifferentiated sarcomas.

Lower Urinary Tract Tumors

Key Features–Lower Urinary Tract Tumors in Dogs

- Tumors of the lower urinary tract in dogs comprise tumors that arise in the bladder or urethra.
- Bladder tumors tend to occur in female dogs and are more common than urethral tumors, which tend to occur in male dogs.
- Bladder tumors tend to arise in older, small terrier breed dogs although any age of dog and any breed can be affected. Scottish terriers may be overrepresented.
- TCC is the most common primary bladder tumor and accounts for approximately two-thirds of all bladder tumors.
- The remaining one-third of primary canine bladder tumors comprises both malignant and benign tumors, although malignant tumors in this category also exceed benign tumors by a ratio of approximately 2:1.
- Herbicides and insecticides have been implicated in the pathogenesis of TCC in dogs.

- The lower urinary tract is an uncommon site of secondary tumor spread, but involvement may be seen in cases of lymphoma.
- Locoregional spread may involve the prostate in male dogs.

Key Features–Lower Urinary Tract Tumors in Cats

- Bladder tumors tend to occur less frequently in cats than in dogs.
- There appears to be no sex predilection in cats.
- TCC of the bladder is the most common tumor type; however, other malignant and benign tumors also occur.
- Urethral tumors have been rarely reported in cats.

Clinical Features Associated with Lower Urinary Tract Tumors in Dogs and Cats

- Although the clinical signs are easily recognized they are variable, and species differences are noted (Table 15.1).
- This is more likely to reflect the behavior of the animal and how closely it is observed than any differences in the disease process.
- Clinical signs may be misdiagnosed as a urinary tract infection (UTI) or, in the case of cats, feline urological syndrome (FUS) in the first instance.
- A UTI may accompany a lower urinary tract tumor, but animals diagnosed with a presumed UTI that do not respond to the symptomatic treatment should be investigated for the possibility of underlying lower urinary tract neoplasia.
- Pollakiuria, stranguria, and dysuria are commonly associated with lower urethral obstruction in neutered male cats; however, when no obstruction can be detected further investigations to exclude a lower urinary tract tumor are warranted.

Investigation of Suspected Lower Urinary Tract Tumors in Dogs and Cats

- When a case presents with the clinical signs listed above, it is important to establish a working diagnosis as quickly as possible (Figure 15.1).

Table 15.1. Clinical features of urinary tract tumors

Dogs	Clinical Sign	Cats
•	Dysuria	•
•	Stranguria	•
•	Pollakiuria	•
•	Hematuria	•
•	PU/PD	
•	Urinary incontinence	
	Tenesmus or constipation	•
	Rectal prolapse	•
	Anorexia	•
	Palpable caudal abdominal mass	•

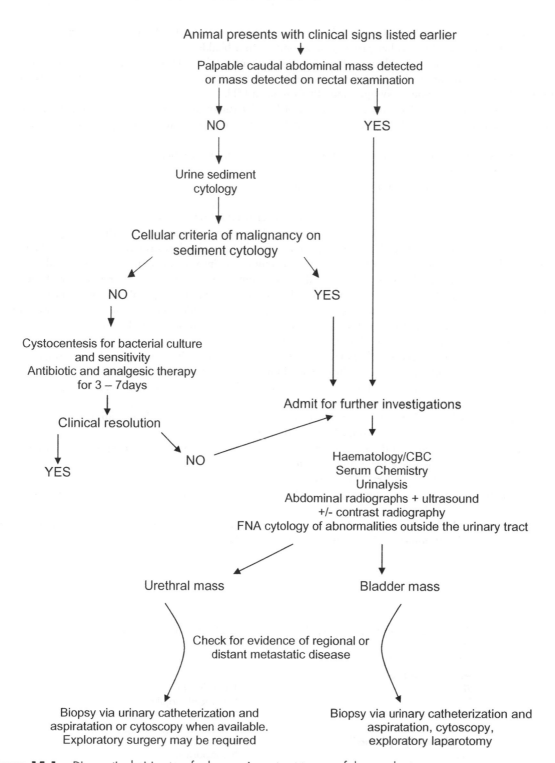

Figure 15.1. Diagnostic decision tree for lower urinary tract tumors of dogs and cats.

- In many cases, the clinician will suspect a lower urinary tract infection (UTI), but it is important to remember that this could be either primary or secondary to a bladder tumor.
- Attempts should be made to exclude malignancy on sediment cytology. However, careful follow-up is required as some tumors will not exfoliate into urine and many cases of lower urinary tract tumors will improve for periods of time on symptomatic therapy for a UTI.
- A urine dipstick test is available for the detection of bladder tumor antigen in dogs, but care should be taken in interpreting the results in the face of hematuria and proteinuria when false positive results are likely.
- Further investigations are warranted if any of the following criteria are met:
  - A mass can be palpated.
  - Sediment cytology indicates abnormal cellular pathology.
  - Symptomatic treatment has been unsuccessful.
  - Initial investigations of a "blocked cat" show no lower urethral obstruction.
- Urine samples should be obtained by free catch or via the placement of a urinary catheter.
- Cystocentesis and diagnostic needle aspirate cytology should be avoided in suspected cases of bladder neoplasia due to the risk of shedding and seeding of tumor cells into the abdomen and body wall.
- Plain abdominal radiography is unlikely to be diagnostic but does help to assess the remainder of the abdomen for abnormalities, such as regional lymph node assessment and regional bony metastasis.
- Contrast radiography, including a double contrast cytogram, retrograde urethrogram/vaginourethrogram may be helpful in delineating a mass lesion involving the bladder wall or mucosal surface.
- Ultrasound is the diagnostic test of choice, especially in female cats.
- Ultrasound will permit guided needle aspirate biopsies of any abnormality **outside** the lower urinary tract.
- Samples from the bladder lumen or urethral urothelium may be obtained in three ways:
  - Pass a urinary catheter and use aspirate techniques under ultrasound guidance to direct the tip of a urinary catheter onto the area of interest.
  - Cystoscopy may be available at referral level for dogs and can be used to obtain samples endoscopically.
  - Exploratory surgery can be used to facilitate incisional biopsy.
- Laparotomy is usually required if lesions do not have a mucosal component, or in cases where urinary catheterization is not possible – for example, in female cats.
- Complete staging should be undertaken (Tables 15.2, 15.3):
  - Regional metastasis. May be suggested by pelvic or medial iliac lymphadenopathy, prostatomegaly or irregularities of the pelvic bones.
  - Distant metastasis. May be suggested by single/multiple mass lesions of the spleen, liver, or thorax using ultrasound for the abdomen and radiography/CT for the thorax.
  - Biopsy all suspected sites of secondary involvement when possible.

Table 15.2. Clinical staging (TNM) of urinary bladder tumors in dogs and cats

Primary tumor	
Tis	Tumor in situ
T1	Superficial, papillary
T2	Invasion of the bladder wall
T3	Invasion of neighboring organs
Regional lymph node	
N0	No metastasis
N1	Regional nodal involvement
N2	Regional involvement
Distant metastasis	
M0	No metastasis
M1	Metastasis

Table 15.3.   Histological classification of lower urinary tract tumors in dogs and cats

	Benign	Malignant
Epithelial	Papilloma Adenoma	Transitional cell carcinoma Squamous cell carcinoma Adenocarcinoma Undifferentiated carcinoma
Mesenchymal	Leimyoma Fibroma Hemangioma	Leimyosarcoma Fibrosarcoma Hemangiosarcoma Rhabdomyosarcoma Undifferentiated sarcoma

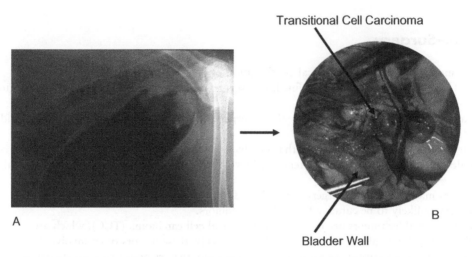

Figure 15.2.   Radiographic features of transitional cell carcinoma of the bladder (A) and associated findings at pathology (B).

Key Features–Treatment of Lower Urinary Tract Tumors

- Surgical intervention to perform a variety of palliative, urinary bypass procedures may be possible in order to relieve urinary obstruction and are better described in dogs than in cats. Examples include cystectomy with ureterocolonic anastomosis or ureterourethral anastomosis, transabdominal cystotomy catheter placement, and transurethral urethrotomy. These are not detailed here.
- Extended survival period can be achieved but the likelihood of a cure is remote unless a benign tumor can be completely excised.
- In general, treatment of lower urinary tract tumors aims to control clinical signs and improve quality of life.
- This is achieved by slowing down the rate of primary tumor growth and/or reducing the bulk of the primary tumor.
- In turn, pelvic outflow obstruction, the likelihood of secondary bacterial infection, and discomfort will be reduced.
- Treatment is unlikely to affect the metastatic rate or alter disease progression and survival times once gross metastasis is detected.
- Treatment may be warranted in the face of metastatic disease in order to control clinical signs associated with the primary tumor (Table 15.4).

Table 15.4. Outcome for treatment of TCC in dogs

Modality	Details of Treatment	Outcome
Surgery	Complete excision	Median survival 12–13 months
Surgery	Incomplete excision	Survival 1–5 months
Surgery + radiotherapy	Intraoperative RT	Median survival 15 months
Surgery + chemotherapy	X	Median survival 11 months
Chemotherapy	Piroxicam (0.3 mg/kg SID, PO) Mitoxantrone (5 mg/m^2 q 21days, IV)	Median survival 12 months
Radiation + chemotherapy	Piroxicam, mitoxantrone plus weekly fractionation	No advantage over chemotherapy alone

Treatment–Surgery

- Before treatment commences, histological confirmation of diagnosis is required.
- The aims of surgery should be clearly defined, i.e., surgery to achieve palliative relief of obstruction versus definitive surgery to attempt a cure.
- Similar, palliative effects can be achieved without surgery in many cases, which avoids the morbidity associated with urinary tract surgery.
- Any tumor type where multifocal disease that involves the trigone is unlikely to be amenable to curative surgery unless transplantation of the ureters is achieved. Consider referral for a specialist surgical opinion.
- Benign tumors may be cured by surgery. Consider referral for a specialist surgical opinion.
- Surgery is very unlikely to be curative for malignant tumors.
- The majority of bladder tumors are malignant transitional cell carcinoma (TCC), which are often multifocal and may also metastasize. In dogs especially, these tumors often involve the trigone making reconstructive surgery problematic. For these tumors nonsurgical treatment is appropriate.
- Adjuvant treatment with chemotherapy and/or radiotherapy may be required for malignant tumors treated with surgery. This will depend on histological assessment of margins.
- Surgical seeding into the abdomen or laparotomy incision site is possible with surgery for TCC. Clean instruments should be used for wound closure, and packing and/or flushing of the surgical site is warranted.

Treatment–Chemotherapy

- Before treatment commences, histological confirmation of diagnosis is required.
- Chemotherapy is relatively well described and established in dogs, but not in cats.
- Chemotherapy avoids the morbidity associated with surgery and radiotherapy, is generally well tolerated, and can improve quality of life and survival times.
- Chemotherapy is the treatment of choice for the majority of dogs with TCC of the bladder or urethra. It may also be used in cats.
- The best results for dogs so far have been obtained with a combination of mitoxantrone given systemically plus a COX-2 inhibitor (such as piroxicam or meloxicam).
- Hematological and GI toxicity may be expected in up to 20% of dogs treated.
- Renal function should be monitored when COX-2 inhibitors are used.
- Platinum-based drugs have no treatment advantage over mitoxantrone and may accelerate renal compromise in patients with preexisting renal disease or pelvic outflow obstruction.

Treatment – Radiotherapy

- Before treatment commences, histological confirmation of diagnosis is required.
- The optimum radiotherapy schedule has yet to be determined.
- Currently, radiotherapy has a limited application in the treatment of lower urinary tract tumors in dogs. Radiotherapy has not been reported in the management of feline bladder tumors.
- Conventional fraction sizes used in most fractionated veterinary treatment protocols and large single intraoperative doses are likely to result in bladder fibrosis and treatment-associated morbidity.
- Studies to date combining radiotherapy with chemotherapy or surgery for canine bladder tumors are disappointing. The addition of weekly fractionated radiotherapy to a standard mitoxantrone plus piroxicam protocol did not improve outcome over that expected with chemotherapy alone.
- Intraoperative therapy with large fractions has little benefit.

Outcome for Treatment of TCC in Cats

- There is a paucity of information describing treatment of feline bladder tumors.
- Surgery has been attempted without long-term survival in malignant disease, but it may be indicated for benign disease that is away from the trigone region.
- Cats will tolerate systemic anticancer treatment with mitoxantrone at a dose rate of 6.5 mg/m^2 q 21 days, IV, which could be used to treat TCC, although reports are anecdotal.
- Similarly there are anecdotal reports of the use of COX-2 inhibitors such as meloxicam and piroxicam in cats with TCC, although care is needed with long-term dosing. The dose of piroxicam in cats is 0.3 mg/kg q 48 hours, PO.

Prognosis – Lower Urinary Tract Tumors in Dogs and Cats

- Without treatment of any kind, survival although variable, is not expected to be beyond a few months in both species.
- Animals are most often euthanized due to progression of the primary tumor when clinical signs cannot be controlled.
- Metastasis from malignant tumors occurs in approximately 30–60% of TCC, but is infrequently detected at presentation in both species.
- For interventional therapy to be deemed effective, survival beyond that expected with the best supportive care must be achieved.
- In dogs, outcome depends on several factors:
  - Size of primary tumor
  - Presence or absence of regional metastasis
  - Presence or absence of distant metastasis
  - Histological grade
- These prognostic factors are also likely to be applicable to cats.
- Response to chemotherapy is another good predictor of outcome, with nonresponders likely to do far worse than dogs that do respond to therapy.

Key Features – Treatment of Urethral Tumors in Dogs and Cats

- These tumors are rarely encountered in both species but the majority are TCC (Figure 15.3).
- Definitive surgery is problematic and rarely attempted.
- Palliative surgery to debulk the lesion may be achieved endoscopically in dogs.

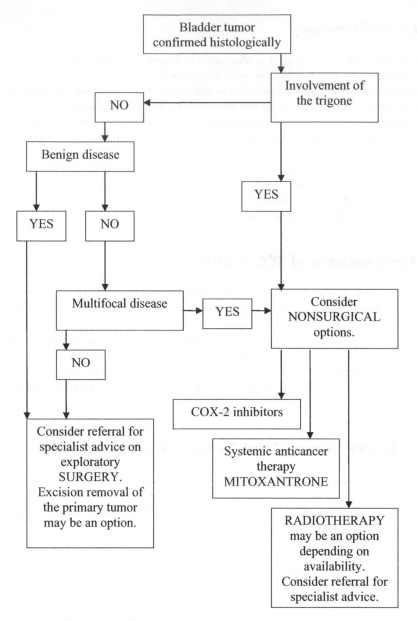

Figure 15.3. Therapeutic decision tree for bladder tumors in dogs and cats.

- Chemotherapy, as outlined for bladder tumors, can be used to debulk the tumor and give control of clinical signs.

Upper Urinary Tract Tumors

Key Features – Renal Tumors in Dogs

- Upper urinary tract tumors are rare in dogs, and comprise tumors of the kidney and ureters.
- Unlike lower urinary tract tumors, tumors of the kidney and ureters are often clinically silent unless the tumor involves the renal pelvis or has a tendency to, in which case hematuria can be recognized clinically.
- When renal tumors are recognized, renal carcinoma and nephroblastoma are most often reported in dogs.
- Renal carcinomas tend to affect older, male dogs.
- Nephroblastoma tends to occur in young dogs of either sex.
- Both renal carcinoma and nephroblastoma are highly metastatic and may have bilateral renal involvement because of de novo disease.
- Metastatic tumors from a variety of sites may affect the kidney.
- German Shepherd dogs have a breed predisposition to renal cystadenocarcinomas, which is recognized in association with multifocal nodular dermatofibrosis.

Key Features – Renal Tumors in Cats

- Renal lymphoma is a well-recognized anatomical form of lymphoma in cats and is often bilateral. Other sites of lymphoma involvement should be investigated if renal lymphoma is confirmed (see Chapters 9 and 10).
- Unlike lower urinary tract tumors, tumors of the kidney and ureters are often clinically silent.
- Azotemia and the associated clinical signs may be more commonly recognized in association with renal tumors in cats than dogs.
- If the tumor involves the renal pelvis or has a tendency to bleed, hematuria can be recognized clinically.
- With the exception of renal lymphoma, primary upper urinary tract tumors are rare in cats.
- There appears to be no sex predilection in cats.
- When renal tumors are detected in cats, they are usually TCC or renal carcinomas.
- Nephroblastoma affects young cats and is very rare.
- TCC, renal carcinoma, and nephroblastoma and are highly metastatic in the cat and may be bilateral either by de novo development or from metastasis.
- It is difficult to distinguish renal adenoma from low-grade renal carcinoma in cats.
- Metastatic tumors from a variety of sites may affect the kidney.

Clinical Features Associated with Renal Tumors in Dogs and Cats

- Renal tumors are often clinically silent.
- When the tumor involves the renal pelvis or has a tendency to bleed, such as a hemangiosarcoma, hematuria may be recognized clinically.
- Preexisting renal compromise may be destabilized by further loss of renal function associated with the tumor, especially if the tumor occurs bilaterally. This may result in clinical signs associated with azotemia such as anorexia, lethargy, polyuria and polydipsia, halitosis, and vomiting.
- An abdominal mass may be palpated in an animal presented for nonspecific clinical signs, especially in cats.

- Metastatic disease is not uncommon at presentation, and signs may relate to other body systems.
- Hypertrophic osteopathy (Marie's disease) may be seen in dogs resulting in a shifting lameness, heat and edema of the limbs, and new bone formation radiographically.
- Polycythemia may be seen in dogs due to excessive renal erythropoietin production. Chronic blood loss anemia is actually much more common.
- German Shepherd dogs with renal cystadenocarcinomas can present with azotemia, weight loss, and lethargy or abdominal signs associated with the tumor, which is bilateral. However, troublesome cutaneous nodules may also be the presenting complaint.

Investigation of Suspected Renal Tumors in Dogs and Cats

- In cats, renal lymphoma should be excluded.
- In GSDs, consider that renal cystadenocarcinoma compels, and check for any cutaneous lesions.
- All animals should have their serum chemistry checked and a CBC performed.
- Abdominal ultrasonography is central to the diagnosis and investigation of suspected renal tumors and has largely replaced contrast radiography (Figure 15.4, Table 15.5).
- Abdominal ultrasound will aid in the detection of bilateral involvement and metastatic involvement of other organs, such as the adrenal glands, liver, or regional lymph nodes, and permit ultrasound guided biopsy of the primary lesion and any suspected metastatic lesions.
- When ultrasound is not available, an intravenous urography can help with the delineation of filling defects and ureteric outflow obstruction.
- Plain radiography of the whole abdomen is useful to delineate the relative positions of abnormal abdominal organs and to detect any extension of the tumor to the vertebrae.
- Thoracic radiographs or CT evaluation will determine metastatic involvement.
- When clinical signs suggest hypertrophic osteopathy, radiography of the long bones is required.
- Ultrasound guided needle aspirates or Tru-cut biopsy can achieve a definitive diagnosis in most cases.
- Laparotomy may be required if ultrasound is not available, guided biopsies are inconclusive, or there is a risk of hemorrhage.
- MRI or CT of the abdomen can facilitate staging and surgical planning.

Key Features – Treatment of Renal Tumors in Dogs and Cats

- Pathological diagnosis and complete staging is mandatory even in the case of bilateral disease in order to exclude lymphoma, which is amenable to systemic anticancer drug treatment (Figure 15.5) (see Chapters 9 and 10).

Table 15.5. Histological classification of renal tumors in dogs and cats

	Benign	Malignant
Epithelial	Papilloma Adenoma	Renal tubular cell carcinoma Transitional cell carcinoma Adenocarcinoma Renal cystadenoma
Mesenchymal	Hemangioma Fibroma	Lymphoma Hemangiosarcoma Histiocytic sarcoma Fibrosarcoma
Pluripotent stem cell origin		Nephroblastoma

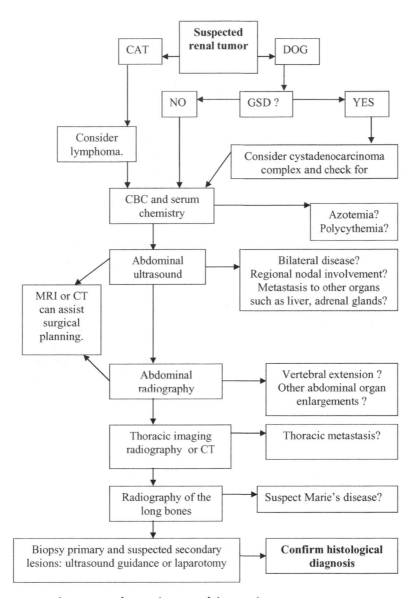

Figure 15.4.   Diagnostic decision tree for renal tumors of dogs and cats.

- Unilateral benign tumors can be cured by nephrectomy.
- **Check function of contralateral kidney by excretion urography BEFORE nephrectomy.**
- Nephrectomy for diagnostic purposes should be avoided and only performed once lymphoma or metastatic disease to the kidney has been excluded from the list of differential diagnoses.
- Assuming lymphoma has been excluded, malignant unilateral disease, in the absence of metastatic involvement, should be treated by nephrectomy.
- For bilateral disease and for the approximate 30–50% of renal tumors that will present with metastatic disease at the time of diagnosis, there is no effective treatment beyond palliative care.
- Adjuvant therapy following nephrectomy for malignant tumors has not been established.
- Nephroblastoma is often unilateral, and although tumors can become very large, they are amenable to nephrectomy if metastatic disease is not detected.

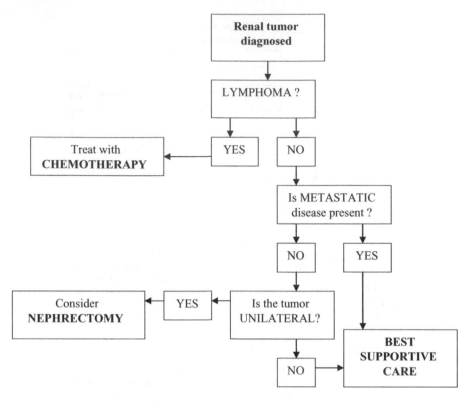

Figure 15.5. Therapeutic decision tree for renal tumors in dogs and cats.

- The dermatological consequences of renal cystadenocarcinoma complex in the GSD are often the rate-limiting factor to quality of life and survival. Skin fibromas may require debulking surgery. Renal disease is very often bilateral and nephrectomy is seldom indicated in these cases.

Prognosis – Renal Tumors in Dogs and Cats

- The majority of renal tumors are malignant, and up to 50% will have metastasized at presentation.
- However, it is important to establish a pathological diagnosis since benign tumors can be cured with nephrectomy.
- Renal lymphoma is very treatable with chemotherapy, and survival times on the order of 12 months are not uncommon. **Nephrectomy is contraindicated in renal lymphoma.**
- Malignant tumors have a range of metastatic potential. If metastasis is not detected at presentation, nephrectomy can result in survival times ranging from a few weeks to up to 4 years in dogs.
- Survival in cats is likely to be shorter than in dogs.
- Perioperative mortality is an issue for both dogs and cats.

Key Features – Treatment of Ureteric Tumors in Dogs and Cats

- Ureteric tumors are rarely reported in dogs.
- These are benign papillomas and present with unilateral hydronephrosis.
- Nephrectomy is indicated and curative.

16
TUMORS OF THE REPRODUCTIVE TRACT

David J. Argyle

Part 1:   The Female Reproductive Tract
Part 2:   Tumors of the Male Reproductive Tract

Part 1: The Female Reproductive Tract

This section will cover tumors of the ovary, uterus, vagina, and vulva.

Key Points: Ovarian Tumors
- These are uncommon tumors.
- They can be categorized as
  - **Epithelial tumors** (account for 40–50% of cases)
    - Papillary adenoma
    - Papillary adenocarcinoma
    - Cystadenoma
    - Undifferentiated carcinoma
  - **Sex cord – stromal** (35–50% of cases)
    - Thecoma
    - Luteoma
    - Granulosa cell tumor
  - **Germ cell tumors** (6–20% of cases)
    - Dysgerminoma
    - Teratocarcinoma
    - Teratoma

Ovarian Tumors

The most common of the three types are epithelial tumors and sex cord tumors (Figure 16.1).

It is rare for any of these tumors to be functional. The exception is granulosa cell tumor, which is functional in around 50% of cases.

Epithelial Tumors

- These are adenomas and adenocarcinomas.
- Carcinomas usually present with ascites after transcoleomic spread of the tumor.
- They can be bilateral.
- Carcinomas can metastasize to renal and paraaortic lymph nodes, liver, and lungs.
- Cystadenomas are thought to arise from the rete ovarii, are unilateral, and consist of multiple thin-walled cysts containing a watery fluid.
- Diagnosis is based upon history, clinical signs, diagnostic imaging, cytology of ascitic fluid, and exploratory surgery.

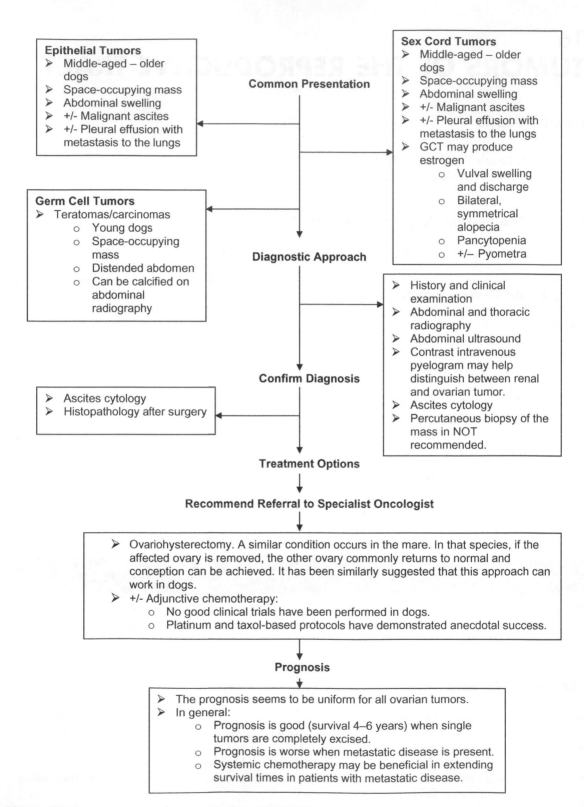

Figure 16.1. Ovarian tumors.

Sex Cord Tumors

- Granulosa cell tumor is the most common sex cord tumor.
- Around 50% of cases are considered active for the production of steroid hormones.
- In steroid (e.g., estrogen) producing tumors, the affected ovary is greatly increased in size and the other ovary atrophied.
- This is the most common ovarian tumor in the bitch and can affect any age of bitch, although more often found in the older animal. The bitch may show either signs similar to cystic ovaries or else anestrus with the time from the previous heat greatly extended.

Germ Cell Tumors

- These comprise dysgerminomas, teratomas, and teratocarcinomas.
- Dysgerminomas are usually unilateral, grow by expansion, and have a metastatic rate of around 20–30% (mainly to abdominal lymph nodes).
- Teratomas/carcinomas contain germ cells that undergo differentiation into two or more germinal layers and can contain a combination of ectoderm, mesoderm, and endoderm.

Feline Ovarian Tumors

- Epithelial, germ cell, and sex cord tumors have been reported.
- Sex cord tumors would appear to be the most common, but all are rare.
- Metastasis can occur.
- Therapy would be as for the dog. **Cisplatin cannot be used in cats.**
- Recommend referral to specialist oncologist.

Uterine Tumors

- These are leiomyoma(sarcoma) or carcinoma.
- They are very rare in the dog and cat with very few case reports in the literature.
- In cats, uterine adenocarcinoma is the most frequently reported with a well-documented metastatic potential (Figure 16.2).

Vaginal and Vulval Tumors

- These are typically benign tumors of the type leiomyoma; fibroleiomyomas, fibromas, and polyps also can occur (Figure 16.3).
- They present as a red mass protruding from vulval lips or a mass distorting the normal outline of the vagina.
- Incidence is higher in nulliparous and entire bitches.

Transmissible Venereal Tumor (TVT) (Figure 16.4)

- TVT is found in imported bitches or bitches living near ports in Britain.
- They can affect males and females.
- They are not common in the Northern states of the U.S.

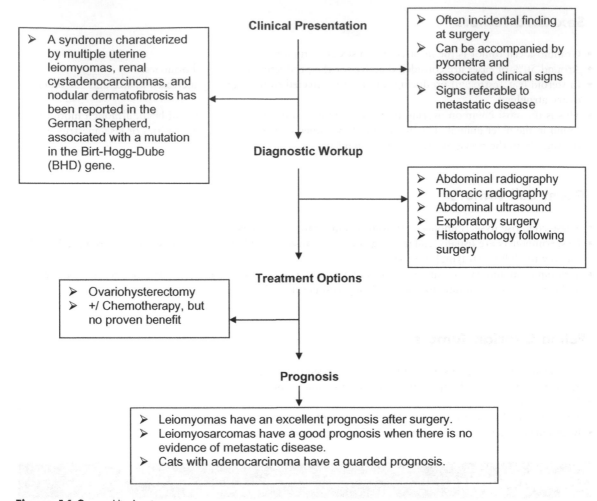

Figure 16.2.   Uterine tumors.

- They are enzootic in southern states of USA, Central and South America, certain parts of Africa, the Far East, the Middle East, and southeastern Europe.
- Route of infection is from the infected penis of the male at intromission.
- TVT is horizontally transmitted irrespective of MHC barriers, allowing transplantation of cells during coitus.

Part 2: Tumors of the Male Reproductive Tract

This section will include diseases of the prostate, testicles, penis, and prepuce.

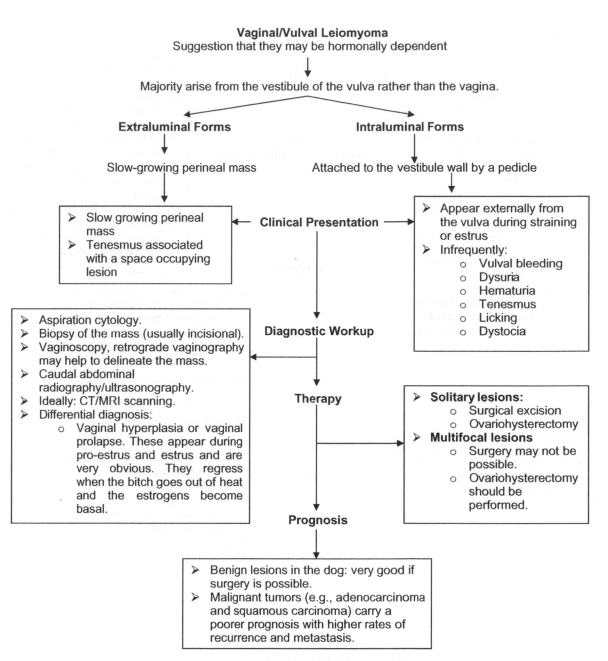

Vaginal/Vulval Leiomyoma
Suggestion that they may be hormonally dependent

Majority arise from the vestibule of the vulva rather than the vagina.

Extraluminal Forms

Slow-growing perineal mass

> - Slow growing perineal mass
> - Tenesmus associated with a space occupying lesion

Intraluminal Forms

Attached to the vestibule wall by a pedicle

> - Appear externally from the vulva during straining or estrus
> - Infrequently:
>   - Vulval bleeding
>   - Dysuria
>   - Hematuria
>   - Tenesmus
>   - Licking
>   - Dystocia

Clinical Presentation

Diagnostic Workup

> - Aspiration cytology.
> - Biopsy of the mass (usually incisional).
> - Vaginoscopy, retrograde vaginography may help to delineate the mass.
> - Caudal abdominal radiography/ultrasonography.
> - Ideally: CT/MRI scanning.
> - Differential diagnosis:
>   - Vaginal hyperplasia or vaginal prolapse. These appear during pro-estrus and estrus and are very obvious. They regress when the bitch goes out of heat and the estrogens become basal.

Therapy

> - **Solitary lesions:**
>   - Surgical excision
>   - Ovariohysterectomy
> - **Multifocal lesions**
>   - Surgery may not be possible.
>   - Ovariohysterectomy should be performed.

Prognosis

> - Benign lesions in the dog: very good if surgery is possible.
> - Malignant tumors (e.g., adenocarcinoma and squamous carcinoma) carry a poorer prognosis with higher rates of recurrence and metastasis.

Figure 16.3. Vaginal and vulval leiomyoma.

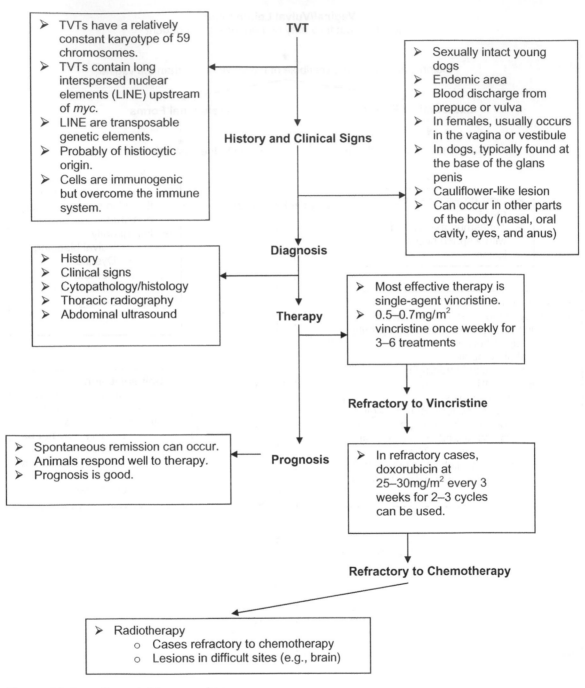

TVT

- TVTs have a relatively constant karyotype of 59 chromosomes.
- TVTs contain long interspersed nuclear elements (LINE) upstream of *myc*.
- LINE are transposable genetic elements.
- Probably of histiocytic origin.
- Cells are immunogenic but overcome the immune system.

History and Clinical Signs

- Sexually intact young dogs
- Endemic area
- Blood discharge from prepuce or vulva
- In females, usually occurs in the vagina or vestibule
- In dogs, typically found at the base of the glans penis
- Cauliflower-like lesion
- Can occur in other parts of the body (nasal, oral cavity, eyes, and anus)

Diagnosis

- History
- Clinical signs
- Cytopathology/histology
- Thoracic radiography
- Abdominal ultrasound

Therapy

- Most effective therapy is single-agent vincristine.
- $0.5-0.7 \text{mg/m}^2$ vincristine once weekly for 3–6 treatments

Refractory to Vincristine

- In refractory cases, doxorubicin at $25-30 \text{mg/m}^2$ every 3 weeks for 2–3 cycles can be used.

Prognosis

- Spontaneous remission can occur.
- Animals respond well to therapy.
- Prognosis is good.

Refractory to Chemotherapy

- Radiotherapy
  - Cases refractory to chemotherapy
  - Lesions in difficult sites (e.g., brain)

Figure 16.4. Transmissible venereal tumors.

Prostatic Carcinoma

Key Points
- Prostatic tumors are rare in the dog, compared to man where it is one of the most common cancers.
- The usual age of presentation in dogs is 9–11 years.
- In man, prostatic intraepithelial neoplasia (PIN) is recognized as a precursor lesion to overt prostatic cancer.
- PIN has been described in dogs, suggesting similar biology to that seen in man.
- Recognized histological subtypes include
  - **Epithelial Tumors**
    - Adenocarcinoma (most common)
    - Squamous cell carcinoma
    - Transitional cell carcinoma
  - **Mesenchymal Tumors** (rarely)
    - Hemangiosarcoma
    - Leiomyosarcoma
- The role of castration in the etiology remains controversial. Recent epidemiological studies have suggested that castration provides an increased risk of prostatic carcinoma.
- Most carcinomas arise from the ductal epithelium, which lacks androgen receptors. This suggests that androgens do not play a part in disease initiation or progression. However, larger studies are required to completely elucidate whether androgens play a role in this disease.

Clinical Features of Prostatic Tumors (Figure 16.5–16.7)

- A reflection of
  - Local invasion and expansion
  - Metastatic spread

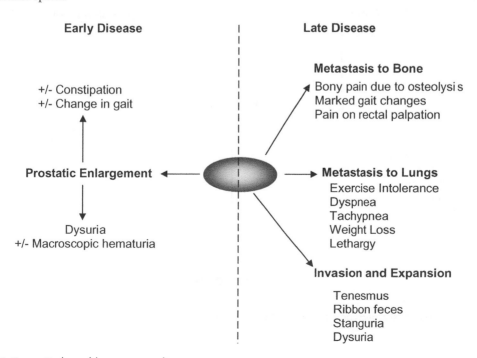

Early Disease

+/- Constipation
+/- Change in gait

Prostatic Enlargement

Dysuria
+/- Macroscopic hematuria

Late Disease

Metastasis to Bone
Bony pain due to osteolysis
Marked gait changes
Pain on rectal palpation

Metastasis to Lungs
Exercise Intolerance
Dyspnea
Tachypnea
Weight Loss
Lethargy

Invasion and Expansion

Tenesmus
Ribbon feces
Stanguria
Dysuria

Figure 16.5.   Early and late prostate disease.

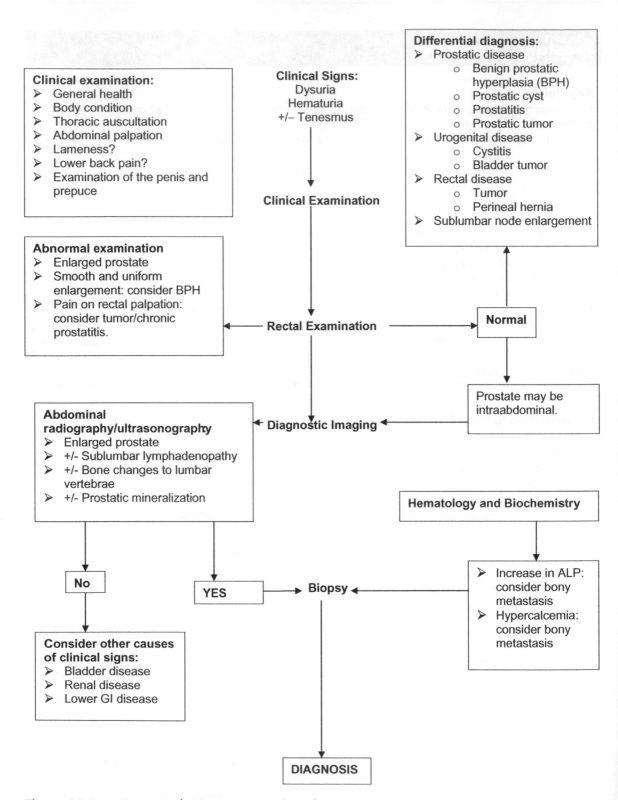

Figure 16.6.   Diagnostic decision tree – prostatic carcinoma.

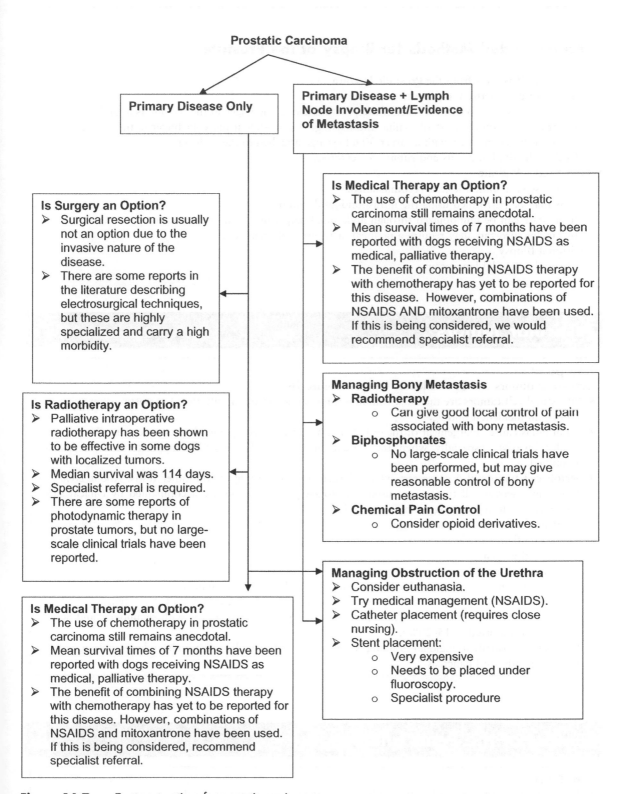

Prostatic Carcinoma

Primary Disease Only

Primary Disease + Lymph Node Involvement/Evidence of Metastasis

Is Surgery an Option?
➤ Surgical resection is usually not an option due to the invasive nature of the disease.
➤ There are some reports in the literature describing electrosurgical techniques, but these are highly specialized and carry a high morbidity.

Is Radiotherapy an Option?
➤ Palliative intraoperative radiotherapy has been shown to be effective in some dogs with localized tumors.
➤ Median survival was 114 days.
➤ Specialist referral is required.
➤ There are some reports of photodynamic therapy in prostate tumors, but no large-scale clinical trials have been reported.

Is Medical Therapy an Option?
➤ The use of chemotherapy in prostatic carcinoma still remains anecdotal.
➤ Mean survival times of 7 months have been reported with dogs receiving NSAIDS as medical, palliative therapy.
➤ The benefit of combining NSAIDS therapy with chemotherapy has yet to be reported for this disease. However, combinations of NSAIDS and mitoxantrone have been used. If this is being considered, recommend specialist referral.

Is Medical Therapy an Option?
➤ The use of chemotherapy in prostatic carcinoma still remains anecdotal.
➤ Mean survival times of 7 months have been reported with dogs receiving NSAIDS as medical, palliative therapy.
➤ The benefit of combining NSAIDS therapy with chemotherapy has yet to be reported for this disease. However, combinations of NSAIDS AND mitoxantrone have been used. If this is being considered, we would recommend specialist referral.

Managing Bony Metastasis
➤ **Radiotherapy**
  o Can give good local control of pain associated with bony metastasis.
➤ **Biphosphonates**
  o No large-scale clinical trials have been performed, but may give reasonable control of bony metastasis.
➤ **Chemical Pain Control**
  o Consider opioid derivatives.

Managing Obstruction of the Urethra
➤ Consider euthanasia.
➤ Try medical management (NSAIDS).
➤ Catheter placement (requires close nursing).
➤ Stent placement:
  o Very expensive
  o Needs to be placed under fluoroscopy.
  o Specialist procedure

Figure 16.7.　Treatment options for prostatic carcinoma.

Recommended Methods for Biopsy of the Prostate

- Cytological Washings from the Prostatic Urethra
  - Sedate or anesthetize the patient.
  - Insert urinary catheter to the level of the prostate (using one finger in the rectum as a guide).
  - Insert a small volume of sterile saline and massage the prostate using your finger in the rectum.
  - Apply negative pressure with a larger 30 ml syringe attached to the catheter.
  - Collect the fluid and cells and submit for cytology.
- Fine Needle Aspirate
  - Heavy sedation/anesthesia is recommended.
  - This may be performed using the ultrasound-guided approach.
  - If prostate can be immobilized through abdominal palpation, it can be performed percutaneous.
  - Intrapelvic prostate may require a perineal or transrectal approach.
- Incisional Biopsy
  - Through a caudal laparotomy

Testicular Tumors

Key point
Testicular tumors can be divided as follows (Figure 16.8):
- **Interstitial cell tumors** are the most common tumors and are often only found at postmortem examination as an incidental finding.
- **Seminomas** cause enlargement of the testicle but are rarely accompanied by systemic signs. They can be locally invasive, especially when they occur in abdominal testes. The opposite testis is usually atrophied.
- **Sertoli cell tumors** also cause testicular enlargement and atrophy of the other testis. About 20% are malignant. Sertoli cell tumors are usually estrogen producers and are accompanied by clinical signs associated with hyperestrogenism. These include
  - Attractiveness to other male dogs
  - Bilateral flank hair loss
  - Preputial edema
  - Gynecomastia
- Cryptorchidism is a risk factor for both seminomas and Sertoli cell tumors.
- Boxers, German Shepherds, and Weimeraners appear to be at increased risk of development.
- All tumor types have a low metastatic potential. The greatest potential is with seminomas and Sertoli cell tumors (reported at 15–20%).
- Metastasis is usually to regional draining lymph nodes and then ultimately to liver, lungs, spleen, kidney, adrenal glands, and pancreas.

Tumors of the Penis and Prepuce

Key Points
- The epithelial surfaces can be affected by any of the tumors found in the skin section.
- Surgery would be the treatment of choice (resection, scrotal ablation, and urethethrostomy).
- The most common tumor is the TVT (see above).

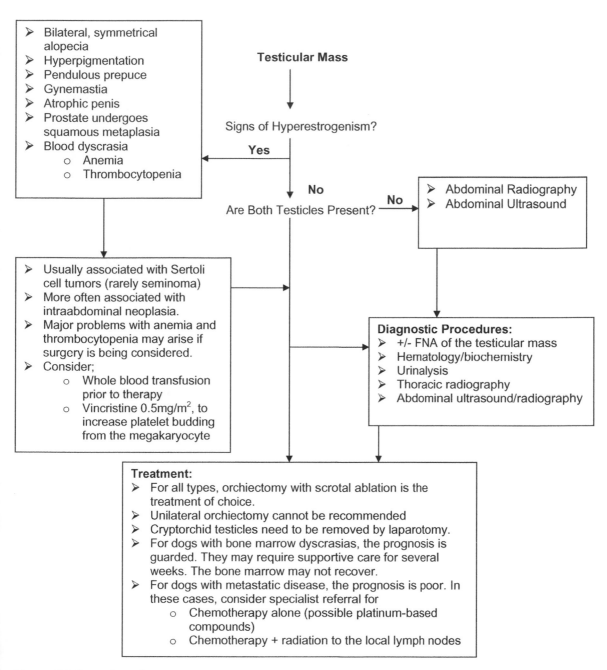

Testicular Mass

Signs of Hyperestrogenism?

Yes →
> - Bilateral, symmetrical alopecia
> - Hyperpigmentation
> - Pendulous prepuce
> - Gynemastia
> - Atrophic penis
> - Prostate undergoes squamous metaplasia
> - Blood dyscrasia
>   - Anemia
>   - Thrombocytopenia

→
> - Usually associated with Sertoli cell tumors (rarely seminoma)
> - More often associated with intraabdominal neoplasia.
> - Major problems with anemia and thrombocytopenia may arise if surgery is being considered.
> - Consider;
>   - Whole blood transfusion prior to therapy
>   - Vincristine 0.5mg/m^2, to increase platelet budding from the megakaryocyte

No

Are Both Testicles Present? — **No** →
> - Abdominal Radiography
> - Abdominal Ultrasound

Diagnostic Procedures:
> - +/- FNA of the testicular mass
> - Hematology/biochemistry
> - Urinalysis
> - Thoracic radiography
> - Abdominal ultrasound/radiography

Treatment:
> - For all types, orchiectomy with scrotal ablation is the treatment of choice.
> - Unilateral orchiectomy cannot be recommended
> - Cryptorchid testicles need to be removed by laparotomy.
> - For dogs with bone marrow dyscrasias, the prognosis is guarded. They may require supportive care for several weeks. The bone marrow may not recover.
> - For dogs with metastatic disease, the prognosis is poor. In these cases, consider specialist referral for
>   - Chemotherapy alone (possible platinum-based compounds)
>   - Chemotherapy + radiation to the local lymph nodes

Figure 16.8.   Testicular tumors.

325

17
CANINE AND FELINE MAMMARY TUMORS

David J. Argyle, Michelle M. Turek, and Valerie MacDonald

This chapter describes the main clinical and pathological features of mammary tumors in dogs and cats.

Canine Mammary Gland Tumors (MGT)

Key Points
- Mammary tumors are the most common neoplasms in intact female dogs; 2/1000 female dogs are at risk.
- Malignant neoplasms represent 50% of all mammary tumors diagnosed (Figure 17.1).
- These tumors affect older dogs (median age: 10–11 years; rare in dogs <5 years).
- Mammary gland tumors are hormonally dependent. Ovariohysterectomy can greatly decrease the risk of developing mammary gland tumors. Dogs spayed before their first estrus have a risk of 0.5%; after their first estrus the risk jumps to 8%, and after their second estrus the risk goes to 26%.
- Estrogen and progesterone receptors have been identified in mammary gland tumors, with up to 50% of malignant tumors and up to 70% of benign tumors expressing receptors.
- Obesity may play a role in canine MGT, as it does with human MGT. In spayed dogs, the incidence of MGT is reduced if dogs are thin (rather than obese) at 9 to 12 months of age.
- Tumors may affect any breed but poodles, English and Brittany spaniels, English setters, pointers, fox terriers, Boston Terriers, and cocker spaniels are overrepresented.
- These are rare in male dogs, but they are reported.
- 50:50 rule: 50% of mammary masses are benign, and 50% are malignant.
- Of the 50% that are malignant, 50% will recur or metastasize following the first surgical resection.
- While epithelial malignancies are most common, multiple histologic types occur.
- Inflammatory carcinomas are red, warm, and edematous and they grow and metastasize **VERY** rapidly.
- The grading scheme for MGT crosses conventional borders and includes distant disease as part of the criteria for a high-grade tumor (Tables 17.1, 17.2).
- After inflammatory carcinomas, sarcomas have a worse prognosis than other carcinomas.

Treatment of Canine MGT

- **Surgery is the treatment of choice** for almost all MGTs unless impossible to remove (Figure 17.3, Table 17.3).
- The goal of surgery is to remove the entire tumor, including microscopic disease, by the simplest procedure.
- Surgical procedures:
  - **Nodulectomy.** This is the simple removal of a small nodule from a mammary gland. It is suggested that this should be undertaken for firm masses smaller than 0.5 cm. It is difficult to justify this type of approach

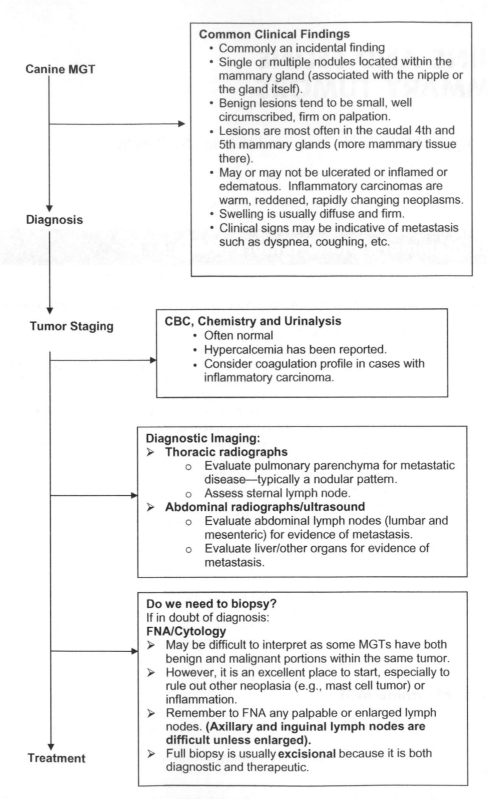

Figure 17.1. Diagnostic decision tree in canine MGT.

Table 17.1. Classification of canine and feline mammary tumors

Malignant Tumors	Benign Tumors
Noninfiltrating (in situ) carcinoma	Simple adenoma
Complex carcinoma	Complex adenoma
Simple carcinoma (Figure 17.2)	Basaloid adenoma
Tubulopapillary carcinoma	Fibroadenoma
Solid carcinoma	Benign mixed tumor
Cribriform carcinoma	Duct papilloma
Anaplastic carcinoma	
Special types of carcinoma	
Spindle cell carcinoma	
Squamous cell carcinoma	
Mucinous carcinoma	
Lipid-rich carcinoma	
Sarcomas	
Fibrosarcoma	
Osteosarcoma	
Carcinosarcoma	
Carcinoma or sarcomas in benign tumor	

Table 17.2. Staging for canine mammary tumors

Stage	T	N	M
I	T_1	N_0	M_0
II	T_2	N_0	M_0
III	T_3	N_0	M_0
IV	Any T	N_1	M_0
V	Any T	Any N	M_1

T = Primary tumor.
T_1 = <3 cm maximum diameter.
T_2 = 3–5 cm maximum diameter.
T_3 = >5 cm maximum diameter.
N = Regional lymph node.
N_0 = No metastasis (histology or cytology).
N_1 = Metastasis present (histology or cytology).
M = Distant metastasis.
M_0 = No distant metastasis.
M_1 = Distant metastasis.

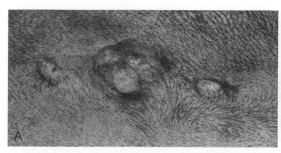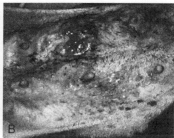

Figure 17.2. Clinical presentation of simple (A) and inflammatory anaplastic (B) canine mammary carcinoma.

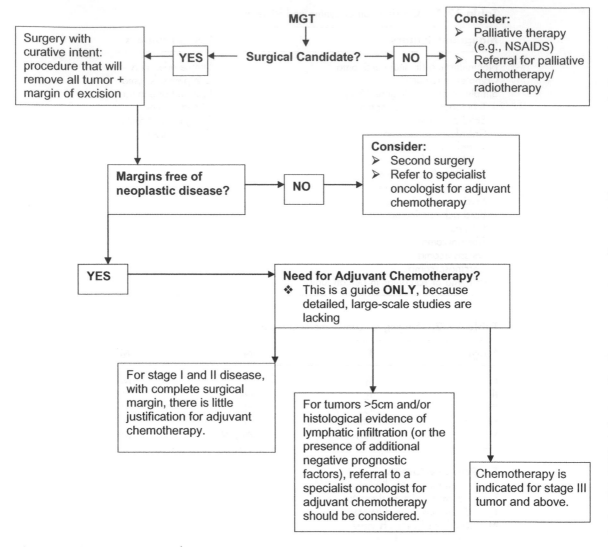

Figure 17.3. MGT treatment decision tree.

Table 17.3. Prognosis factors in canine MGT

Factors Associated with a Good Prognosis	Factors Associated with a Poor Prognosis
Size: <3 cm	Size: >3 cm
Well-circumscribed tumors	Invasive tumors
Stage of disease: no evidence of metastasis	Stage of disease: evidence of metastasis
Well-differentiated tubular/papillary carcinomas (lower grade)	Anaplastic carcinomas (higher grade)
No evidence of vascular or lymphatic invasion on biopsy	Estrogen receptor negative
Estrogen receptor/progesterone receptor positive	Histologic type: inflammatory carcinoma or sarcoma
Sex: it appears that male dogs have a higher incidence of benign tumors; hence, prognosis associated with mammary masses in male dogs is generally favorable.	Ulceration
	Evidence of vascular or lymphatic invasion on biopsy

due to the limitation of the surgical procedure in achieving appropriate surgical margins. Consider this as a biopsy procedure only.

- **Mammectomy.** This is the removal of a single gland from the chain.
- **Partial mastectomy or regional mastectomy.** This is the removal of >1 gland in one region of the mammary chain.
- **Unilateral radical mastectomy.** This is the removal of the entire chain on one side of the bitch. The elimination of the entire chain is indicated where there are multiple tumors in most if not all the glands. Technically this is a simple surgical procedure that removes all the affected tissue in one incision rather than attempting several mammectomies.
- **Bilateral radical mastectomy.** This is the removal of both the left and right mammary chains where there are multiple masses in both in the chains. A simultaneous bilateral procedure is not recommended due to the difficulty in closing the wound appropriately. There are techniques to leave tissue at the cranial end of the incision over the sternum to provide supportive tissue. If this type of procedure is advised it is recommended that the most important side is dealt with first and the other side completed in 3 to 4 weeks.

Key Points in Surgical Excision

- The use of radical versus conservative excision has been debated, with little differences in recurrence rates and survival times. Consequently, the current advice is when choosing a surgical procedure, **the main goal of surgery is to remove all tumor using the simplest procedure possible (and gaining a complete surgical excision).**
- Where there is involvement of the underlying fascia and muscle, this must be removed at the time of the surgery whatever technique is employed. A radical unilateral mastectomy is, however, advised in such circumstances.
- **Removal of lymph nodes:** The superficial inguinal lymph node is always removed with gland 5 since it lies nearly within the substance of the fat associated with the gland, but the axillary node is removed only if it is enlarged or there is cytological evidence that there are metastases present.
- Concurrent **ovariohysterectomy (OHE)** at the time of mammary surgery is controversial. However:
  - Spaying removes the possibility of pyometra, uterine or ovarian tumors and unwanted pregnancies.
  - Because up to 50% of malignant MGTs express estrogen or progesterone receptors, spaying has theoretical therapeutic benefit. However, clinical studies have shown **NO** anticancer benefit with OHE once the tumors have developed.
  - If OHE is to be performed, do it BEFORE tumor removal to prevent seeding of the abdomen with the tumor.

Key Points: The Role of Chemotherapy

- This has not been thoroughly investigated in dogs with MGT.
- With tumor types in which metastases or recurrence is likely (see prognostic factors below), adjuvant therapy is recommended.
- Protocols are extrapolated from human medicine.
- Chemotherapy options include
  - Single-agent doxorubicin (25–30 mg/m^2 every 14–21 days for 4–5 cycles)
  - Combined doxorubicin/cyclophosphamide
  - Single-agent carboplatin (300 mg/m^2 every 21 days for 4–5 cycles)
  - Taxol derivatives (specialist referral only)
- Piroxicam may be of some benefit in the palliative setting, but no large-scale studies have been performed.
- Providing accurate survival estimates is not possible.
- The use of hormonal therapy (e.g., antiestrogen drugs) has no proven benefit.

Key Point: Factors NOT Associated with a Prognosis
- Age
- Breed
- OHE status
- Weight
- Type of surgery
- Number of tumors
- Glands involved
- History of pregnancy

Feline Mammary Tumors

Key Points
- These are the third most common tumor, accounting for 17% of all neoplasms in female cats.
- Tumors occur in cats with a mean age of 10 to 12 years, range of 9 months to 23 years.
- Siamese cats are at risk, but any breed can develop MGTs.
- Hormonal influence is likely.
  - Intact cats are more likely to develop mammary tumors.
  - Cats spayed at <6 months of age have a 91% reduction in risk of development of MGTs.
  - Cats spayed at <12 months of age have an 86% reduction in risk.
  - Parity does not seem to affect MGT development,
  - There is a strong association between the use of progesterone-like drugs and the development of benign or malignant mammary masses in cats.
  - Few (<10%) MGT are estrogen receptor positive.
- Tumors are rare in male cats; however, they are more common as compared to male dogs.

Classification and Biological Behavior

- 80:20 rule: 80% of mammary masses are malignant and 20% are benign (some studies suggest that 90:10 is a more appropriate ratio of malignant to benign) (Tables 17.4, 17.5).
- Most are commonly classified as adenocarcinomas (tubular, papillary, and solid), and most have regions of different differentiation (i.e., mixed tumors).
- Disease-free and overall survival depend on size of tumor at time of diagnosis (<2 cm is good), histologic grade (degree of differentiation), and extent of surgical resection.

Common Clinical Findings

- Tumors are often advanced at the time of diagnosis.
- Tumors may adhere to overlying skin but rarely adhere to underlying abdominal wall.
- Tumors are usually firm and nodular.
- Tumors may be ulcerated, be associated with discharge from the nipple, or involve multiple glands.
- Acute respiratory distress secondary to malignant pleural effusion is also possible.

Table 17.4.   Minimum diagnostic database and tumor staging for feline MGT

Diagnostic Test	Justification
CBC/chemistry and urinalysis	Investigate any concurrent disease. Results are often normal.
Thoracic radiography	Evaluate pulmonary parenchyma for metastatic disease. Cats can develop pleural effusion or interstitial changes rather than the typical nodular metastatic lesions. Assess sternal lymph node.
Abdominal imaging	Evaluate abdominal lymph nodes (lumbar and mesenteric) for evidence of metastasis. Evaluate liver/other organs for evidence of metastasis.
FNA/cytology	MGT may be difficult to interpret because some MGTs have both benign and malignant portions within the same tumor. This is an excellent way to rule out other neoplasia (e.g., mast cell tumor) or inflammation.
Biopsy	Excision is preferred because it is both diagnostic and therapeutic.

Table 17.5.   Staging for feline MGT

Stage	T	N	M
I	T_1	N_0	M_0
II	T_2	N_0	M_0
III	$T_{1,2}$	N_1	M_0
	T_3	$N_{0,1}$	M_0
IV	Any T	Any N	M_1

T = Primary tumor.
T_1 = <2 cm maximum diameter.
T_2 = 2–3 cm maximum diameter.
T_3 = >3 cm maximum diameter.
N = Regional lymph node.
N_0 = No lymph node metastasis (histology or cytology).
N_1 = Lymph node metastasis present (histology or cytology).
M = Distant metastasis.
M_0 = No distant metastasis.
M_1 = Distant metastasis.

- Do not confuse with **benign fibroepithelial hyperplasia:**
  - In young cats after a silent estrus, or continuously calling.
  - It has been associated with chronic progestin therapy.
  - One or more glands are involved.
  - Ovariohysterectomy is the treatment of choice, but resolution may take several months.

Surgery

- This is the TREATMENT OF CHOICE for almost all MGTs unless impossible to remove (Figure 17.4).
- Radical mastectomy with lymph node excision is recommended. Some oncologists will recommend bilateral radical mastectomy. In this case, staged mastectomies are ideal.

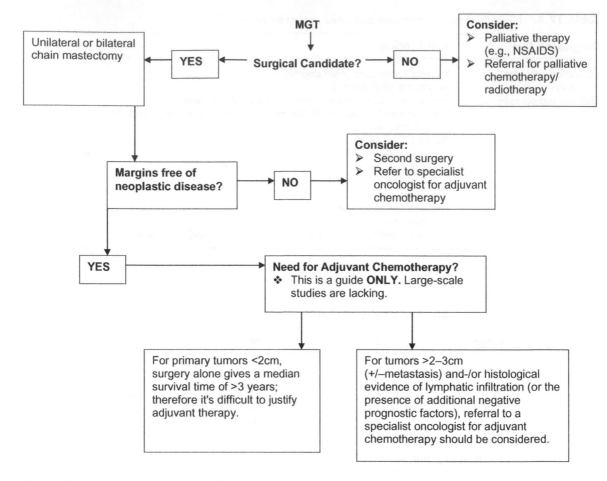

Figure 17.4. Feline MGT treatment decision tree.

Radiation Therapy

- There is a lack of clinical information regarding efficacy of radiotherapy for feline MGT.

Chemotherapy

- Generally recommended, although effectiveness varies from study to study.
- Doxorubicin/cyclophosphamide therapy has been described, although the efficacy of each drug as a single agent is largely unknown due to the lack of large-scale clinical trials.
- Doxorubicin given at 1 mg/kg IV for 5 cycles has demonstrated benefit in some cats, but large studies are required to confirm efficacy.
- Where cats have compromised renal function, mitoxantrone can be used as an alternative to doxorubicin.

Prognosis

- Average survival is 10 to 12 months.
- Prognosis in male cats is similar to prognosis in female cats.
- Tumor size is the most important prognostic factor.
  - For tumors <2 cm, MST is >3 years.
  - For tumors 2–3 cm, MST is ~2 years.
  - For tumors >3 cm, MST is 4–6 months.
- Other prognostic factors include
  - Histologic type and grade (degree of differentiation, number of mitoses, and amount of necrosis)
  - Old age associated with unfavorable prognosis
  - Stage of disease (cats presenting with distant metastasis rarely survive >2 months)
  - Evidence of vascular/lymphatic invasion associated with worse prognosis
  - Extent of surgical resection:
    - 2/3 of MGTs will recur following conservative surgery.
    - Cats undergoing uni- or bilateral mastectomies have a longer disease-free interval but the same survival time as cats undergoing simpler surgical procedures.
    - Even with aggressive surgery, metastatic disease is still a concern.

18
TUMORS OF THE MUSCULOSKELETAL SYSTEM

Malcolm J. Brearley and Alison Hayes

This section describes the main clinical and pathological features of musculoskeletal system tumors in dogs and cats. It includes bone tumors and tumors of the noncutaneous, soft tissues such as connective tissues and muscles.

Key Points
- Primary tumors of the musculoskeletal system originate from mesenchymal cells and comprise tumors of bone and soft tissues such as muscle, joints, and other associated connective tissue structures.
- The musculoskeletal system can be affected by a large number of secondary tumors, which metastasize to the bone or soft tissues or involve these structures by local extension.
- The presenting signs differ according to the species, tumor location, and biological behavior of the tumor.
- Although primary bone tumors and tumors of the soft tissues are largely malignant, their metastatic potential is variable among tumor types.
- Previous trauma, radiotherapy, or implants may be associated with primary malignant bone tumor development.
- Careful staging and diagnostic histopathology is required, sometimes alongside immunohistochemistry, in order to accurately diagnose the disease, offer predictive information, and formulate a treatment plan.
- There are certain species and breed associations in the development of some tumor types in this group.
- There are certain predilection sites for the development of some tumors in this group.
- Large- and giant-breed dogs are predisposed to the development of malignant bone tumors.
- Bernese Mountain dogs, retriever breeds, and Rottweilers are overrepresented in the breeds developing histiocytic sarcomas.
- In cats, an aggressive form of soft-tissue sarcoma is recognized, which appears to develop at the site of injection or trauma (FISS, feline injection-site sarcoma – formerly VAFS, vaccine associated feline sarcoma).
- Histiocytic diseases and FISS are covered in Chapters 8 and 6, respectively.

Bone Tumors

Key Points – Bone Tumors in Dogs
- Primary bone tumors can arise in the axial and appendicular skeleton.
- Appendicular tumors are more commonly encountered than axial tumors.
- Osteosarcoma is the most common tumor of both the axial and appendicular skeleton and is highly malignant, although metastatic rates are regarded as lower in axial cases.

- Regardless of site, primary tumor excision and adjuvant chemotherapy is required for all cases of canine osteosarcoma.
- Other tumor types are far less common and include other malignant tumors and a range of benign tumors.
- Appendicular osteosarcomas affect middle-aged to older large- and giant-breeds most commonly.
- Predilection sites are the metaphyseal areas of the distal femur, proximal tibia, proximal humerus, and distal radius. The forelimb is more commonly involved compared to the hindlimb.
- Secondary bone tumors affecting the appendicular skeleton tend to be located in the diaphyseal regions.
- Axial osteosarcoma can arise in the cranial bones, mandible, spine, pelvis, and ribs.
- Tumors occur in middle-aged to older dogs of any breed.
- Tumors of the rib tend to affect younger animals.
- Locoregional spread of tumors arising outside bone is common in the mandible and maxilla.

Key Points – Bone Tumors in Cats

- Primary bone tumors are less common in cats than dogs.
- Tumors arise in the axial and appendicular skeleton in approximately equal numbers.
- Osteosarcoma is the most common tumor of both the axial and appendicular skeleton.
- Osteosarcomas, regardless of site, are considered to be less malignant in cats compared to dogs.
- Regardless of site, primary tumor excision is indicated.
- Adjuvant chemotherapy is rarely recommended for cats.
- Other tumor types are far less common, and include other malignant tumors and a range of benign tumors.
- Appendicular osteosarcomas affect middle-aged to older cats without breed association.
- Predilection sites are the metaphyseal areas of the distal femur, proximal tibia, and proximal humerus. The hindlimb is more commonly involved compared to the forelimb.
- Secondary bone tumors affecting the appendicular skeleton may be recognized.
- Axial osteosarcoma can arise in the cranial bones, mandible, spine, pelvis, and ribs.
- Locoregional spread of tumors arising outside bone is common in the mandible and maxilla, especially with oral squamous cell carcinoma.

Clinical Features Associated with Bone Tumors in Dogs and Cats

- Appendicular bone tumors often present with pain and lameness.
- Dogs may present with acute, non–weight-bearing lameness or have a more insidious lameness that does not respond to simple analgesic regimens commonly used for suspected trauma or osteoarthritis over a 1–3 month period.
- Cats may present with a more chronic, lower grade of discomfort, which may have been present for several months.
- Either species may suddenly decompensate and develop a non–weight-bearing lameness following pathological fracture.
- Localized swelling at the site of the tumor may be detectable, although this may be absent or overlooked with early lesions or in heavily muscled areas such as the proximal forelimb.

Investigation of Suspected Bone Tumor in Dogs and Cats

- Radiography is indicated when a dog or cat presents with an acute lameness, and although a primary bone tumor may not be suspected, many cases will be diagnosed in the search for a traumatic lesion.
- Cats with unresponsive, chronic low-grade lameness or large and giant canine breeds with sudden onset lameness should be investigated promptly with a view to excluding a primary bone tumor.
- Any cat or dog presenting with an obvious bony swelling, with or without pain, should undergo diagnostic radiography.
- Radiographically, bone tumors are often mixed (lytic and proliferative), although one type may predominate. The zone of transition to normal bone, the degree of cortical disruption, and periosteal reaction are taken into account when deciding whether the lesion has an aggressive appearance or not.
- Primary bone tumors do not cross to both sides of a joint.
- Complete staging should be undertaken and will include the following (Tables 18.1, 18.2):
  - A thoracic study (radiographic or CT) to determine metastatic involvement.
  - An abdominal ultrasound examination, particularly with primary disease caudal to the diaphragm to detect locoregional lymph node involvement and distant metastasis to parenchymal organs
  - Needle aspirate cytology or regional lymph nodes, where accessible
  - Needle aspirate cytology of any cutaneous masses
- Scintigraphy to search for other occult bony secondary tumors can be helpful in certain cases.
- When metastatic disease has been excluded, needle aspirate cytology can be utilized successfully in the diagnosis of primary and secondary bone tumors (Figures 18.1–18.4). This will reduce the trauma of an incisional biopsy and accelerate the diagnostic processes by avoiding the requirement for decalcification. Ultrasound guidance is desirable to locate a bony window, although radiography can be used in a similar way.
- When this is not possible, a core biopsy using a Jamshidi-style instrument or bone marrow core biopsy punch is performed. Samples should be taken from the center and margins of the lesion, in tangential planes, taking into consideration any later limb salvage surgery that may be attempted.
- It is important to exclude bacterial, fungal, and secondary neoplasia prior to excisional surgery. This may be achievable on radiography alone, particularly in areas that do not encounter fungal diseases of bone.
- A definitive diagnosis of exact tumor type may not be obtainable on these small samples, and should not be expected. However, if primary neoplasia is suspected based on these preliminary findings, and lymphoma is excluded, the whole lesion should be submitted for confirmation of diagnosis once surgical excision is performed.
- CT or MRI of the primary tumor type may assist with surgical planning if lesions are large and/or affect the proximal limb.

Table 18.1.   Clinical staging (TNM) of bone tumors in dogs

Primary Tumor	
T1	Tumor remains within the medulla or cortex
T2	Tumor extends beyond the periosteum
Regional Lymph Node	
N0	No metastasis
N1	Regional nodal involvement
Distant Metastasis	
M0	No metastasis
M1	Metastasis

Table 18.2. Histological classification of bone tumors in dogs and cats

Dogs	Malignant	Cats
•	Osteosarcoma	•
•	Parosteal osteosarcoma*	•
•	Chondrosarcoma	•
•	Fibrosarcoma	•
•	Plasma cell tumors	•
•	Hemangiosarcoma	•
•	Multilobular tumor of bone**	
	Benign	
•	Osteoma	•
	Osteochondroma	•
•	Osteochondromatosis	•
	Bone cysts	•

*Synonyms include periosteal osteosarcoma, juxtacortical osteosarcoma, surface osteosarcoma, extraossous osteosarcoma.
**Synonyms include chondroma rodens, multilobular osteochondrosarcoma, multilobular osteoma, multilobular osteosarcoma, multilobular chondrosarcoma.

Key Points – Treatment of Bone Tumors in Dogs and Cats

- For primary malignant bone tumors, surgery to remove the primary tumor is the goal of therapy once lymphoma has been excluded.
- Lymphoma and plasma cell tumors can be treated with chemotherapy. Radiation therapy can be used in solitary cases with curative intent.
- When secondary disease is detected, definitive therapy to excise the primary tumor is rarely warranted. Palliative options should be considered.
- Analgesia can be difficult to achieve for malignant bone tumors.
- Radiotherapy can be used to boost analgesia, but care is needed to prevent pathological fracture following radiation therapy.
- Adjuvant chemotherapy is indicated in dogs with osteosarcoma.
- A variety of limb salvage procedures may be achievable in specialist settings. However, the complication rates can be high and adjuvant chemotherapy is still required for canine osteosarcoma. These procedures are not detailed here.
- Extended survival period can be achieved but the likelihood of a cure is remote with canine osteosarcoma.
- Benign bone tumors, chondrosarcoma, and osteosarcoma in cats carry a better prognosis, and long-term survival and cure may be achievable.
- Treatment may be warranted in the face of metastatic disease in order to control clinical signs associated with the primary tumor (Figure 18.5).

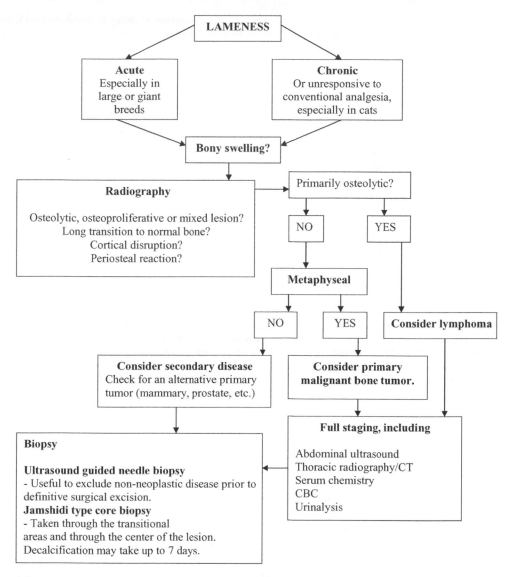

Figure 18.1. Diagnostic decision tree for bone tumors of dogs and cats.

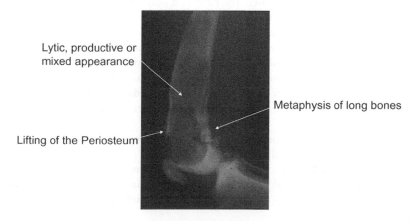

Figure 18.2. Radiograph of an osteosarcoma of the femur.

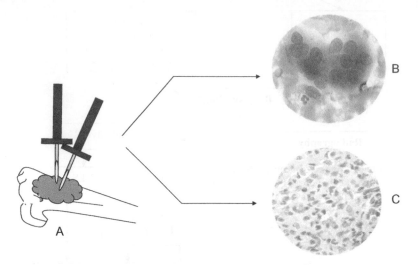

Figure 18.3. Biopsy of primary bone tumors. In some cases where the tumor is soft enough, it is possible to gain a fine needle aspirate showing evidence of mesenchymal neoplasia (B). In most cases a core biopsy is retrieved using a Jamshidi needle (A). To maximize the possibility of gaining a good quality sample, the core is taken from the center of the lesion (as measured on a radiograph). Multiple cores are taken to improve yield. The core samples can be used to make a cytological roll preparation (B) and then submitted in formalin for histopathology (C).

Treatment – Surgery

- Amputation or extensive surgery to remove a primary tumor is not indicated in the face of metastatic disease.
- Before treatment commences, histological confirmation of malignancy is desirable.
- Amputation is the mainstay of treatment for primary malignant bone tumors of the appendicular skeleton in dogs and cats.
- Chemotherapy should be discussed ahead of surgery and implemented once a definitive diagnosis is confirmed.
- In certain circumstances, e.g., when the animal has not originated or traveled through an area where fungal disease is endemic diagnosis, and where the pain of a suspected primary malignant bone tumor of the appendicular skeleton cannot be controlled by other means, then amputation without prior confirmation by biopsy may be acceptable.
- Limb salvage procedures may be considered in cases where amputation is contraindicated due to other orthopedic or neurological problems. Only selected centers have this level of surgical expertise, and a bone banking facility is often required for limb tumors. Exceptions to this include partial scapulectomy and distal radial tumors where an allograft is not required. Specialist advice should be sought to explore limb preservation techniques. Recovery can be prolonged and complication rates are high even in experienced hands.
- Primary bone tumors of the axial skeleton are rarely amenable to surgery, with the exception of tumors involving the mandible and certain maxillary tumors.
- Benign tumors of the appendicular and axial skeleton may be amenable to surgery with curative intent.
- Often the definitive diagnosis is achieved only after the entire primary tumor has been excised. The provisional diagnosis obtained on preoperative bone assessments should always be confirmed with submission of the whole lesion.

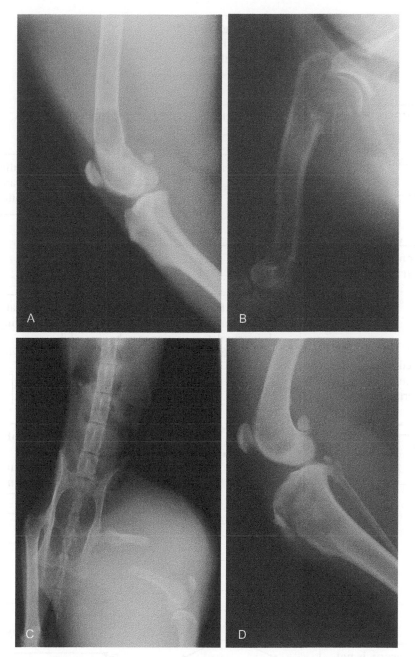

Figure 18.4. Lytic osteogenic osteosarcoma of the distil femur (A), metastatic lesion in the proximal humerus of a small breed dog (B), large soft tissue sarcoma of the hindlimb causing pathological fracture of the femur (C), and lytic bone tumor of the proximal tibia causing pathological fracture (D).

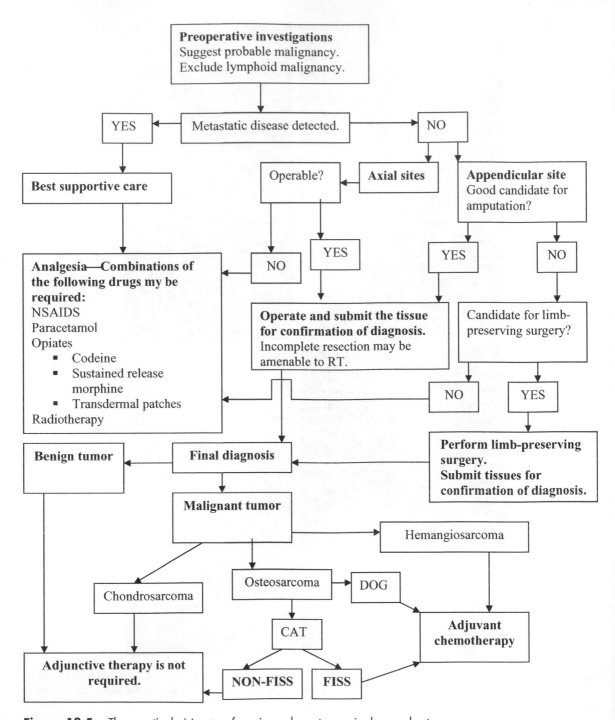

Figure 18.5. Therapeutic decision tree for primary bone tumors in dogs and cats.

Treatment – Chemotherapy

- Before treatment commences, histological confirmation of diagnosis is required.
- Chemotherapy is most often used in combination with surgery for appendicular osteosarcoma, and has been shown to significantly improve survival over cases treated by surgery alone (Table 18.3). For axial tumors (with only 20% metastatic rate), the value of adjuvant chemotherapy is yet to be proven.
- Chemotherapy is relatively well described and established in dogs with osteosarcoma, but not in cats.
- Treatment is usually instituted between 14 and 21 days postsurgery.
- Chemotherapy in the face of macroscopic metastatic disease will not improve survival outcome and is contraindicated.
- Adjuvant treatment with single-agent platinum drugs (cisplatin and carboplatin) or doxorubicin results in similar survival advantages over surgery alone.
- **Carboplatin** given at 300 mg/m^2 IV every 21 days for 4 cycles results in a median survival of approximately 10.5 months with a 1-year survival of 35%. This can be given without premedication or fluid therapy on an outpatient basis and for this reason is the drug of choice for many veterinary oncologists.
- **Cisplatin** given at 60 mg/m^2 IV every 21 days for 4 cycles results in a median survival of 10.5 months with a 1-year survival of 46%. This regimen requires concomitant saline diuresis starting before and after drug administration plus a rigorous antiemetics regimen. This results in patient therapy often necessitating overnight hospitalization.
- Doxorubicin is associated with an irreversible, cumulate, and dose-related myocardial toxicity. Care is required when using doxorubicin in the large and giant breed predisposed to developing osteosarcoma because these breeds may also have a preexisting cardiac disease, e.g., the Doberman, Irish wolfhound, and Great Dane.
- Various combination drug therapies have been attempted. Survival advantages over surgery plus single-agent chemotherapy have not been established.
- Biphosphenates such as pamidronate (dose, 1 mg/kg) inhibit osteoclast activity and can be used to palliate osteosarcoma in the palliative setting. Other pain relief is likely to be required.
- Chemotherapy can also be used with curative intent for osseous plasmacytoma and lymphoma. See Chapters 9 and 10.

Treatment – Radiotherapy

- Radiotherapy can help with the provision of balanced analgesia for primary malignant tumors of the appendicular skeleton in dogs and cats that are inoperable or when metastatic disease has been discovered.

Table 18.3. Outcome for treatment of primary appendicular osteosarcoma in dogs

Treatment	Details	Median Survival (Months)	1-Year Survival (%)	2-Year Survival (%)
Palliative care	With metastatic disease	2.5 (variable)	–	–
Radiotherapy alone	Strategic single doses or planned coarse-fractionation protocol	4 (variable)	–	–
Surgery alone	Complete excision	4.3	12	2
Surgery + chemotherapy	Cisplatin	10.7	45	21
	Carboplatin	10.5	35	–
	Cisplatin and doxorubicin together	11	48	28
	Cisplatin and doxorubicin alternating	10	37	26
	Carboplatin and doxorubicin together	7.8	–	–
	Carboplatin and doxorubicin alternating	10.5	48	18

- Radiotherapy can be used as sole modality therapy with curative intent for lymphoid solitary lymphoma and osseous plasmacytoma.
- Radiotherapy can be used for palliation of inoperable axial tumors, particularly of mandible and maxilla, and tumors arising in the facial bones or nasal cavities.
- Radiotherapy can be used for treatment of incompletely resected tumors of the mandible and maxilla.
- Care should be taken when irradiating benign tumors, such as juvenile jaw tumors in young dogs, due to the possibility of second malignancy at the site of radiation.
- Intraoperative therapy during limb salvage procedures has been reported.

Outcome for Treatment of Bone Tumors in Cats

- There is a paucity of information describing treatment of feline bone tumors.
- Surgery to remove appendicular osteosarcoma can result in extended survival (in excess of 5 years) without the use of adjuvant chemotherapy.
- Metastatic disease is reported, and may present early in the disease course, but it is less likely in cats than in dogs.
- Axial sites such as the skull, spine, and pelvis are more difficult to treat surgically. However, prolonged survival in excess of 1 year can be expected with debulking surgery alone, or in combination with radiotherapy, or with palliative treatment alone in certain cases.
- The requirement for adequate analgesia should not be overlooked in these cases.
- Osteosarcomas arising outside the skeletal system may occur. These can often be in sites traditionally associated with injection-site sarcomas and as such are often associated with a poorer prognosis due to extensive local invasion and a higher chance of metastasis.
- Benign bone tumors can be treated with surgical excision in cats. Repeated surgeries may be necessary over time to achieve control in a case of osteochondromas and osteochondromatosis.

Prognosis – Bone Tumors in Dogs and Cats

- The outcome in dogs and cats with osteosarcoma is governed both by the location and behavior of the primary tumor and the development of metastatic disease. Elevated levels of bone-specific ALK phosphatase is a negative prognostic indicator in dogs.
- Without treatment of any kind, survival, although variable, is not expected to be beyond a few months in dogs and cats with appendicular osteosarcoma. Dogs and cats are most likely to be euthanized due to our inability to achieve good palliative care and pain control.
- Dogs receiving adequate local disease control for a primary osteosarcoma of either the appendicular or axial skeleton are most likely to be euthanized following the development of secondary tumors. Despite adjuvant chemotherapy, the 2-year survival is 20–30%.
- The type and duration of chemotherapy can have a bearing on the survival postsurgery, although the differences between published protocols are not great.
- Secondary disease can occur in a variety of locations, including the thorax, regional nodes, skin, and other bony sites.
  - In cats, surgery to remove appendicular osteosarcoma can result in extended survival (in excess of 5 years) without the use of adjuvant chemotherapy.
  - Cats with inoperable or incompletely excised axial osteosarcomas can survive for extended periods, on the order of 1 year.
- For malignant tumors other than osteosarcoma (and the rare primary osseous hemangiosarcoma), the prognosis is much better since the metastatic potential is less and survival hinges more on adequacy of local disease control than the control of metastatic spread.
- Beware: The diagnosis of fibrosarcoma or chondrosarcoma cannot be made on a biopsy specimen – it can be made only on the large surgical specimen with multiple sections.

- Osseous hemangiosarcoma is rare in both cats and dogs and carries a guarded prognosis. Metastatic disease is often detected at presentation. Chemotherapy is not well documented for cases presenting without metastatic disease, although doxorubicin would be a logical choice.
- Chondrosarcoma treated with complete surgical excision in dogs and cats is often cured since the metastatic potential is low (less than 5%).

Soft-Tissue Sarcomas in Dogs and Cats

Key Points – Soft-Tissue Sarcomas in Dogs

- These comprise a diverse group of malignant tumors representing the components of the nonbony musculoskeletal system, none of which can be categorically distinguished clinically.
- Light microscopy may need to be augmented with immunohistochemistry and special staining techniques in some cases when the exact cell of origin needs to be determined.
- Tumors comprised of cells that are spindle-shaped may be referred to as spindle cell sarcomas, but this does not imply a precise tumor type.
- Soft-tissue sarcomas tend to affect middle-aged to older dogs. They are rarely encountered in the young.
- They often present as single masses located beneath the skin, which are relatively immobile, poorly circumscribed, and varying in size and growth rate.
- Tumors may invade and/or ulcerate through the overlying skin.
- Most soft-tissue sarcomas have a tendency to slow, localized, but invasive growth patterns and a relatively low metastatic potential. These are often but not exclusively located on the subcutaneous tissues of the distal limb.
- Other tumors can be more aggressive in terms of their rapid growth patterns and metastatic potential. These tumors can arise in a variety of soft-tissue locations, and they include the histiocytic sarcoma group and some synovial cell sarcomas.
- A pseudocapsule comprising a part of the tumor with a very active growth fraction is often encountered during conservative surgeries, leading to a high rate of local recurrence with conservative resections.
- A malignant phenotype may not confer a more guarded prognosis since wide local resections are required for most benign and malignant tumors. Local recurrence rather than metastasis is more important for long-term survival and quality of life for the majority of soft-tissue sarcomas. Exceptions to this are outlined in Table 18.4, with further details on specific tumor types.

Investigation of Suspected Soft-Tissue Sarcomas in Dogs and Cats

- These tumors rarely exfoliate well, and routine needle aspirate cytology often results in a low yield and a nondiagnostic sample. There are two exceptions to this scenario:
  - Lipomas can usually be confirmed on needle aspirate cytology. Provided the lesion is smooth, and relatively mobile, without signs of localized invasion (thus lowering the suspicion of an infiltrating lipoma or liposarcoma), then proceed to conservative, excisional biopsy without further investigations.
  - Histiocytomas are usually able to be diagnosed on needle aspirate cytology when features of malignancy are absent. The majority of histiocytomas will spontaneously resolve within days or weeks of presentation. If this does not occur or when there is a clinical indication to do so, these can be removed with a conservative, excisional biopsy.
- When a nondiagnostic sample is taken or when features of malignancy are observed, an incisional biopsy is performed (Figure 18.6).
- The site of incision should be carefully placed so that the biopsy tract may be easily removed if a later, definitive excision is performed.

Table 18.4. Commonly recognized benign and malignant soft-tissue tumors in dogs

Tissue of Origin	Tumor Benign	Tumor Malignant	Key Features
Fat	Lipoma	Liposarcoma Infiltrative lipoma	Benign tumors are common and easily controlled with conservative resection, when required. Despite the name, infiltrative lipomas require wide surgical resection and careful preoperative planning to achieve local control, and metastasis may (rarely) be recognized. Radiotherapy can be used to augment local control following incomplete surgical resection. Liposarcomas have a typical pattern of local invasion and rare metastasis.
Fibroblasts	Fibroma	Fibrosarcoma	Derived from cells capable of producing a collagen matrix. Most are slow growing and approximately half are found on the distal limb. Typical pattern of local invasion and rare metastasis. Some may be more invasive and have a rapid growth potential.
? cells surrounding vessels	–	Hemangiopericytoma	Controversial cell of origin. May arise from the cell's supporting and surrounding vessels. In health, the hemangiopericyte is not, however, recognized. Often appear histologically as whorls of cells. Despite the name, these tumors require wide surgical resection to achieve local control and metastasis may (rarely) be recognized.
Blood vessels	Hemangioma	Hemangiosarcoma	The benign form is often present as small, blood-filled masses on the skin surface. For the malignant form, tumor grade is prognostic. The metastatic potential is much less than is found in the visceral form, and it increases with depth from the skin surface. It is vital that a primary musculoskeletal hemangiosarcoma is not in fact a secondary tumor from a visceral hemangiosarcoma with careful staging.
Lymphatic vessels	Lymphangioma	Lymphangiosarcoma	Tumors are comprised of lymph vessels and have an invasive growth pattern. Rare tumors. The skin of the abdominal wall and hindlimbs seem to be most commonly affected. Adjacent or surrounding lymphedema often recognized. The less common, malignant phenotype is highly metastatic.
Langerhans and dendritic cells	Histiocytoma	Histiocytic sarcoma	Spontaneous regression of the benign form, histiocytomas in most cases. The histiocytic sarcoma group encompasses a number of tumors types with varying pathogenesis, and breed associations. All types carry a guarded prognosis. Further detail in Chapter 8.
Muscle	–	Rhabdomyosarcoma	Derived from cells that produce muscle filaments. Many tumors are capable of a more invasive and rapid growth pattern and higher metastatic potential.
Mucin-producing cells	Myxoma	Myxosarcoma	Infiltrative growth pattern producing an ill-defined mass with pockets of thick-, pale-, or amber-colored fluid present. Rarely metastasize.
Smooth muscles	Leiomyoma	Leiomyosarcoma	Small and slow growing. Rarely metastasize. Located on the trunk and neck.
Nerve sheath	Neurofibroma	Neurofibrosarcoma	Synonyms include nerve sheath tumor, schwannoma, perineural fibroblastoma, neurilemmoma. Rare tumors that often occur in the distal limb and infrequently metastasize. Rarely, multiple nodules may occur along a nerve (termed *neurofibromatosis*). Typical pattern of local invasion and rare metastasis.
Synovium	–	Synovial cell sarcoma	Synovial sarcomas comprise a number of histological types, based on the relative amounts of the epithelial and fibroblastic components. The higher the grade and epithelial component, the poorer the prognosis. Metastatic rates are relatively high (30%). Large breeds and male dogs are overrepresented; predilection site is the stifle. Secondary, bony pathology is typically on both sides of a joint. There is a requirement to perform immunohistochemistry to differentiate synovial cell sarcoma from joint-based histiocytic sarcoma.

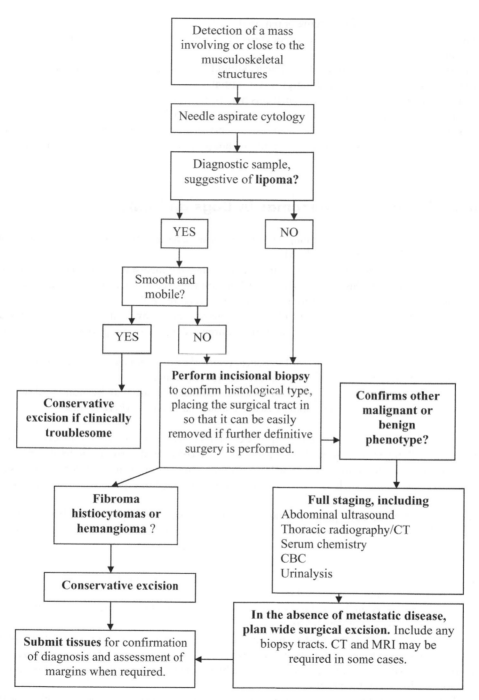

Figure 18.6. Diagnostic decision tree for canine and non-FISS feline cases of soft-tissue sarcomas.

- Once malignancy is confirmed, full staging is required.
- CT and MRI can be valuable tools in the preoperative assessment of some tumors, particularly proximal limb tumors and in cases of FISS.
- All excised tissues from investigations of treatments should be submitted for histopathology service. Information on tumor type, grade, and margins is essential.
- In order to assist the histopathology service, margins may be marked by painting with ink (allow to dry for 20 minutes prior to formalin fixation) or tagging with suture material. Snips of tissue submitted from the tumor bed, obtained prior to closure using clean instruments, can also be useful in assessments of margins.
- Immunohistochemistry or other specialized staining techniques may be required for assessment of tumor type.

Treatment of Soft-Tissue Sarcomas in Dogs and Cats

- Regardless of the exact tumor type, the majority of soft-tissue sarcomas require wide surgical excision to avoid local regrowth (Figure 18.7 – Table A).
- Adequate local control will result in a cure in most cases, since the metastatic potential is relatively low for most tumors of this type. The histiocytic group and FISS are the exceptions to this general rule.
- Careful staging is required before attempting any treatment (Figure 18.8 – Table B).
- In the face of gross metastatic disease, control of the primary tumor may confer little or no survival advantage since adjuvant chemotherapy is likely to be unrewarding. Two exceptions to this rule may be encountered.
  - If the primary tumor is causing quality of life issues, removal of the primary (± the secondary masses) may improve quality of life, but it is unlikely to improved life expectancy.
  - If the primary tumor is not limiting quality of life, the secondary disease may be monitored, with intervention to address the primary and secondary disease considered in cases where metastatic disease is slowly progressing.
- In the absence of metastatic disease, the best approach is a single, definitive surgical procedure to remove the primary tumor. Referral to a surgical specialist should be considered early in the treatment plan.
- In some situations complete tumor removal will necessitate amputation or major reconstructive surgery. Advanced imaging techniques such as CT and MRI can be very helpful, especially when amputation of a high, proximal tumor is performed.
- At all times avoid repeated, inadequate surgical resections. Repeated attempts at marginal resection reduce the likelihood of complete local control with increasing likelihood of further local contamination.
- Consider referral to a surgical specialist – first chance is their best chance.
- When an incomplete or *dirty* excision takes place, a second or subsequent surgery may be required. If repeat surgery is required, all scar tissue must be viewed as potentially capable of harboring residual tumor cells, and the entire scar must be removed en bloc.
- With all attempts at surgery, margins should be considered on three dimensions. The deep margin is often the rate-limiting factor to a complete, *clean* resection.
- When it is impossible to achieve tumor-free margins at surgery, consider the requirement for postoperative radiotherapy. A conservative surgical approach followed by a planned course of radiation therapy is preferable to a large reconstruction, which does not achieve complete surgical excision. This approach can result in prolonged local control or cure.
- Radiation planning is best done at the preoperative stage. Large reconstructions and the placement of contaminated scar tissue in certain locations may make postoperative radiotherapy impossible.
- There is a finite window of time in which to perform radiation therapy after an incomplete surgical resection. Consult your provider for specific information.
- Neoadjuvant therapy with doxorubicin prior to surgical resection can reduce the size of the tumor facilitating adequate local control. Careful surgical timing is required in order to avoid tumor regrowth following an initial response, or rapid tumor growth if the tumor is unresponsive. Specialist referral should be advised to optimize management of such cases. Adjuvant chemotherapy has a limited application.
- Consider this for high-grade soft-tissue sarcomas and cases of FISS.

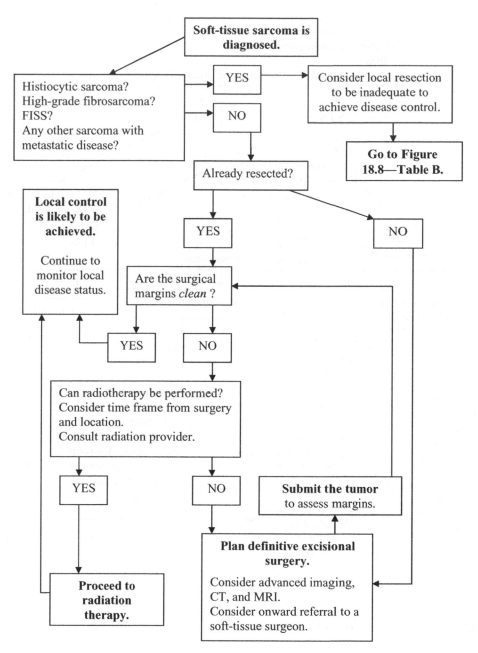

Figure 18.7. Decision tree for treatment of soft-tissue sarcomas in dogs and cats – Table A.

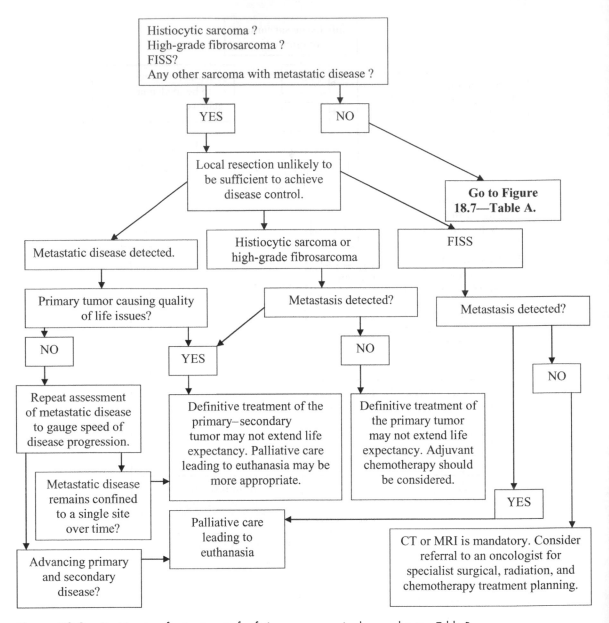

Figure 18.8. Decision tree for treatment of soft-tissue sarcomas in dogs and cats – Table B.

Prognosis – Soft Tissue Sarcomas in Dogs and Cats

- When local disease control can be achieved, the prognosis is very good for the majority of soft-tissue sarcomas in dogs and cats since the metastatic rates are low, typically in the order of 15% or less. Many dogs and cats will go on to enjoy extended periods of remission.
- Continued vigilance is, however, required to check for local disease recurrence after complete resection and following radiation therapy. Local recurrence can be seen many months or years following an apparent successful local treatment.
- In the case of canine histiocytic sarcoma, high-grade fibrosarcoma, and FISS, the prognosis should remain guarded since there are much higher expectations of metastasis, which is likely to be unresponsive to chemotherapy.
- In cases of FISS treated by carefully planned, radical surgery, the expected disease-free interval is approximately 12 months. However, with marginal (incomplete) resection, the disease-free intervals can be as short as 2 months. The 2-year survival for all cats treated is in the order of 10–15%. When surgery can be combined with radiation therapy, the survival may be extended to approximately 2–2.5 years. The usefulness of chemotherapy in the adjuvant setting is still debated.
- The prognosis for cases of canine fibrosarcoma is difficult to predict because so much depends on the adequacy of the primary tumor resection. However, with metastatic rates being up to three times higher for high-grade tumors, compared to low-grade tumors, the outlook has to be more guarded for the higher-grade malignancy. Median survival times of approximately 3–8 months for high-grade tumors has been reported, compared to periods of up to 4 years for low-grade tumors. Controlled studies comparing the effects of chemotherapy are lacking, but it is regularly used in the treatment of high-grade cases.

The prognosis for cases of localized canine histiocytic sarcoma is largely determined by the presence or absence of metastatic disease. If the disease presents and remains localized, and surgery to remove the tumor is complete, survival times can be prolonged. However, metastatic rates approach 90% for periarticular tumors, meaning that the prognosis must remain guarded in these cases. When treated with surgery and chemotherapy, survival on the order of 12 months can be expected. For localized cutaneous histiocytic sarcomas, the metastatic rates appear to be lower, and thus the survival times may be longer.

References and Selected Further Reading

Bentel, G.C. 1995. Radiation Therapy Planning, 2nd edition. McGraw-Hill Medical, New York.

Bomford, C.K., Kunkler, I.H. 2002. Walter & Miller's Textbook of Radiotherapy: Radiation Physics, Therapy and Oncology, 6th edition. Churchill Livingstone/ Elsevier, Amsterdam.

Dobson, J.M., Lascelles, B., Duncan, X. 2003. BSAVA Manual of Canine and Feline Oncology (British Small Animal Veterinary Association), 2nd edition. British Small Animal Veterinary Association.

Fossum, T.W. 2006. Small Animal Surgery Textbook, 3rd edition. Mosby College Publishing, St. Louis, Missouri.

Saunders, D.S. 2003. Textbook of Small Animal Surgery: 2-Volume Set, 3rd edition. W.B. Saunders, Encinitas, California.

Withrow, S.J., Vail, D.M. 2007. Small Animal Clinical Oncology, 4th edition. W.B. Saunders, Encinitas, California.

19

TUMORS OF THE BRAIN, SPINAL CORD, PERIPHERAL NERVES, AND SPECIAL SENSES

Malcolm J. Brearley and David J. Argyle

Brain Tumors

Incidence and Risk Factors

- Uncommon; estimates 14.5/100,000 dogs, 3.5/100,000 cats
- Dogs: middle-aged all breeds, (more common in brachycephalics, especially boxers), no sex predilection
- Cats: no breed predilection but may be male predominance and tend to be older age group
- Possible association between mucopolysaccharidosis type 1 and meningiomas in young cats

Pathology and Behavior

- The tumor types encountered in the central nervous system are given in Table 19.1.
- Often divided into extra-axial or intra-axial based on anatomical site as described by imaging (Figure 19.1, Table 19.2)
  - Extra-axial includes meningiomas, schwannomas (neuromas), choroid plexus tumors
  - Intra-axial includes gliomas, ependymomas
- Other tumors – intracranial extension of skull tumors (osteoma/sarcoma, chondrosarcoma) or caudally from nasal chamber
- Pituitary-based tumors (adenomas, adenocarcinomas) may mushroom into the hypothalamic region.
- Dogs – meningiomas and gliomas in approximately equal proportion (30–45% each)
- Cats – meningiomas (which may be multiple) predominate; lymphoma and gliomas uncommon
- Young individuals (<1-year-old dogs) may be affected by embryonal tumors e.g., medulloblastoma.

Pathogenesis

- Pathological effects of brain tumors can be divided into primary and secondary effects.
- Primary effects caused by direct compression and invasion of brain tissue.
- Secondary effects include adjacent vasogenic edema, CSF flow disturbance (hydrocephalus).
- Meningiomas in dogs are superficial invasive; in cats they tend not to be.
- Gliomas are invasive and destructive.

Clinical Presentation

- Often vague and progressive; may be months
- May progress/deteriorate acutely

Table 19.1. Tumors of the brain and spinal cord

Cell of Origin	Tumor Type	Comments
Glial cells	Astrocytoma Oligodendroglioma Oligoastrocytoma	Brachycephalic breeds. Oligodendrogliomas tend to arise in the frontal and pyriform lobes of the cerebrum. Astrocytomas are common in the brachycephalic breeds and tend to occur in the cerebellum.
Ependyma and choroid plexus	Ependymoma Choroid plexus papilloma Choroid plexus adenocarcinoma	Ependymoma is an aggressive and infiltrative tumor (brachycephalic breeds). Papilloma is slow growing and well defined. Carcinomas are more aggressive.
Neuronal cell	Gangliocytoma Ganglioglioma	Rare. Tends to be in older dogs and located in the cerebellum.
Embryonal tumors	Medullablastoma Neuroblastoma Intradural, extramedullary spinal cord tumor of young dogs	Occur in young dogs. Aggressive tumors.
Meninges	Meningioma	Common in cats and dogs Base of the brain and cerebral hemispheres
Lymphoid	Lymphoma (T or B cell)	Need to use drugs that cross the blood brain barrier
Histiocytic	Histiocytic sarcoma	Poor prognosis

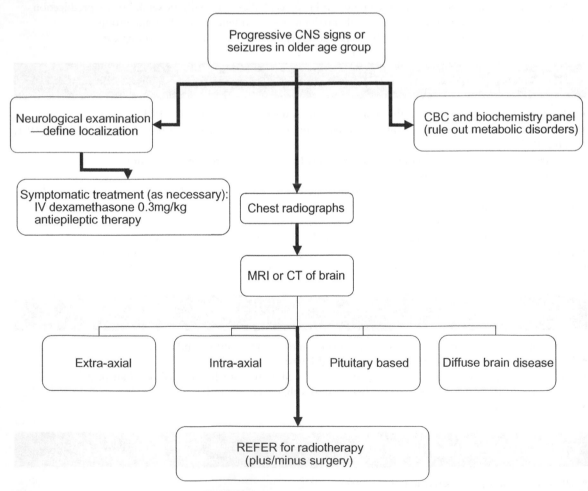

Figure 19.1. Diagnostic decision tree for dogs or cats presenting with progressive CNS clinical signs and/or seizures.

Table 19.2.   The diagnosis of brain tumors based upon MRI

MRI Feature	Comment	Likely Diagnosis
Extra-axial	Mass located outside of the brain parenchyma	Meningioma (most likely) Schwannoma Choroid plexus tumor
Intra-axial	Mass located within the brain parenchyma	Glial tumor
Pituitary	Mass involving the pituitary gland with extension dorsally	Pituitary macroadenoma

- Character changes (mimicking "old age"), vacant walking/circling, standing in corners
- Seizures developing in middle to old age, warranting imaging investigation
- Cranial nerve deficits
- Lateralized central neurological signs
- Clinical signs of brain tumors also site-dependent (Figure 19.2)

Differential Diagnosis

- Other generalized brain diseases
  - Meningitis
  - Hepatic encephalopathy
  - GME
  - Distemper
- Other focal brain diseases
  - Abscess
  - GME

Diagnostic Investigations and Staging

- CBC and biochemistry – to rule out metabolic causes
- Chest radiographs as part of routine health assessment
  - Skull radiographs of limited value but may demonstrate tumors arising from skull
- Advanced Imaging – MRI and CT (Figure 19.3, see also Table 19.2)
  - Extra-axial
    - Broad-based + surface contact (dural tail)
    - Mild mass effect and edema
    - Variable enhancement often homogeneous
  - Intra-axial
    - Within brain parenchyma
    - Moderate mass effect and edema
    - Heterogeneous enhancement
  - Pituitary-based
    - Mushrooming from pituitary fossa
    - Usually homogeneous enhancement but sometimes cystic and heterogeneous
- CSF sampling – BEWARE of sudden alteration CSF dynamics following cisternal pressure may cause cerebellar herniation and acute medullary compression leading to respiratory arrest.
  - Hyperventilation under anesthesia may reduce ICP by reducing CSF pressure secondary to reduced pCO_2.
  - CSF may be altered but often nonspecific.

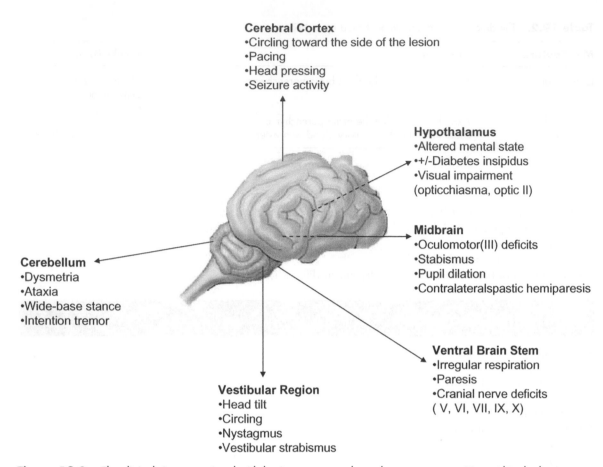

Cerebral Cortex
•Circling toward the side of the lesion
•Pacing
•Head pressing
•Seizure activity

Hypothalamus
•Altered mental state
•+/-Diabetes insipidus
•Visual impairment
(opticchiasma, optic II)

Midbrain
•Oculomotor(III) deficits
•Stabismus
•Pupil dilation
•Contralateralspastic hemiparesis

Cerebellum
•Dysmetria
•Ataxia
•Wide-base stance
•Intention tremor

Ventral Brain Stem
•Irregular respiration
•Paresis
•Cranial nerve deficits
(V, VI, VII, IX, X)

Vestibular Region
•Head tilt
•Circling
•Nystagmus
•Vestibular strabismus

Figure 19.2. The clinical signs associated with brain tumors are dependent on tumor position within the brain.

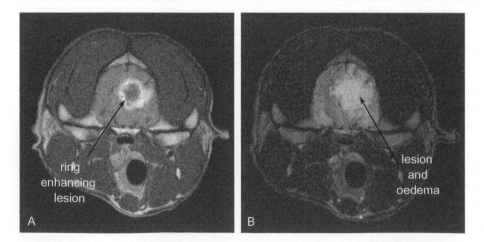

ring
enhancing
lesion

lesion
and
oedema

A

B

Figure 19.3. MRI images of a canine brain tumor (glial tumor). (A) Glial tumor with gadolinium enhancement and (B) glial tumor showing marked edema of the local tissue.

Staging

- Rarely metastasize to the distant organs.

Prognostic Factors

- Tentative diagnosis of tumor type
- Site of tumor – ventral brain stem and cerebellar-pontine angle tend to respond poorly.
- Neurological status – however, with aggressive support some with severe central signs can improve dramatically.

Treatment Options

Palliative Therapy

- Antiepileptic drugs as appropriate
- Corticosteroids – dexamethasone 0.25 mg/kg intravenously
- If comatosed: intubate and hyperventilate to reduce pCO_2 and thereby reduce intracranial pressure.

Definitive Treatment

- Surgery
  - Specialist surgical procedure requires specialist anesthesia support and perioperative intensive care.
  - May be curative for meningiomas in cats, especially on more accessible convex surfaces of cerebrum.
  - Unlikely to be curative for canine meningiomas and gliomas due to invasive nature of tumors.
  - Cytoreductive surgery may be beneficial prior to radiation therapy.
- Radiation therapy
  - Fractionated and coarse-fractionated protocols are described as sole therapy with similar response rates and survival times. Coarse-fractionated protocols have potentially more side effects (e.g., ischemic necrosis) but reported less than 10%.
  - Adjuvant radiation following surgery gives better survival times, especially for meningiomas.
- Chemotherapy
  - Blood brain barrier limits brain penetration by most drugs.
  - None proven.
  - There are anecdotal reports of lomustine (CCNU), carmustine (BiCNU), and hydroxyurea.

Outcome of Therapy (MST = Median Survival Time)

- No treatment or palliative therapy only – days to a few months; rare cases of many months with corticosteroids alone
- Surgery alone
  - MST ~5 months
  - Cats meningiomas – MST ~2 years
- Radiotherapy alone
  - Canine meningiomas – MST ~12–15 months
  - Canine gliomas – MST ~9–10 months

- Surgery + radiotherapy
  - Canine meningiomas – MST ~18 months
  - Canine gliomas – MST as radiotherapy alone
- Pituitary macrotumors
  - Mild neurological at presentation MST ~21 months
  - Severe neurological at presentation MST ~13 months

Spinal Cord Tumors

Incidence and Risk Factors

- Uncommon
- Mostly large-breed dogs
- Middle age (average 5–7 yo)
- Young age (<3 yo) accounts for significant minority (up to 25%)
- Rare in cats with exception of lymphoma

Pathology and Behavior

- Classified on histology and on anatomical basis; latter is more useful (Figure 19.4, Table 19.3).
- Intramedullary tumors are rare in dogs and cats.
- Intradural-extramedullary tumors account for 35%.
  - Meningiomas, peripheral nerve sheath tumors

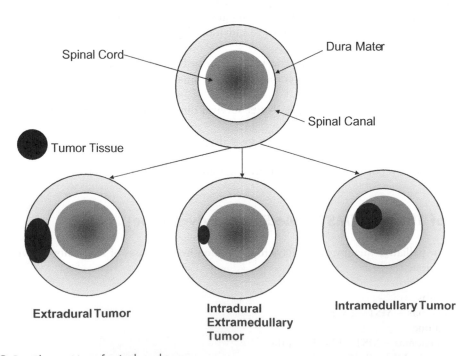

Figure 19.4. The position of spinal cord tumors.

Table 19.3. Tumors of the spinal cord

Location	Comment	Tumor Types
Intramedullary	Arise within the spinal cord	Glial tumors Metastatic tumors Lymphoma
Intradural extramedullary	Arise from the connective tissue of the dura mater	Meningioma Poorly differentiated tumor of young dogs Peripheral nerve sheath tumors Ependymoma (neuroepithelioma)
Extradural	Arise from connective tissue in the spinal canal/column	Primary bone tumors Metastatic tumors Lymphoma Multiple myeloma

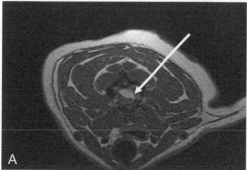 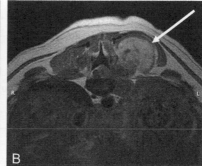

Figure 19.5. MRI images of spinal cord tumors.

- Extradural tumors account for up to 50%.
  - Primary bone tumor of vertebra (osteosarcoma, plasmacytoma)
  - Metastatic involvement of vertebra
- Compression of cord is common to all types of spinal cord tumors.

Clinical Presentation

- Often vague and slowly progressive over a few months
  - Intramedullary tumors are more rapid – a few weeks.
  - Ischemic and hemorrhagic events will give acute deterioration.
- Progressive pain and paresis
- Acute paralysis

Diagnostic Investigations and Staging

- Neurological evaluation to localize where possible.
- Survey radiographs of vertebral column.
- CSF may contain lymphoblasts associated with lymphoma.
- CT and MRI are the most useful imaging techniques (Figure 19.5).
- Surgical exploration and biopsy can be used.

Prognosis

- Prognosis is generally poor because the treatment options are very limited.
- Euthanasia due to uncontrollable pain and/or paraplegia may be best option.

Treatment

Surgery

- Intraoperative cytology may identify lymphoma.
- Extradural malignant tumors may be cytoreduced but rarely cured.
- Intradural extramedullary tumors, in particular meninigioma, can sometimes be completely removed.
- Involvement of the cord limits any attempts for wide excision.

Radiation Therapy

- The spinal cord is prone to radiation-induced ischemic damage and therefore rarely performed.
  - Solitary lymphoma or solitary plasmacytoma of vertebra can be responsive to radiation at nontoxic doses.

Chemotherapy

- For lymphoma, standard protocols can be used.

Tumors of Peripheral Nerves

Incidence and Risk Factors

- Uncommon

Pathology and Behavior

- Generic term is peripheral nerve sheath tumors. **Detailed classification is widely disputed.**
  - Tumors arising from periaxonal Schwann cells = schwannomas.
  - Tumors arising from perineural fibroblasts = neurofibroma/sarcoma.
- Brachial plexus is the most common site in dogs.
  - Extension proximally into spinal canal is common.
- Other tumors can affect the brachial plexus, e.g., lymphoma.

Clinical Presentation

- Often vague and slowly progressive
- Present with variable lameness with no defined focus

- Paresis and muscle atrophy in later stages
- Pain on passive manipulation of limb
- Pain on deep palpation into axilla
- Edge of mass may be palpable in deep axilla

Diagnostic Investigations and Staging

- Deep palpation of axilla under anesthesia
- Electromyography (EMG)
- Survey radiographs of vertebral column
- CT and MRI
- Surgical exploration and biopsy

Prognosis

- Prognosis is generally poor because the treatment options are very limited.
- Euthanasia due to uncontrollable pain may be best option.

Treatment

Surgery

- Involvement proximally into spinal canal limits opportunity for wide excision.

Radiation Therapy

- The spinal cord is prone to radiation-induced ischemic damage and therefore rarely performed.

Chemotherapy

- Following cytoreductive surgery, anthracycline based protocols (doxorubicin ± cyclophosphamide) have been suggested but with unproven benefit.

Tumors of the Eye and Associated Structures

Introduction

Ocular tumors may involve
- Eyelids, third eyelid, and conjunctiva
- Globe
- Orbit and optic nerve

An overview of ocular tumors is given in Table 19.4 and Figure 19.6.

Table 19.4. Tumors affecting the eye and associated structures

Site	Structure	Tumor Types
Intraocular	Cornea and sclera	Melanoma
	Ciliary body and iris	Squamous carcinoma
	Retinal and choroid	Ciliary body adenoma
		Melanoma
		Intraocular sarcoma of cats
		Metastatic tumors
		Lymphoma
		Melanoma
		Retinoblastoma
Extraocular	Eyelids	Squamous cell carcinoma
	Third eyelid	Basal cell carcinoma
	Conjunctiva	Meibomian (sebaceous) gland adenoma in dogs
	Orbit	Melanoma
	Optic nerve	Mast cell tumor
		Squamous cell carcinoma
		Melanoma
		Papilloma
		Adenoma/adenocarcinoma
		Secondary lymphoma
		Squamous cell carcinoma
		Melanoma
		Lymphoma
		Histiocytic disease
		Mesenchyma tumors or extension from tumors of the nasal or frontal sinuses
		Meningioma

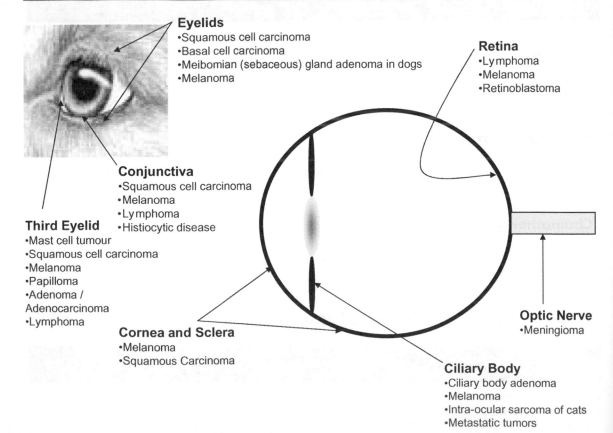

Eyelids
•Squamous cell carcinoma
•Basal cell carcinoma
•Meibomian (sebaceous) gland adenoma in dogs
•Melanoma

Retina
•Lymphoma
•Melanoma
•Retinoblastoma

Conjunctiva
•Squamous cell carcinoma
•Melanoma
•Lymphoma
•Histiocytic disease

Third Eyelid
•Mast cell tumour
•Squamous cell carcinoma
•Melanoma
•Papilloma
•Adenoma /
Adenocarcinoma
•Lymphoma

Cornea and Sclera
•Melanoma
•Squamous Carcinoma

Optic Nerve
•Meningioma

Ciliary Body
•Ciliary body adenoma
•Melanoma
•Intra-ocular sarcoma of cats
•Metastatic tumors

Figure 19.6. Tumors of the eye and associated structures.

Part 1: Tumors of the Eyelid, Third Eyelid, and Conjunctiva

Incidence and Risk Factors

- Benign tumors of the eyelids are common in dogs.
- Squamous cell carcinoma of the eyelid in white-faced cats is associated with UV-light exposure.

Clinical Presentation

- Mass on lid
- Ulcerative erosive lesion
- Rarely metastasize

Diagnostic Investigations and Staging

- Clinical appearance
- Biopsy – incisional or excisional

Surgery

- Small tumors are removed by wedge-shaped excisional biopsy.
- Large tumors require wide excision with flaps to reconstruct.
- Large excisions may result in nonfunctional lids requiring enucleation.

Radiation Therapy

- Strontium-90 plesiotherapy is used for superficial squamous cell carcinoma and mast cell tumors of lids.

Chemotherapy

- None proven

Outcome

- Benign and early malignant tumors carry fair to good prognosis with adequate local treatment.
- Large invasive malignant tumors have high local recurrence rate unless wide excision (plus enucleation) is performed.

Part 2: Tumors of the Globe

Incidence and Risk Factors

- Generally uncommon tumors
- Intraocular sarcoma of cats associated with previous ocular trauma

Pathology and Behavior

- Limbal melanoma – essentially benign
- Melanoma arising from iris or ciliary body
  - Dogs – locally invasive but low metastatic rate
  - Cats – locally invasive and high metastatic rate
- Ciliary body adenocarcinoma
  - More common in dog than cat
  - Locally invasive but low metastatic rate
- Intraocular sarcoma of cats
  - Locally invasive and high metastatic rate
- Metastatic tumors (osteosarcoma)
- Lymphoma
  - As part of multicentric lymphoma – (indicative of stage V)

Clinical Presentation

- Varied clinical signs:
  - Conjunctivitis, obvious mass bulging from globe or distorting iris and pupil
  - Secondary uveitis and glaucoma

Diagnostic Investigations and Staging

- Ophthalmic examination
- Chest radiographs
- Ultrasound of the globe
- MRI
- FNA, especially of regional lymph nodes

Prognosis

- Canine intraocular tumors generally carry a good prognosis following enucleation.
- Feline intraocular tumors generally carry a guarded prognosis following enucleation.
- Feline intraocular sarcomas carry a poor prognosis due to high metastatic rate.
- Intraocular lymphoma is a poor prognostic factor for multicentric lymphoma.

Surgery

- Limbal melanoma may be treated by local excision and adjuvant Sr-90 radiation.

Chemotherapy

- Chemotherapy is indicated for lymphoma.

Part 3: Tumors of the Orbit and Optic Nerve

Pathology and Behavior

- Various tumor types may expand into/invade retrobulbar space, e.g.:
  - Osteosarcoma of bones of orbit
  - Maxillary sarcomas
  - Intranasal malignant tumors
  - Intranasal lymphoma (cats especially)
- Meningioma arises from optic nerve sheath.

Clinical Presentation

- Exophthalmus
- Protrusion of third eyelid
- Deviation of eye
- Unable to retropulse eye
- Loss of vision/light reflexes
- Pain (more common with retrobulbar abscess)

Diagnostic Investigations and Staging

- Radiographs (intraoral).
- Ultrasound.
- CT or MRI imaging is best.
- Ultrasound-guided FNA or core biopsy, but <80% definitive diagnosis.
  - FNA useful to differentiate tumor from abscess.

Prognosis

- Bone invasion and limited options for wide excision give poor prognosis.

Surgery

- Orbit exenteration is the treatment of choice.

Radiation Therapy

- Adjuvant radiotherapy following surgery may improve local control.
- Primary radiotherapy may be useful in cats to control intranasal lymphoma with extension into retrobulbar space.

Chemotherapy

- Lymphoma invading retrobulbar space can be treated with standard protocols.

Outcome

- Metastases are rare for most tumor types (varies with type).
- Local recurrence is common.

References and Selected Further Reading: Oncological Surgery

Saunders, D.S. 2003. Textbook of Small Animal Surgery: 2-Volume Set, 3rd edition. W.B. Saunders, Encinitas, California.

Withrow, S.J., Vail, D.M. 2007. Small Animal Clinical Oncology, 4th edition. W.B. Saunders, Encinitas, California.

20
MISCELLANEOUS TUMORS

David J. Argyle

Part 1: Cranial Mediastinal Mass

Signs Referable to a Cranial Mediastinal Mass

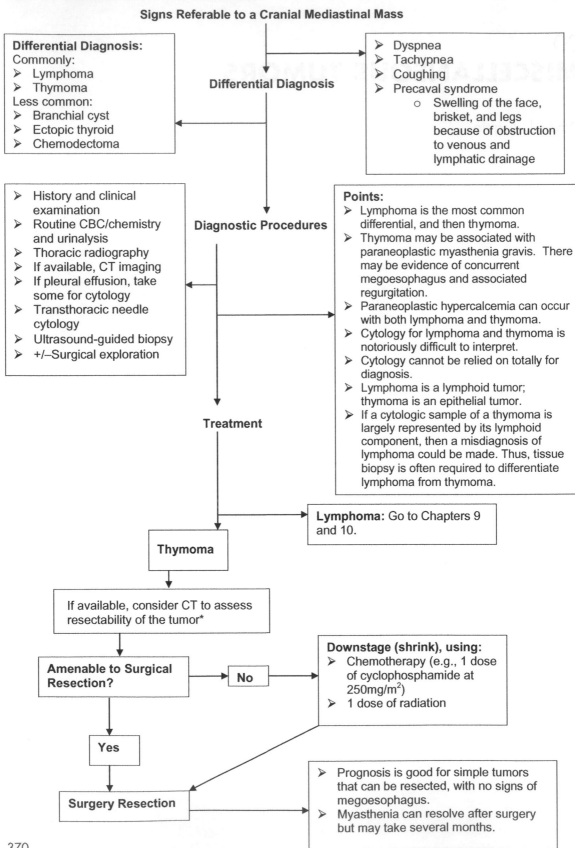

Differential Diagnosis:
Commonly:
➢ Lymphoma
➢ Thymoma
Less common:
➢ Branchial cyst
➢ Ectopic thyroid
➢ Chemodectoma

Differential Diagnosis

➢ Dyspnea
➢ Tachypnea
➢ Coughing
➢ Precaval syndrome
   o Swelling of the face, brisket, and legs because of obstruction to venous and lymphatic drainage

➢ History and clinical examination
➢ Routine CBC/chemistry and urinalysis
➢ Thoracic radiography
➢ If available, CT imaging
➢ If pleural effusion, take some for cytology
➢ Transthoracic needle cytology
➢ Ultrasound-guided biopsy
➢ +/–Surgical exploration

Diagnostic Procedures

Points:
➢ Lymphoma is the most common differential, and then thymoma.
➢ Thymoma may be associated with paraneoplastic myasthenia gravis. There may be evidence of concurrent megoesophagus and associated regurgitation.
➢ Paraneoplastic hypercalcemia can occur with both lymphoma and thymoma.
➢ Cytology for lymphoma and thymoma is notoriously difficult to interpret.
➢ Cytology cannot be relied on totally for diagnosis.
➢ Lymphoma is a lymphoid tumor; thymoma is an epithelial tumor.
➢ If a cytologic sample of a thymoma is largely represented by its lymphoid component, then a misdiagnosis of lymphoma could be made. Thus, tissue biopsy is often required to differentiate lymphoma from thymoma.

Treatment

Lymphoma: Go to Chapters 9 and 10.

Thymoma

If available, consider CT to assess resectability of the tumor*

Amenable to Surgical Resection?

No

Downstage (shrink), using:
➢ Chemotherapy (e.g., 1 dose of cyclophosphamide at 250mg/m^2)
➢ 1 dose of radiation

Yes

Surgery Resection

➢ Prognosis is good for simple tumors that can be resected, with no signs of megoesophagus.
➢ Myasthenia can resolve after surgery but may take several months.

Part 2: Malignant Effusions

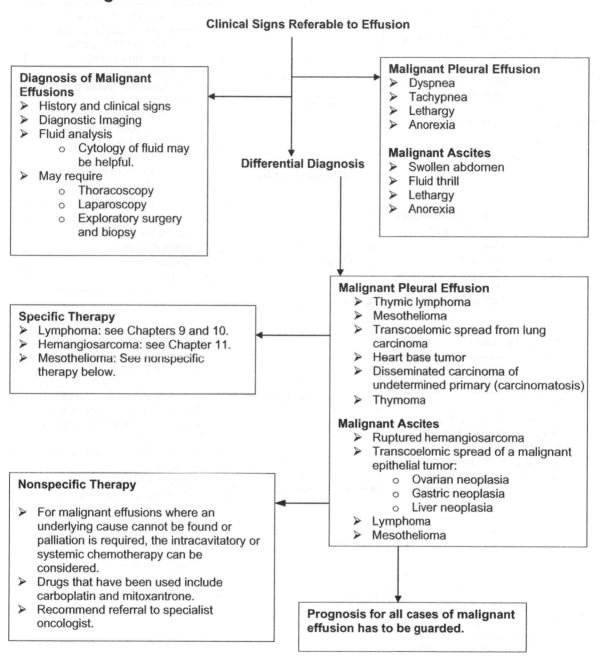

Clinical Signs Referable to Effusion

Diagnosis of Malignant Effusions
- History and clinical signs
- Diagnostic Imaging
- Fluid analysis
    - Cytology of fluid may be helpful.
- May require
    - Thoracoscopy
    - Laparoscopy
    - Exploratory surgery and biopsy

Differential Diagnosis

Malignant Pleural Effusion
- Dyspnea
- Tachypnea
- Lethargy
- Anorexia

Malignant Ascites
- Swollen abdomen
- Fluid thrill
- Lethargy
- Anorexia

Malignant Pleural Effusion
- Thymic lymphoma
- Mesothelioma
- Transcoelomic spread from lung carcinoma
- Heart base tumor
- Disseminated carcinoma of undetermined primary (carcinomatosis)
- Thymoma

Malignant Ascites
- Ruptured hemangiosarcoma
- Transcoelomic spread of a malignant epithelial tumor:
    - Ovarian neoplasia
    - Gastric neoplasia
    - Liver neoplasia
- Lymphoma
- Mesothelioma

Specific Therapy
- Lymphoma: see Chapters 9 and 10.
- Hemangiosarcoma: see Chapter 11.
- Mesothelioma: See nonspecific therapy below.

Nonspecific Therapy

- For malignant effusions where an underlying cause cannot be found or palliation is required, the intracavitatory or systemic chemotherapy can be considered.
- Drugs that have been used include carboplatin and mitoxantrone.
- Recommend referral to specialist oncologist.

Prognosis for all cases of malignant effusion has to be guarded.

Part 3: Cardiac Tumors

Tumors of the Heart

Tumor Types

- Can be
  - Within the heart
  - Intramural
  - Within the pericardium
  - At the heart base
- Right atrial hemangiosarcoma (most common)
- Aortic body tumor
  - Chemodectoma
  - Paraganglioma
- Lymphoma
- Ectopic thyroid tumor
- Myxoma

Clinical Features

- Hemangiosarcoma most commonly associated with hemorrhagic pericardial effusion and cardiac tamponade
- Obstruction of blood flow out of the heart:
  - Murmur
  - Jugular distension
  - Ascites
  - Pleural effusion
  - Pulmonary edema
  - Cranial vena cava (or precaval) syndrome
- Distruption to electrical conduction leading to dysrhythmias
- Cough
- Dyspnea

Diagnostic Workup

- History and clinical examination
- CBC/chemistry/urinalysis
- Thoracic radiography
- Electrocardiography
- Echocardiography
- Ideally thoracic CT
- Cytology of effusions is usually of little value.
- Main aim is to determine the extent of disease.

Treatment

- Initial medical management:
  - Stabilize cardiac function e.g., dysrhythmias
  - Emergency drainage of pericardium if required
- For solitary lesions that can be surgically excised, surgery is the treatment of choice.
- Surgery should be performed by a recognized specialist.
- Surgery should always include a subphrenic pericardectomy.
- All procedures must be considered palliative.
- The value of chemotherapy is limited but may be considered for lymphoma, hemangiosarcoma and mesothelioma.
- Radiotherapy may be considered for aortic body tumors.

Prognosis

- For right atrial hemangiosarcoma, the prognosis is poor. Surgery, including pericardectomy, combined with chemotherapy offers the longest survival times, with median survival times reported between 5–8 months.
- Aortic body tumors are usually nonresectable, but dogs may benefit from a sub-total pericardectomy. There may be a role for radiotherapy but this has not been proven.
- Due to the rarity of other tumor types, prognosis is difficult to predict accurately in these cases. In general, prognosis is guarded to poor.
- Tumors detected incidentally (i.e. no clinical signs) may in some cases have a more favorable prognosis if they are associated with slow growth (e.g., ectopic thyroid tumor)

Index

Printed and bound by CPI Group (UK) Ltd, Croydon, CR0 4YY

27/10/2024

14580250-0005